Myofascial Massage

Myofascial Massage

Marian Wolfe Dixon, MA, NCTMB, LMT

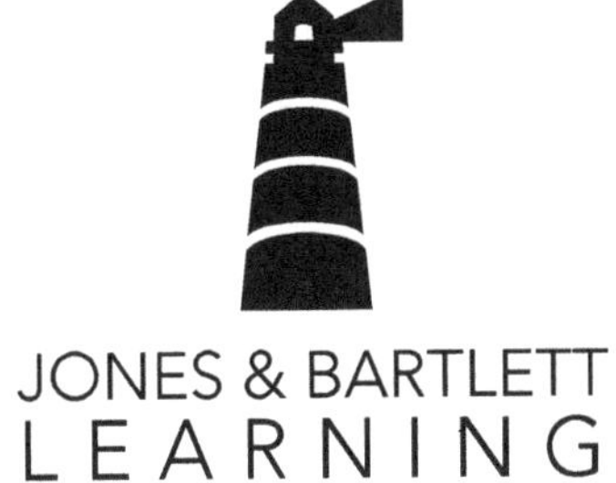

JONES & BARTLETT
LEARNING

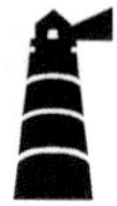

World Headquarters
Jones & Bartlett Learning
5 Wall Street
Burlington, MA 01803
978-443-5000
info@jblearning.com
www.jblearning.com

Jones & Bartlett Learning books and products are available through most bookstores and online booksellers. To contact Jones & Bartlett Learning directly, call 800-832-0034, fax 978-443-8000, or visit our website, www.jblearning.com.

Substantial discounts on bulk quantities of Jones & Bartlett Learning publications are available to corporations, professional associations, and other qualified organizations. For details and specific discount information, contact the special sales department at Jones & Bartlett Learning via the above contact information or send an email to specialsales@jblearning.com.

ISBN: 978-1-284-21024-8

Production Credits
VP, Product Management: Amanda Martin
Director of Product Management: Cathy L. Esperti
Product Manager: Sean Fabery
Product Specialist: Andrew LaBelle
Product Coordinator: Elena Sorrentino
Manager, Project Management: Kristen Rogers
Project Specialist: Brooke Haley
Director of Marketing: Andrea DeFronzo
Marketing Manager: Dani Burford
VP, Manufacturing and Inventory Control: Therese Connell
Cover Design: Kristin E. Parker
Printing and Binding: Lighting Source, an Ingram Company

Library of Congress Cataloging-in-Publication Data unavailable at time of printing.

6048

Printed in the United States of America
24 23 22 21 20 10 9 8 7 6 5 4 3 2 1

I dedicate Myofascial Massage *to my beloved family:*
Art, my kind and multitalented husband;
Roy, my brilliant and compassionate son;
and Sophie, our sweet family dog.

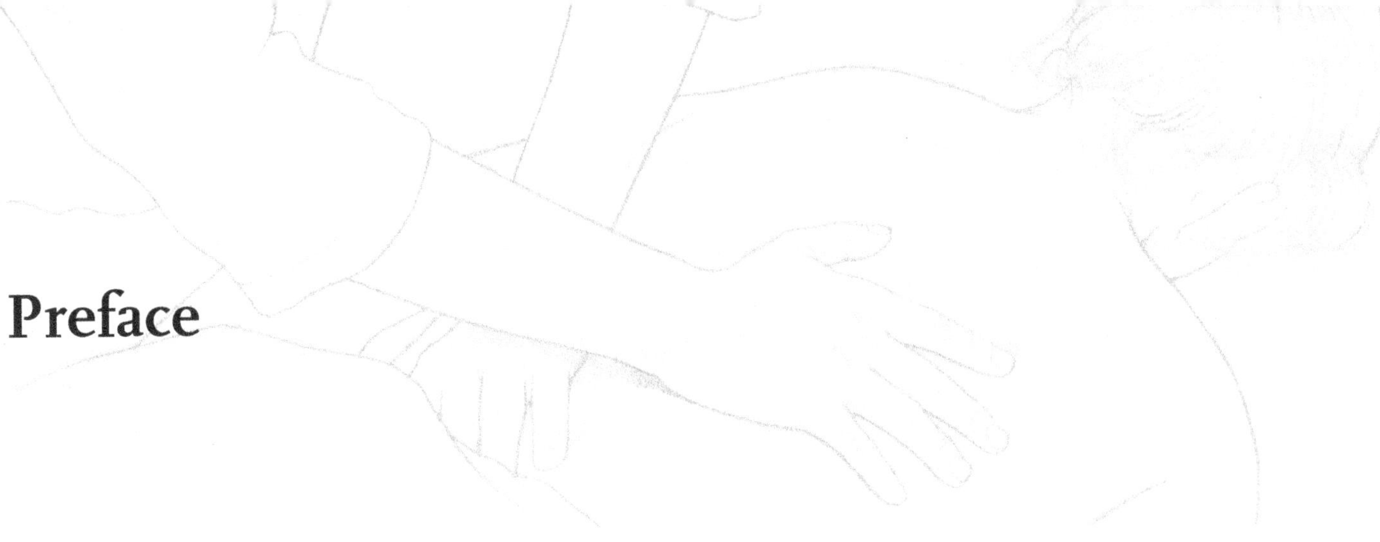

Preface

Myofascial Massage is written primarily for students and practitioners of massage therapy, physical therapy, nursing, and for other hands-on healthcare providers who have an introductory knowledge of massage and are interested in pursuing training in myofascial massage. It can be used for prelicensing or continuing education courses in myofascial techniques, as well as for stand-alone courses at massage schools. Currently, a wide variety of dissimilar techniques and skills are presented to bodyworkers as myofascial techniques. Each specialized institute promotes its own brand of myofascial work as the standard (and purports to teach the true myofascial therapy). This book clearly organizes and teaches key myofascial techniques that make up the diverse bodywork styles presented as myofascial massage.

Myofascial Massage will help licensed massage therapists, physical therapists, chiropractors, osteopaths, and other bodyworkers sort out the advantages and disadvantages of different approaches to myofascial massage. Descriptions of myofascial techniques are grounded in the fascinating story of soft tissue anatomy and physiology. Bands of connective tissue (CT) known as fascia surround and profoundly affect viscera as well as muscular, neural, vascular, and osseous tissues. Explanations of physiological processes for muscles, nerves, and CTs will help readers understand how myofascial (soft) tissue functions as a unit and how to apply bodywork to enhance CT functioning.

GOALS

Myofascial Massage has five primary goals:

1. **To relate the anatomy and physiology of connective tissue to the practice of myofascial massage.** Not only will readers see how the myofascia functions, but they will also get an appreciation of functionality that can improve the application of manual techniques.
2. **To relate the anatomy and physiology of muscle and nerve tissue to connective tissue.** The firm understanding that myofascia operates as a unit of muscle surrounded by CT and innervated by nerves further refines the practitioner's application of myofascial techniques.
3. **To expose practitioners to a variety of myofascial techniques.** This text provides a broad overview of myofascial massage, with language that clearly conveys what is being done to the body (e.g., longitudinal friction, fascial stretching, rocking). Clear terminology facilitates learning in the classroom. Practitioners who use this book should come away with a clear understanding of such terms as *myofascial release, trigger point work,* and *craniosacral therapy.*
4. **To help practitioners identify suitable fields of advanced myofascial work.** The book provides a theoretical overview of myofascial massage approaches and exposes readers to options for specialization and further investigation. The aim is to help practitioners make informed decisions when pursuing continuing education hours and advanced courses of study.
5. **To enhance the bodyworker's toolbox.** *Myofascial Massage* is designed to help bodyworkers expand their repertoire of manual tools for working with myofascial conditions. Sample protocols and practice guides, detailed charts and descriptions of techniques, illustrations, and discussion materials refine the practitioner's ability to sense and respond to problems in the myofascial network. The classroom provides a supervised environment where students can practice the different myofascial approaches and techniques introduced in *Myofascial Massage.* Combined with classroom practice time and discussion, the text provides basic training in the neuromuscular, direct CT, indirect CT, and craniosacral approaches to myofascial massage.

Overall, *Myofascial Massage* consolidates anatomy and physiology, intent, and technique into a unified presentation that offers massage practitioners a better grasp of the myofascial massage field and its implications for massage practice in general. In a single volume, *Myofascial Massage* bridges the gap between an introductory Swedish massage class and the vast array of advanced myofascial study programs offered by diverse institutions. The organization of the chapters provides a logical method of learning the basic anatomy, techniques, and adjunctive exercises of myofascial massage.

ORGANIZATION

The main parts of the book are as follows:

- An Introduction to Myofascial Massage (Chapter 1)
- The Anatomy and Physiology of Myofascial Massage (Chapters 2 to 4)
- Direct Methods Used in Myofascial Massage (Chapters 5 to 7)
- Indirect Methods Used in Myofascial Massage (Chapters 8 to 10)
- Integrating Myofascial Massage into Practice (Chapter 11)

Chapter 1 broadly defines myofascial massage to draw an umbrella wide enough to harbor the diverse styles of myofascial bodywork currently in practice. Chapters 2 to 4 describe the anatomical and physiological underpinnings of myofascial work and the general effect on muscle, CT, and the nervous system.

Subsequent chapters focus on specific myofascial approaches. Chapter 5 covers direct methods such as myofascial trigger point massage, neuromuscular therapy, and muscle energy techniques. Chapter 6 addresses Rolfing and structural integration. Indirect methods include Hanna Somatics Education, Trager, and Barnes' Myofascial Release in Chapter 8 and subtle therapies such as craniosacral therapy in Chapter 10. The bodywork chapters provide a sample protocol for the specific approach discussed, and when appropriate, indicate similarities to commonly used Swedish massage applications.

Chapters 7 and 9 provide direction for supplementing myofascial therapies with hatha yoga and exercise guidelines to speed client progress.

The final chapter, Chapter 11, "Putting It All Together," encourages readers to integrate myofascial skills into their current practices and to use myofascial bodywork to broaden their perspectives of massage. The underlying logic of the sequencing of chapters is further discussed in Chapter 1.

Overall, the organization of the chapters provides students with a logical method of learning the subtleties of myofascial massage. The text will help students learn the basics and select advanced courses that best reflect their own approach to myofascial study.

FEATURES

Chapters include the following special pedagogical features to support the book's purpose as the primary reference and teaching resource on myofascial massage fundamentals:

- **Key terms** (in boldface) are defined at the beginning of each chapter and are included in a glossary at the end of the book.
- **Massage Implications**, which are included in each anatomy chapter (Chapters 2 to 4), bridge the gap between knowledge of structure and function and an understanding of the influence of anatomy and physiology on practice.
- **Sample Protocols** are provided for a typical session or series of sessions in each myofascial approach (except for the neuromuscular approach in which protocols are injury driven and there is no typical all-over body treatment).
- **Guidelines** for critical thinking strategies, improved body mechanics, and communication skills during sessions are provided for each myofascial approach (neuromuscular, direct CT, indirect CT, and craniosacral) and for recommendations about exercise and hatha yoga.
- **One Therapist's Experience boxes** present testimonials from novices or students about what it feels like to use the myofascial approach covered in that chapter. These are provided for each myofascial approach and for recommendations about exercise and hatha yoga.
- **Chapter Summaries** are included at the end of each chapter to highlight major concepts presented in each section.
- **Review Questions** are provided at the end of each chapter as guides for study.

ARTWORK AND TABLES

To illustrate the text, figures have been chosen to enhance the reader's understanding of the anatomy under study or the technique being described and the mechanics of correct application. The technique illustrations include arrows that show the direction of the component forces, the resulting direction of force, and/or myofascial stretching.

Although generously illustrated, *Myofascial Massage* is not a primer in anatomy and physiology. Rather, the book assumes that massage students have a basic grasp of both. Readers who discover that certain aspects of anatomy or physiology are unclear should consult a basic text.

For expeditious reviews of techniques and to help categorize and consolidate the techniques by intent, tables are included throughout the book. Tables also provide quick and easy access to essential information about any technique for first-time students or to refresh the memory of experienced practitioners. The tables are intended for review or conceptual purposes only, not to learn the techniques at the outset. Detailed descriptions and illustrations of the techniques are given in the narrative text.

CLASS TESTING

Most of the material in *Myofascial Massage* is derived from lectures I delivered from 1996 to 2004 in a variety of massage II, myofascial, and craniosacral courses. In all of these classes, the material has received consistently high reviews from preprofessional students, as well as from experienced massage therapists and physical therapists. Classes were filled or overflowing. Students who enrolled in these classes had heard of myofascial techniques but did not have a clear idea of what they were. Clients who have experienced any form of myofascial massage are enthusiastic and seek out myofascial practitioners. Myofascial therapies are generally perceived to be extremely effective and their benefits long lasting. Therapists seek out myofascial courses because they know that clients value practitioners who can make them feel and function better.

Since 2003, selected chapters of this text have been distributed as study aids, and student feedback on the accuracy and helpfulness of this information has been incorporated into the text. The students providing this feedback have included a good mix of beginning and intermediate massage students as well as seasoned professionals (primarily massage therapists but also nurses, chiropractors, physical therapists, physical therapy assistants, and dentists).

PROFESSIONAL TERMINOLOGY AND GENDER

In this text, the terms *therapist* and *practitioner* are synonymous and refer to the person performing bodywork. Sometimes *bodyworker* is also used. The people who receive myofascial massage are called *clients*. Clients are referred to as *he* or *she* more or less randomly. There is no hidden meaning behind any gender designation.

NOTES TO STUDENTS AND INSTRUCTORS

Myofascial Massage is geared toward schools that include myofascial massage training in their standard curriculum but that do not promote one specialized myofascial approach to the exclusion of others. In my experience, students want exposure to a wide variety of approaches, styles, and techniques; this book presents the broadest overview of myofascial theories and techniques currently available. The book enables instructors to create or supplement an existing myofascial program with a theoretical framework and practical descriptions of the art and practice of myofascial massage.

Although selected chapters (Chapters 5, 6, 8, and 10) stand on their own as references for neuromuscular, direct CT, indirect CT, or craniosacral classes, I recommend that readers proceed through the text in the order indicated in the table of contents. Just as training for Swedish massage progresses from a full-body orientation to more specific areas of focus and from superficial stroking to deep, myofascial massage is easier to assimilate when proceeding from general to specific and from superficial to deep intent. Paradoxically, sequential chapters require access to deeper and deeper structures with successively more and more subtle contact requiring less and less pressure. Thus, in the craniosacral approach to myofascial massage, students access the deepest, most internal structures—the dura mater and the cerebrospinal fluid—that flow within the specialized CT sac.

I recommend that practitioners not combine myofascial and Swedish (or other) approaches while still learning myofascial techniques. Massage sessions can become confusing and muddled if therapists are not really clear about what structures they intend to access and the manipulations they are trying to perform. After therapists become skilled in myofascial work and their intent is clear, they can mix and match myofascial techniques with Swedish or any other type of bodywork.

Proficiency in myofascial work requires an investment of practice, experience, and time. As with any endeavor, *practice* builds proficiency. Developing manual skills requires more than reading words in print, no matter how enlightening and inspiring they may be. Methods need to be practiced so therapists can see what happens. But constant repetition of drills without time to assimilate new skills is not enough. It takes *time* to integrate kinesthetic learning. The *experience* therapists need to master myofascial massage can only be partially acquired by practice and time. Experience also means receiving the kind of myofascial bodywork the therapist wishes to practice.

One important component of the myofascial massage experience can be obtained by enrolling in a myofascial course. Training is invaluable for the interaction it provides with peers and an instructor who is there to demonstrate the skills, guide students' practice, and answer questions firsthand. Practice time in and out of the classroom is well spent; it will deepen the therapists' experience of the different myofascial approaches by allowing them to feel the effects of myofascial bodywork for themselves.

Finally, the reader should recognize that *Myofascial Massage* is not an in-depth manual on any of the specific modalities. However, it provides enough detail about concepts and practices for readers to learn the basics as well as the resources readers needed to "get their hands wet" and make sound choices for deeper study.

I wish every reader success and hope that this textbook finds a prominent place in your library for many years to come. I welcome suggestions, corrections, and criticisms, as well as compliments, about *Myofascial Massage*.

Acknowledgments

First in my heart is my gratitude to my family for being here on earth with me. Thank you, Art, Roy, and Sophie, for all that you are.

This text could not have been completed without the support of KriyaYoga practice and the Multnomah Monthly Meeting of Friends.

Professionally, thanks to Pete Darcy for having the confidence in me to undertake the publication of *Myofascial Massage*. I wish to thank my development editor, David Payne, for his support throughout the project and especially his extra efforts and time spent photographing and conferring with me about the art program. A huge thank you to freelance editor Laura Bonazzoli for her sheer genius in editing and in helping me, without judging, to more clearly articulate what I wanted to say. Thanks also to production editor Eve Malakoff-Klein for her thoroughness and clarity during the production process.

I am grateful especially to Gayle MacDonald for her generosity in introducing me to Pete Darcy and to Thierry Bogliolo, my editor at Findhorn (*Bodylessons, 2005*). Thank you also to Leslie Stager, Diana Thompson, and Marybetts Sinclair for the enlightening professional and personal conversations about massage and writing about massage.

Reviewers

Christopher Alvarado, BA, NCTMB
Chicago School of Massage Therapy
Chicago, IL

Kate Anagnostis, MS
Downeast School of Massage
Brunswick, ME

Joanne Braun, BSEd
Kinnelon, NJ

Betsy Krizenesky, WRMT
Neenah, WI

Claudette C. Laroche, BSN
Hooksett, NH

Debra Stell, MA, BA, CMT
Bryman College
Anaheim, CA

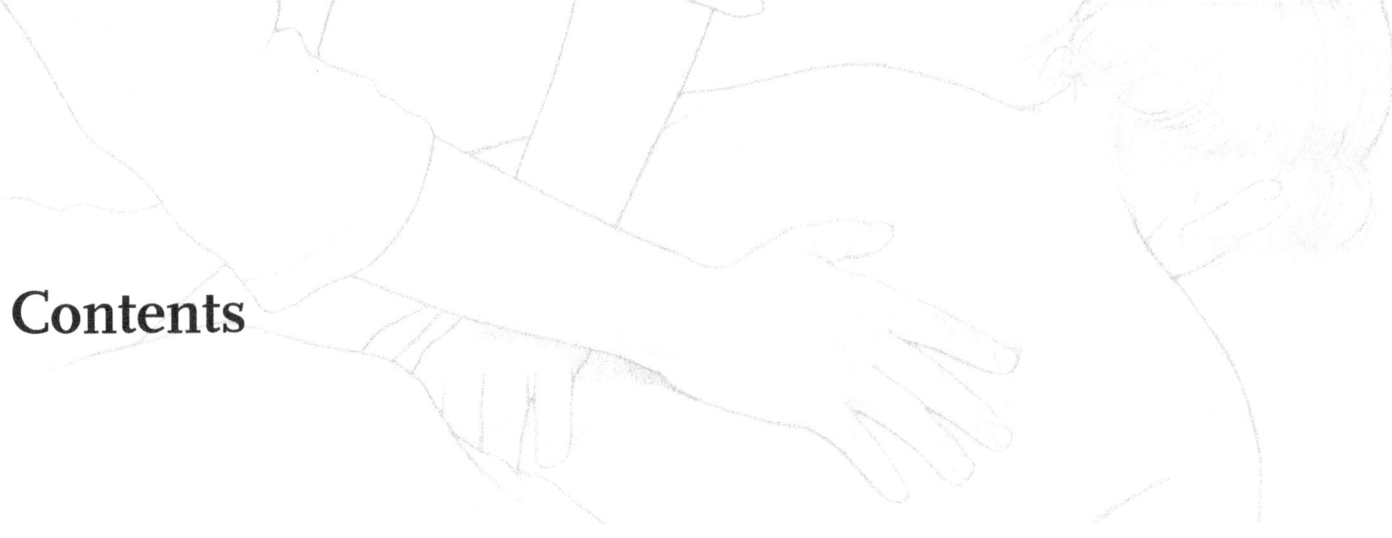

Contents

Chapter 1

An Introduction to Myofascial Massage

OBJECTIVES

- Define myofascia and myofascial massage.
- Describe the components of myofascia.
- Explain the purpose of myofascial massage.
- List the primary objectives of this text and the rationale behind the sequencing of its chapters.

CHAPTER OUTLINE

KEY TERMS

Myofascial (MF) massage: A type of bodywork that focuses on the myofascial unit, including muscle, connective tissue, and the neuromuscular junction.

Connective tissue (CT): Tissue that provides structure and holds the body together. CT is composed of a small number of cells embedded in a matrix (mother substance) of fibers and a solid, semisolid, or liquid ground substance. The five types of CT are loose CT, dense CT, cartilage, bone, and blood.

Fascia: Two specific types of connective tissue: loose connective tissue (superficial fascia) and dense connective tissue (deep fascia).

Superficial fascia (loose connective tissue): Fascia that lies just beneath the surface of the skin.

Deep fascia (dense connective tissue): Fascia that surrounds individual muscle fibers, fiber bundles, and whole muscles, as well as tendons attaching muscles to bones and ligaments joining together bones.

Myofascia: A type of deep fascia that is bound to muscle tissue. The term is sometimes used to specify only the fascia that is bound to the muscles and is sometimes used to refer to the entire unit of muscle and fascia.

Dura mater: The outermost band of the three-layered connective tissue sac (meninges) that surrounds the brain and spinal cord. Sometimes refers to the entire sac. Also known as the dura.

Technique: Massage stroke or manipulation. A mechanical description of what is actually being performed on the client's body.

Style: A bodywork modality that is trademarked or so popular in massage culture as to be designated by a unique brand name (e.g., Myofascial Release, Trager, or Swedish massage).

Direct method: A myofascial massage approach or technique that focuses on meeting resistance in the tissues with an equal and opposite force.

Indirect method: A myofascial massage approach or technique that focuses on meeting a resistance by softening into a sense of ease.

Neuromuscular approach: An orientation to myofascial massage in which the therapist focuses on local muscular or neural dysfunctions, including trigger points, ischemia, inflammation, hypertonia, and neural impingement. The thumb or finger glides or drags to detect taut bands or muscular nodules and ischemic compression to treat trigger points. Also called neuromuscular therapy (NMT) or neuromuscular techniques.

Direct CT approach: An orientation to myofascial massage in which the therapist releases muscle tissue by using sustained pressure with coached micromovements on the connective tissue (or fascia).

Indirect CT approach: An orientation to myofascial massage in which the therapist releases muscle tissue with movement in the form of jostling, compression, or traction applied to the connective tissue (or fascia). Indirect techniques move up to a restricted point (but not beyond) and then move back from that boundary.

Craniosacral approach: An orientation to myofascial massage in which the therapist applies very light pressure at the cranium, sacrum, and spine to free restrictions in the dura mater, and balance the flow of cerebrospinal fluid. Used to relieve pain in the head, spine, and pelvis, and to release trauma throughout the body. Also called craniosacral technique, Craniosacral Therapy, sacrocranial work, CS, and CST.

Proprioception: Information about the position of muscles, tendons, and ligaments in space. Relayed by nerve receptors in the muscles, joints, and fascial sheaths.

This chapter provides an orientation for students and practicing bodyworkers who wish to embark on the fascinating study of myofascial massage. The chapter begins by defining myofascial massage and describing the components that make up myofascia. It then provides a rationale for using myofascial massage, including its historical context, guiding principles, supporting research, and benefits for the therapist. The final sections of the chapter expand on the Preface's explanation of the objectives of the text and the rationale behind the sequencing of its chapters.

Definitions of Myofascial Massage

Broadly defined, myofascial (MF) massage is any type of bodywork that focuses on the myofascial unit, including muscle, connective tissue (CT), and the neuromuscular junction. In addition, the targeted tissue can encompass CT areas of attachment, where there is no longer any muscle tissue and the CT fibers become tendons, or ligaments, when CT connects bone to bone. Myofascial massage can also include simple self-care suggestions for stretching, self-massage, the use of cold packs and heat, and relaxation to improve the effects of massage.

EXPLAINING "MYO"

The "myo" in myofascial refers to the muscles. (The prefix itself comes from the Greek word for muscle, *myo*.) Students of massage well know muscles as the primary movers and stabilizers of the body. All functions requiring movement, from the pulsing of the heart to the expansion of the ribcage to take in a breath, require muscle activity. Muscles are the largest energy consumers in the human body. Healthy muscles respond to signals from the nervous system with coordinated and complex movements.

EXPLAINING "FASCIA"

Fascia generally refers to two specific types of CT, loose CT (superficial fascia) and dense CT (deep fascia).

Superficial fascia (loose CT) is attached to the underside of the skin. Capillary channels and lymph vessels run through this layer, as do many nerves. Subcutaneous fat is attached to it. Superficial fascia has a great potential to store excess fluid and metabolites, the breakdown products of hormones, neurotransmitters, and other chemicals in the body.

Deep fascia (dense CT) is much tougher and denser material. Sheets of deep fascia separate large sections in the body, such as the abdominal cavity. Deep fascia also separates and defines muscles and organs. The covering around the heart (pericardium) and the lining of the chest cavity (pleura) are both made of specialized deep fascia.

Myofascia is a specific type of deep fascia that is bound to muscle tissue. Sometimes the term is used to specify the fascia that is bound to the muscles and sometimes it refers to the entire unit of muscle and fascia. Healthy myofascia can absorb a fair degree of compression and tensile stress, as well as relaxation.

Myofascia is also the tendons and ligaments that bind the muscle and bone. Cellular membranes in fascial areas of attachment (muscle to tendon, tendon to bone, ligament to bone) can become twisted and convoluted, increasing the total surface area for attachment. This increases the potential for tissues to get stuck together or torn (Travell and Simons, 1999).

Another deep fascial structure is the dura mater, or dura. This is the outer layer of the three-layered CT sac (meninges) that surrounds the brain and spinal cord. Sometimes the terms *dura* or *dural tube* refer to the entire container that holds and protects the craniosacral system.

Serous fascia is loose tissue covering the internal organs (viscera); it holds a rich network of blood and lymph vessels. Even cells have a cytoskeleton connected to a fascial network, which gives cells shape and enables them to function as a unit.

The Rationale for Myofascial Massage

Myofascial massage provides benefits for the both the practitioner and receiver. The historical roots of myofascial massage lie in the field of osteopathy, and research to date is encouraging of its use.

HISTORICAL CONTEXT

Many myofascial techniques originated within American osteopathy (Rubik, 1992). Some examples of myofascial techniques with an osteopathic origin include muscle energy techniques (METs) originally developed and codified by Fred Mitchell, Sr., and Paul Kimberley; myofascial release techniques, originally developed by A. T. Still and Charles Neidner; and craniosacral techniques, advanced by William Sutherland, Hugh Milne, and John Upledger (Rubik, 1992).

GUIDING OSTEOPATHIC PRINCIPLES

Because contemporary myofascial massage is largely an extension and refinement of osteopathic practices, it is important to acknowledge certain guiding osteopathic principles, stated below.

Structure and Function Are Interdependent

A change in form affects function. For example, if the vertebrae are pulled out of line by a contracted muscle, their capacity to support the body will be compromised. Conversely, if the constricted back muscle is relaxed enough so that the vertebrae can move back into alignment, the back can be reasonably expected to move more easily, continuously, and freely.

The Body Has the Ability to Heal Itself

Myofascial massage therapists perform more as facilitators than "fixers." This principle does *not* imply that myofascial bodyworkers do not need to acquire clear and explicit manual techniques with a keen understanding of when and how to use them. Myofascial massage therapists acknowledge, however, that they cannot "make" any individual client "get better." The client accomplishes the true work of healing, with assistance from the practitioner of myofascial massage.

The Body Is a Whole

Myofascial therapists understand and conceptualize the principle of wholeness even more graphically than other manual therapists. The myofascial vision of the body is a network, united by fascia (Figure 1-1). This theme will recur and be developed further throughout the text.

RESEARCH

Myofascial pain is a common cause of musculoskeletal pain in medical practice and is one of the most commonly encountered problems in the outpatient setting (Auleciems,

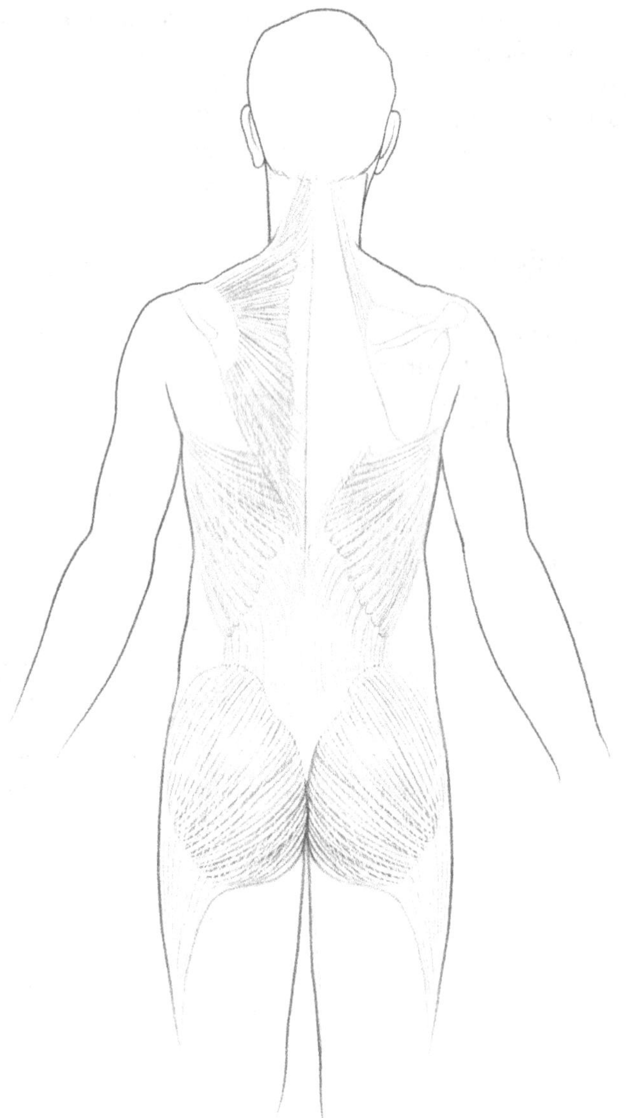

FIGURE 1-1 **The fascial web.** This illustration provides a visual picture of the seamless integration functioning in a living body. When one part moves or is moved, the body as a whole responds.

1995; Skootsky, Jaeger, and Oye, 1989). A small change in the myofascia can cause great stress to other parts of the body (Myers, 2001). It is not surprising, therefore, that clients consistently highly rate the effectiveness of myofascial massage (*The Mainstreaming of Alternative Medicine,* 2000). In addition, case studies indicate that myofascial massage appears to achieve more swift-acting and long-lasting therapeutic change than other types of bodywork (Barnes, 1997; Ezzo, 1994; Upledger, 1987; Upledger and Vredevevoogd, 1983).

These subjective reports certainly support the effectiveness of myofascial massage. The field is still new, however, and a body of rigorous research to back up every point is not yet available. The effectiveness of massage in general has been supported by the findings of several massage studies (Field, 1998; Rich, 2002), but bodywork practice cannot limit itself to what has been scientifically verified by experimental trials. Scientific research is currently too formulaic and too limiting to stand as the ultimate validation of bodywork. Furthermore, the scientific "gold standard" of randomly controlled experimental trials may not be equipped to deal with some of the most basic aspects of therapeutic massage (e.g., what qualifies as "placebo" massage?).

The first step in establishing scientific rigor is laying out the field as it stands. This is what this text aims to do. Because the myofascial playing field can be a confusing jumble of names and styles, systems, orientations, and beliefs, this text attempts to categorize the ideas accurately and to more clearly organize and make sense of the jumble. (A popular saying in the research field is that new ideas are first ignored, then ridiculed, then challenged, and eventually accepted enthusiastically.) Although a research-only account might generate more intellectual endorsement, my hope is to convey my fascination and love for myofascial massage and instill some curiosity in the reader to test concepts through firsthand experience.

BENEFITS FOR THE THERAPIST

In addition to having practical value as a healing tool, myofascial massage can prove advantageous for massage practitioners. Benefits myofascial therapists can expect include a "wholistic" orientation, increased body–mind awareness and improved body mechanics, refined communication skills, a kinesthetic feel for movement, and the challenge of self-acceptance and personal growth.

A "Wholistic" Approach to the Body

Myofascial massage approaches are whole-system approaches. Focusing on the myofascia requires practitioners to treat the body as a whole. Myers (2001) and Barnes (1997) have both declared that there is really only one muscle in the body, which is held in 600 or more fascial pockets. When practitioners visualize the widespread fascial network, they no longer find it sufficient or desirable to view a client as just a "psoas problem." Myofascial massage therapists recognize that pain in the psoas muscle is transferred through the CT and may affect or be affected by adjacent or distant muscles, CT, nerves, circulatory vessels, and organs.

Increased Body–Mind Awareness

Myofascial methods affect both the body and the mind by incorporating both a physiological precision and attention to subtle sensations. In this way, myofascial massage helps heal a split that has emerged in massage therapy between the medical model and energy-based systems. People are not just bodies—they have thoughts, emotions, dreams, and worries, too.

Improved Body Mechanics

Myofascial approaches require careful attention to body mechanics, which, in turn, requires mindfulness during therapy sessions. In the direct method, the therapist cannot sustain both compressive and shearing forces without being attentive to his or her own body to keep from falling or causing injury. In the indirect method, the therapist must let go of subtle tensions in his own body to sense the very small movements that signal subtle tissue release in the client.

Refined Communication Skills

Myofascial approaches require listening to the client's verbal and nonverbal cues and communicating clearly about the techniques as they are applied. Open communication between therapists and their clients enables clients to take an active role in their own healing without fear of pain. "When a patient is sore after a session, you need to rethink the technique, especially the touch experience of the muscles you focused on" (Alexander, 2003). Simply teaching clients how to rate their pain on a number scale (where 10 is excruciating pain, 0 is no pain, and 3 or 4 is a "good hurt") can be an excellent communication tool in itself. With such a tool, trigger point release, stripping (a charged name in itself), and skin rolling do not have to be excruciating to be effective.

Another example of the refined communication skills that myofascial work inspires is in the indirect CT approach, in which therapists learn to focus on the range of ease—the range of movement that feels easy, comfortable, continuous, and smooth. Listening to a client's pain tolerance is a tool for effective work.

A Kinesthetic Feel for Movement

Myofascial work entails a focus on movement, as you will see when you progress through the text. In trigger point massage and the neuromuscular approach, the recommendation is to follow compressive trigger point release with strategic stretching. With the direct CT approach, coached micromovements are essential. Ease of movement is at the heart of the indirect CT approach. In the craniosacral approach, sensitivity to subtle movements is essential.

Personal Growth

My own experience with myofascial massage has been integrative, entailing transformative change for me as well as for my clients. Work with the CT can reveal and heal hurts deep in the body. Myofascial massage can also transform stuck energy into vitality. Myofascial methods require both the client and therapist to internally process (apart from the session) physiological and accompanying psychological changes. This may mean talking with a mentor, counselor, colleague, or peer group to integrate the changes.

Objectives of the Text

This text aims to expose the reader to a variety of myofascial approaches while developing a classification system that clearly states what is actually being done to the body.

SIMPLIFYING AND MAKING SENSE OF MYOFASCIAL TECHNIQUES

A medley of seemingly inconsistent techniques and styles share the term "myofascial." This can present problems for the prospective myofascial massage therapist. For example, a client may have been successfully treated with myofascial trigger point work in the past, and she may be expecting that kind of myofascial bodywork every time. She may quickly become disappointed in a new therapist who specializes in myofascial release because the style is different, not because the work is less effective. It is important for therapists to have an appreciation of the different routes of specialization to inform clients about what they are offering.

When pursuing advanced courses in myofascial therapies, it can be difficult to know just what a certain workshop has to offer. The massage profession as a whole and the subfield of myofascial massage lack clear and consistent terminology to describe methods, approaches, styles, and techniques. Even those words are sometimes used interchangeably and, until now, have not been consistently defined.

In part, the lack of clarity results from the "brand name" modalities (i.e., styles) that use unique but imprecise language to describe what may be common approaches, styles, or techniques. Some myofascial massage styles with different names may be essentially the same (e.g., Rolfing and structural integration). In addition, the same technique included in multiple styles may be given different names (e.g., deep effleurage, muscle sculpting, stripping, and longitudinal friction are essentially the same; skin rolling is a type of pétrissage).

To remedy this problem, this book provides some operative definitions. Myofascial massage **techniques** are massage strokes or manipulations. The techniques are described using neutral language that clearly states what is being done to the body (e.g., longitudinal friction, fascial stretching, rocking). The techniques used in myofascial massage can be categorized in numerous ways, but this text deliberately bypasses styles as a way of grouping techniques and instead classifies techniques into "approaches," which are distinguished by intent.

Style refers to modalities that have become so popular in massage culture as to be commonly referred to by a unique brand name (e.g., Myofascial Release, Trager, or Swedish massage). Many techniques may be grouped together in a style but may not necessarily be unified by intent (other than the intent to work on the myofascia). A mystique surrounds brand name styles, with numerous and fantastic claims about specific modalities being used to cure everything from multiple sclerosis to birth defects. Paradoxically, there can be much duplication of techniques between styles and also much variation, with little clarity about how to select a modality (i.e., style) that reflects a therapist's characteristic touch.

This book arranges techniques into one of two methods and, within those methods, one of two approaches (subcategories of methods). Each method and approach has unique and identifiable intentions with respect to the myofascia. The first conceptual division is between the direct method, which includes approaches and techniques that focus on meeting resistance in the tissues with an equal and opposite force, and the indirect method, which includes approaches and techniques that meet resistance by softening into a sense of ease.

Within the direct method, there is one more conceptual division between the neuromuscular approach, which focuses on the muscles and how they are innervated to contract, and the direct CT approach, which focuses on the fascia. Similarly, within the indirect method, there is a conceptual division between the indirect CT approach, which focuses on the fascial network and fluid that permeates the body, and the craniosacral approach, which focuses on the fascia of the dural tube and the cerebrospinal fluid (CSF) that lies within. The distinction between the direct and indirect methods is shown in Figure 1-2.

FOCUSING ON MYOFASCIAL ANATOMY TO GUIDE THE APPLICATION OF TECHNIQUE

In prelicensing massage programs, classes traditionally focus on muscles (one portion of the myofascia) and Swedish massage (one of a large proliferation of bodywork styles). Students learn where muscles are located, including origins, insertions, and their actions, and how to apply massage to muscles. Yet CT is more prevalent in the body; it comprises the majority of soft tissue and makes up more mass and body weight than any other tissue type, including muscles. A fascial web connects, defines, separates, and carries movement and repair to every corner of the body. Fascia also provides form and definition for every organ by surrounding groups of cells that work together for a unified goal. Myofascia ("muscle/fascia") is inseparable anatomically, with CT surrounding every muscle fiber, every group of muscle fibers, and whole muscles.

The presence of nerve receptors in tendons and in fascial pockets within muscles indicates that myofascia is also involved in nerve receptivity—namely propriocep-

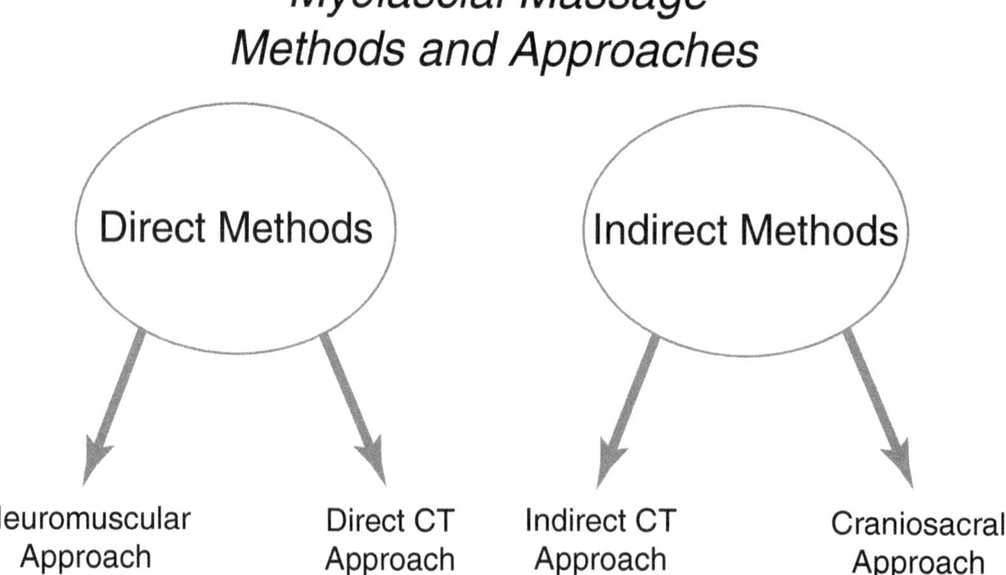

FIGURE 1-2 Direct and indirect myofascial techniques. The primary operative distinction for myofascial techniques is between direct and indirect methods.

tion. Proprioception relays information about the position of muscles, tendons, and ligaments in space. In addition, Earl (1965) and Wilson (1966) claim that, after muscle and joint receptors, fascial sheaths are the most common sites of proprioception. Electron microscope research seems to substantiate that fascia alone contains numerous myelinated sensory neural structures that appear to receive proprioceptive and pain signals (Staubesand, 1996, in Chaitow and DeLany, 2002). Just as muscle is inseparable from fascia, neurons are inseparable from neural CT, which surrounds every nerve fiber and every group of neurons and outlines whole nerves.

Bodywork that takes the interrelated anatomy and physiology of muscles, fascia, and nerves into account has an intellectual "elegance," even apart from a practical value. The body functions as a unit, as a whole, as a living matrix. When muscles are separated out as the only important component of soft tissue, musculoskeletal anatomy becomes divorced from its function. Techniques are reduced to mechanical manipulations. In contrast, working from the myofascial perspective leads to an organic respect for the body as a living, breathing "whole."

EXPANDING THE BODYWORKER'S TOOLBOX

Bodyworkers, like other manual laborers, use their hands as tools to repair, maintain, and build. These skills are improved when principles guide intent (e.g., *listening* to the CSF rhythm or *following* a resistance until it softens). For this reason, *Myofascial Massage* emphasizes both the mechanical ability to execute manipulations and pressures upon the client's soft tissues and the ability to perform these techniques wisely.

To accomplish this end, each of the technique and supplemental activity chapters provides sample protocols. (Given the nature of the neuromuscular approach presented in Chapter 5, a general protocol is not warranted; however, clear guidelines are provided for the use of neuromuscular techniques). The chapters provide recommendations for adapting basic protocols to particular conditions and complaints. In addition, because listening to and following the myofascia depends on a clear knowledge of the structure underneath the therapist's hands (anatomy) and how it functions (physiology), what the therapist is trying to do (intent), and how the therapist plans to carry through (technique), all of these elements are addressed in the book. Covering the basics of all three elements—anatomy or physiology, intent, and technique—provides you with a good understanding of how to apply myofascial massage and massage in general.

To optimize the use of myofascial techniques, the therapist broadens his or her focus to assess a client's whole being in a relaxed, holistic way. This expanded attention can prevent the pitfall of narrowly focusing on simply "fixing what's wrong." Instead of the session's being limited or constricted, with one massage stroke used to "fix" a muscle complaint, leading to a counteraction, and so on, the session can be viewed as a journey that leads the client toward individual goals.

ENCOURAGING EXPERIENTIAL CHOICE

Myofascial Massage provides a theoretical and practical overview of myofascial massage approaches and presents options for specialization and further study. Even more importantly, the text enables you to experience a variety of myofascial approaches by furnishing detailed technique descriptions, illustrations, sample protocols, and personal accounts of what it feels like to put the approach into practice. Combined with classroom practice time and discussion, the text provides basic training in the neuromuscular, direct CT, indirect CT, and craniosacral approaches to myofascial massage.

The book sequentially introduces four distinct approaches to *listening to and following* clients' body signals. Each of the four approaches provides distinctly different sensory information and unique ways of responding to that information. Readers can experiment to find out which approaches best suit their bodywork style.

The Sequencing of Chapters

Intention in manual therapy requires an understanding of how the structure underneath the therapist's hands can optimally function. Thus, an understanding of basic anatomy and physiology of the myofascial unit (CT, muscle, and nerve) is crucial to the proficient application of myofascial massage. Part I of this book is devoted to the anatomy and physiology of the myofascia, concentrating on muscle in Chapter 2, CT in Chapter 3, and the nerve tissue as it relates to myofascia in Chapter 4.

The organization of hands-on therapies in Parts II and III follows a logical progression from the most direct and tangible myofascial approach (and the easiest to apply correctly) to increasingly indirect and subtle approaches requiring more advanced palpatory and treatment skills, including ever-increasing levels of sensitivity and specificity. Table 1-1 presents this progression.

Neuromuscular therapy, the subject of Chapter 5, requires the most tangible or least subtle palpation skills because it concentrates on muscle that is relatively easy to palpate and pushes against resistance manifested in the tissue. Great sensitivity and specificity are not required.

TABLE 1-1 The Progression of Techniques from Tangible to Subtle

Approach	Target Tissue	Level of Palpatory Sensitivity and Specificity of Technique
Neuromuscular and trigger point massage	Muscle, bones (as landmarks)	Grossest (direction of resistance), focusing on muscle resistance
Direct CT	Tendons, ligaments, superficial and deep fascia	Gross (direction of resistance), focusing on line of fascial resistance surrounding muscles
Indirect CT	Superficial and deep fascia; patterns and movement within fascial network; some fascial fluid movement (blood)	Subtler (direction of ease), focusing on movement in direction of ease
Craniosacral	Dura mater and CSF	Subtlest (direction of ease) and most specific, focusing on movement of CSF

The direct CT approach, discussed in Chapter 6, requires a refined touch so the therapist can feel and match resistance in the deep and superficial fascia and hold that edge while following the movement of the CT. The touch is more sensitive and specific than that of neuromuscular therapy because the therapist works with the resistance in the client's body without poking or pushing. Thus, direct CT massage necessitates refining both method and perceptiveness to a higher level.

Even though the approaches are different, neuromuscular and direct CT techniques both meet resistance in the tissues with a direct counterforce. It is an art to find the right amount of resistance to meet soft tissues where they are without giving in or overpowering the tissues. With the skillful application of direct method tablework, the client learns kinesthetically to soften rather than to react by further tightening the muscles. Client awareness can be enhanced through self-care strategies (e.g., movement, stretching, breathing, and visualization) that strengthen the client's intention and reinforce the ability to let go. In Chapter 7, practitioners are introduced to the practice of hatha yoga as an aid to such kinesthetic learning.

The therapist's sensitivity and specificity must become even more sophisticated to sense and return from movement barriers in the indirect CT approach, the subject of Chapter 8. It takes insight and skill to find the fullest arc of *comfortable* range of motion without moving past the point of ease. Indirect therapists help clients replace difficult, jerky, and painful reactions with easy, smooth, and pain-free motion.

As just noted, indirect methods respond to resistance in the tissues by shifting back toward the direction of ease. Because client awareness can be enhanced with exercise that reinforces letting go, feeling the support of the body's weight and gravity, and searching for ease, guidelines for exercise as a supplement to indirect methods are provided in Chapter 9.

In the craniosacral approach to myofascial massage, discussed in Chapter 10, the practitioner uses the subtlest level of perception, palpation, and technique. Craniosacral therapy requires responding to the tiniest dural tube movements as they reflect the flow of the CSF. It thus requires the greatest sensitivity and specificity of all the approaches described in this text.

SUMMARY

Myofascia is a specific type of deep fascia that is bound to muscle tissue. Myofascial massage focuses on the myofascial unit, including muscle, CT, and the neuromuscular junction. Myofascial massage derives from an osteopathic tradition and relies on at least three osteopathic principles. These are 1) the structure and function of the body are interrelated; 2) the body can heal itself; and 3) the body is a whole, united by fascia. Surveys support the popularity of myofascial massage and case studies support the effectiveness of its use. Clients seem to respond more quickly and results last longer. Learning and practicing neuromuscular, direct CT, indirect CT, and craniosacral approaches to myofascial massage is also rewarding for students and therapists, who seem to thrive on listening to and following the myofascia to release discomforts and promote the body's sense of ease. Practicing myofascial techniques can, in itself, improve body mechanics and communication skills for the therapist and provide a kinesthetic sense of the juncture between body, mind, and spirit. It also can promote personal growth.

A comparison of the terms *method, approach, style,* and *technique* can clarify and simplify the learning of myofascial theory and techniques. *Method* specifies whether the therapist meets resistance in the body tissues with an opposing force (direct methods) or faces resistance by giving way to a sense of ease (indirect methods). The two *approaches* to the direct method are distinguished by whether the therapist focuses his or her efforts on the muscle and nerve (neuromuscular) or on the CT (direct CT) aspects of the myofascia. The two approaches to the indirect method are distinguished by whether the therapist focuses his or her efforts on the larger movements of the myofascia as a whole (indirect CT) or on the subtle movements of the dura (craniosacral).

Style designates popular "brands" of myofascial massage, which can be repetitive, confusing, and misleading. For this reason, the term is rarely used in this text. *Techniques* are the actual physical manipulations of the body tissue. Descriptions of technique must be complemented with an increasing awareness and sensitivity to client signals and a clearer sense of what the therapist wants to do.

The ordering of chapters was intentionally planned to lead the reader into successively more subtle and specific intents, palpatory and communications skills, and manipulations.

Review Questions

1. __________ is defined as releasing the muscle via the CT.
   a. Myofascial massage
   b. Myofascial release
   c. Myofascial trigger point work
   d. Connective muscle massage
2. The __________ method of myofascial massage is exemplified by meeting resistance in the body tissues with an opposing force.
   a. indirect
   b. neuromuscular
   c. direct
   d. direct CT
3. The __________ method of myofascial massage is exemplified by meeting resistance in the body tissues with a sense of ease.
   a. indirect
   b. neuromuscular
   c. direct
   d. indirect CT
4. True or false: The direct CT approach to myofascial massage applies sustained pressure to the client's CT while coaching the client in specific micromovements.
5. The __________ approach to myofascial massage focuses on a specific aspect of the CT, that is, the dura mater and the CSF movements within the sac.
6. State four reasons for studying myofascial techniques.
7. List three osteopathic principles that guide the practice of myofascial massage.

REFERENCES

Alexander D. Soft tissue resistance barriers. Massage Therapy Journal 2003;42(1):96–112.

Auleciems LM. Myofascial pain syndrome: a multidisciplinary approach. Nurse Pract 1995;20(4):18, 21–22, 24–28.

Barnes JF. The basic science of myofascial release. Journal of Bodywork and Movement Therapies 1997;1(4):231–238.

Chaitow L, DeLany JW. Clinical Application of Neuromuscular Techniques. Vol. 1: The Upper Body. Edinburgh, UK: Elsevier Science, 2002.

Earl E. The dual sensory role of the muscle spindles. Physical Therapy Journal 1965;45:4.

Ezzo J, ed. Neuromuscular Therapy Update, 1987–1994. Baltimore: 1994.

Field T. Massage therapy effects. American Psychologist 1998;53(12): 1270–1281.

Myers, TW. Anatomy Trains: Myofascial Meridians for Manual and Movement Therapists. London, England: Churchill Livingstone, 2001.

Rich GJ, ed. Massage Therapy: The Evidence for Practice. New York: Mosby, 2002.

Rubik B. Manual healing methods. In: Alternative Medicine: Expanding Medical Horizons. Washington, DC: U.S. Government Printing Office, 1992.

Skootsky SA, Jaeger B, Oye RK. Prevalence of myofascial pain in general internal medicine practice. West J Med 1989;151(2):157–160.

Staubesand J. Zum Feinbau der fascia cruris mit Berucksichtigung epi- und intraszialar Nerven. Manuella Medezin 1996;34:196–200.

The mainstreaming of alternative medicine. Consumer Reports 2000; May:17–25.

Travell JG, Simons DG. Myofascial Pain and Dysfunction: The Trigger Point Manual. Vol. 1: The Upper Extremities. Baltimore: Lippincott Williams & Wilkins, 1999.

Upledger JE. Craniosacral Therapy II: Beyond the Dura. Seattle, WA: Eastland Press, 1987.

Upledger JE, Vredevevoogd JD. Craniosacral Therapy. Seattle, WA: Eastland Press, 1983.

Wilson V. Inhibition in the CNS. Scientific American 1966;5:102–106.

Part

I

The Anatomy and Physiology of Myofascial Massage

Chapter 2

The Anatomy and Physiology of Muscle Tissue

OBJECTIVES

- Explain the relationship of skeletal muscle to connective tissue and nerve tissue.
- Provide an overview of the anatomy and physiology of the muscular system as it is affected by myofascial massage.
- Describe the implications of myofascial massage for muscle tissue.

CHAPTER OUTLINE

KEY TERMS

Muscle fibers: Individual muscle cells.
Fascicles: Bundles of muscle fibers.
Endomysium: Thin connective tissue sheath that wraps each muscle fiber.
Perimysium: Connective tissue sheath that wraps groups of muscle fibers (fascicles).
Epimysium: Connective tissue sheath that wraps an entire muscle.
Aponeuroses: Flattened sheaths of connective tissue that connect muscle to flat bones.
Skeletal muscle tissue: Muscle that is attached to the skeleton through the connective tissue. It moves bones and stabilizes the body.

Excitability: Reactive quality of all muscle tissue in response to an electrical or chemical stimulus.
Contractility: Shortening of muscle tissue in response to stimulation by an electrical charge.
Extensibility: Stretchability beyond a muscle's normal, resting length.
Elasticity: Ability of a muscle to return to its normal resting length after being stretched.
Myofilaments: Microscopic threads that make up the myofibrils of muscle fibers. There are two types, thick and thin.
Myosin: Primary protein component of thick myofilaments.
Actin: Primary protein component of thin myofilaments.
Sliding-filament theory: Description of skeletal muscle contraction as a chain of physical and chemical reactions ending in actin and myosin myofilaments sliding toward each another.
Sarcomeres: Functional (contracting) units of a muscle fiber.
Latent: Short period of time that elapses after the initial nerve impulse and before the muscle begins to shorten.
Contraction: Period during which the thick (myosin) and thin (actin) myofilaments slide past each other.
Relaxation: Period during which the myofilaments return to their separated state.
Refractory: Period when a new nerve impulse cannot cause the muscle to contract again.
Neuromuscular junction: Region at which an electrical impulse is transferred into a muscle.
Ratchet model: Model attributing to myosin a swiveling head that acts like a ratchet to pull the sarcomere together and cause muscles to contract.
Somatic motor neurons: Nerve cells that carry impulses related to muscle movement or glandular secretion.
Motor end plate: Location on the sarcolemma where the somatic motor neurons meet the muscle.
Synaptic cleft (synapse): The extracellular space between two neurons or between a neuron and the muscle fiber or gland it affects.
Motor unit: A somatic motor neuron and all of the muscle fibers to which it connects.
Muscle spindles: Spindle-shaped proprioceptors within skeletal muscles that monitors the muscles' degree of stretch.

Muscles are the primary movers and stabilizers of the body. Indeed, muscle actions are so specific and varied that they are best described in a textbook devoted to kinesiology. Even involuntary movements, from the pulsations of the heart to the expansion of the ribcage during breathing, require muscle activity. In turn, muscle activity requires energy. Thus, it is not surprising that the musculoskeletal system is also the largest consumer of energy in the body.

Healthy muscles move in response to a variety of signals from the nervous system. Trauma, disease, overuse, disuse, or misuse, however, can interfere with this communication. When this happens, even simple movement can become restricted, difficult, painful, or impossible.

It is important for myofascial therapists to consider how the muscular system is affected by the manipulation of soft tissue, especially through myofascial massage. Muscles together with their fascial binding are the media that are molded and shaped by myofascial therapies. Therefore, this chapter focuses on the relationship of skeletal muscle tissue to connective tissue (CT), the innervation of skeletal muscles by nerve tissue, and skeletal muscle physiology. The first section reviews the anatomy of muscle tissue, focusing on its structure and component parts. The second section examines muscle physiology, emphasizing how skeletal muscles contract. The chapter closes with a discussion of the implications of myofascial massage for muscle tissue.

This chapter discusses muscle cells and tissue insofar as they relate to CT. It is not intended to teach the entire muscular system. Much of the information in this chapter is presented in summary form, with some specific topics (e.g., skeletal muscle tissue) receiving a fuller discussion because of the significance they have in respect to myofascial massage. Whole sections relating to cardiac and smooth muscle, muscle location, and other important topics are omitted from the discussion here. Please consult an anatomy and physiology text for a complete discussion of the human muscular system.

Muscle Tissue Anatomy

The structure of muscle tissue establishes conditions that influence how muscle can contract and relax.

THE INTERRELATEDNESS OF MUSCLE TISSUE AND CONNECTIVE TISSUE

Living muscles are inseparable from CT. **Muscle fibers**, individual muscle cells, are held in place by CT, which also surround bundles of muscle fibers called **fascicles** and, finally, entire muscles (Figure 2-1). The CT that surrounds an individual muscle is called endomysium. The perimysium brings nerve fibers and capillaries to the muscle fibers as it binds them into fascicles. Whole muscles are collections of fascicles surrounded by a CT sheath known as the epimysium. Part of the deep fascia, epimysium separates individual muscles with different actions from one another and from surrounding organs. The epimysium is also continuous with the rope-like tendons or sheet-like aponeuroses of CT.

Muscle acts on bones through CT. Tendons connect muscle to the periosteum of long bones such as the humerus or femur. Aponeuroses (flattened sheathes of CT) weave muscles into the periosteum of flat bones such as the skull. Thus, CT conveys the action generated by muscle contraction to the bones, so that we can move. In addition, CT separates muscle from the skin (superficial fascia) and holds groups of muscles with similar actions together (deep fascia) (Premkumar, 2004). These CT delineations allow muscles to act on the skeletal system with less interference from other structures and with more power.

TYPES OF MUSCLE TISSUE

Three types of muscle tissue perform the various activities of the body: skeletal, cardiac, and smooth (Figure 2-2). Each has a different structure and purpose. Muscle types also

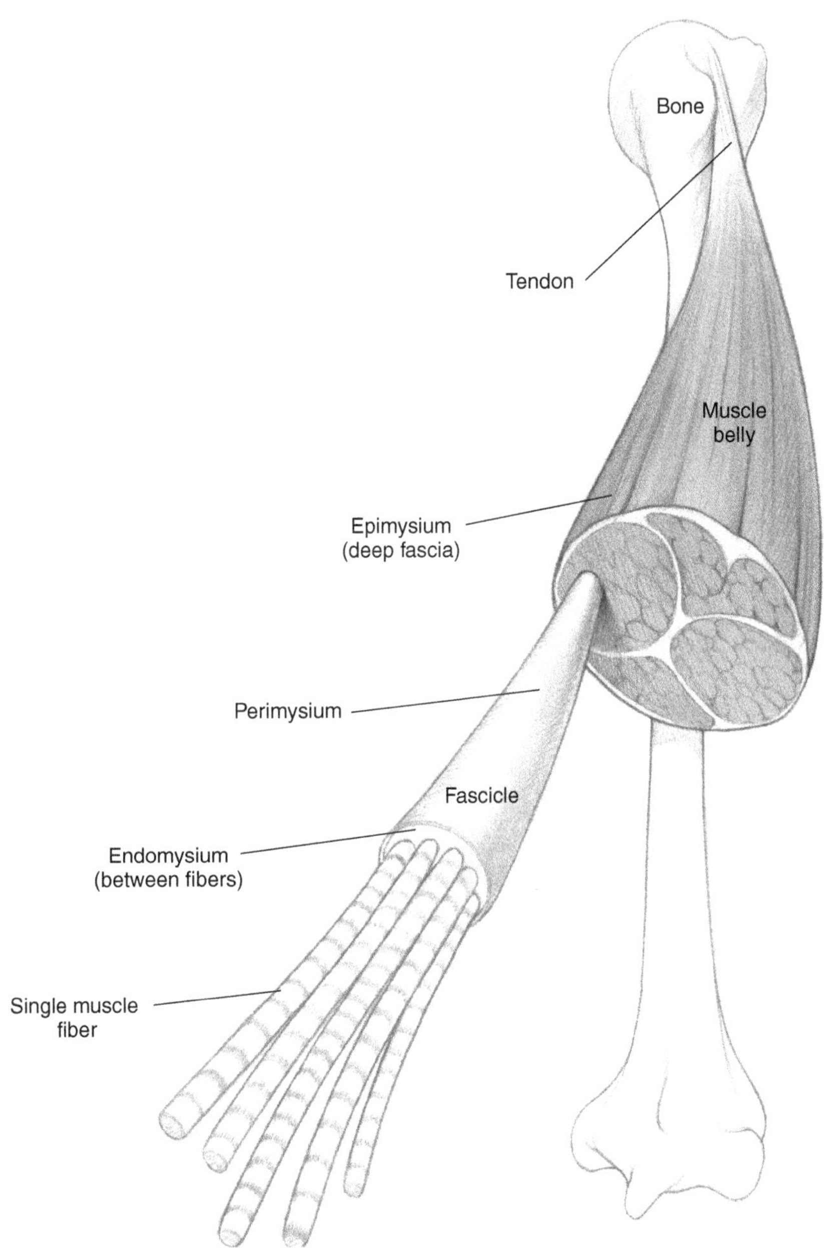

FIGURE 2-1 **Structure of skeletal muscle.** Notice the complex interweaving of CT and muscle tissue.

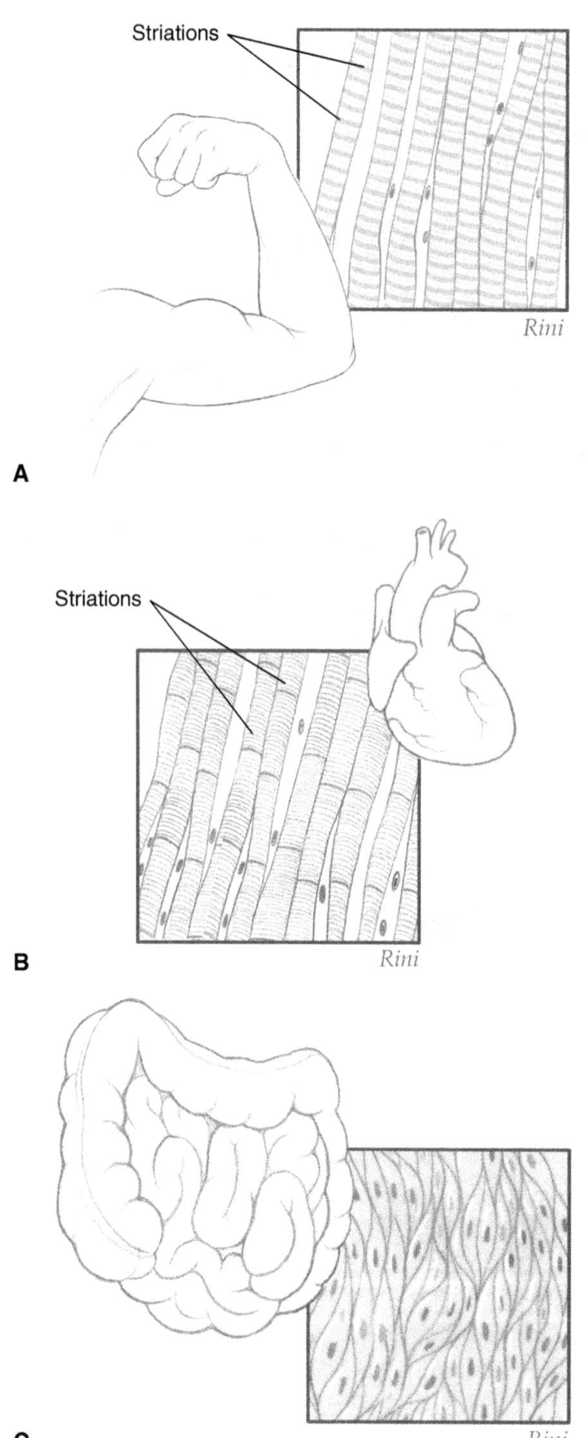

FIGURE 2-2 **Types of muscle tissue.** (**A**) Skeletal, (**B**) cardiac, and (**C**) smooth muscle vary in structure, function, and location.

vary in microscopic appearance, strength, and duration of contraction and in how they are controlled by the nervous system.

Skeletal muscle tissue is attached to the skeleton through the CT and is responsible for moving bones and stabilizing body position. Skeletal muscle movement is voluntary (i.e., controlled by the central nervous system [CNS]). Under a microscope, skeletal muscle tissue is clearly striated (i.e., striped in light and dark bands).

Cardiac muscle forms the wall of the heart and needs no stimulation from the CNS to contract and relax. It has a long resting period (several tenths of a second) between contractions, which serves to move blood through the body. Cardiac muscle is striated.

Smooth muscle is found within the walls of tubes such as blood vessels and the digestive tract. As indicated by their name, smooth muscle fibers are not striated. They are involuntary, responding to impulses from the autonomic nervous system (ANS), to changes in levels of hormones (i.e., specific chemicals produced by endocrine glands and delivered by the blood), and to changes in other chemicals such as hydrogen, oxygen, and carbon dioxide. Smooth muscle also responds to temperature changes and to being stretched (e.g., by the presence of food in the gastrointestinal [GI] tract). It helps to move fluid and food through the GI tract and to regulate the flow of fluid out of other organs (e.g., the bladder).

COMMON CHARACTERISTICS OF MUSCLE TISSUE

All three types of muscle tissue share four characteristics: excitability, contractility, extensibility, and elasticity.

Excitability means that muscle tissue responds to a stimulus (i.e., changes in the environment, either inside or outside the body). Stimuli may be electrical (e.g., originating from a nerve impulse) or chemical (e.g., originating from a hormone released by the endocrine system and reaching the muscle through the blood). In contrast, neither epithelial tissue nor CT has been shown to respond when exposed to electricity or chemicals.

Contractility means that when stimulated by an electrical charge, muscle tissue "contracts" or shortens. The contractile mechanism is the same for all three types of muscle and is described in the physiology section of this chapter.

Muscle tissue can be stretched beyond its normal, resting length. This property is called extensibility.

After muscle tissue is released from a stretch, it returns to its original length, similar to an elastic band. This property is called elasticity.

SPECIAL CHARACTERISTICS OF SKELETAL MUSCLE TISSUE

Skeletal muscle moves the bones of the skeleton, allows the body to stand erect or resist movement, and produces heat (e.g., through shivering). Because we consciously control muscle actions, skeletal muscle movement is said to be voluntary. As noted earlier, skeletal muscle cells cannot contract without a stimulus from the CNS.

Observed under a microscope, skeletal muscle fibers are striated in light and dark bands. Fibers may have more than one nucleus and vary in length from microscopic to 12 inches, depending on their location.

Because muscles are the body's force generators, they require a source of power. Glucose and lipids are processed in the mitochondria to produce the energy needed to permit skeletal muscle contraction and to prevent movement and maintain stability. Some of the energy produced in the mitochondria is stored as glycogen inside the muscles for later use.

Skeletal muscle fibers relax briefly between contractions. Paradoxically, this relaxation allows us to maintain strong contraction. When a contraction involves more than 70% of the available strength, however, blood flow is reduced and oxygen availability diminishes (Chaitow and DeLany, 2002). This means that strong muscle contractions cannot be sustained indefinitely.

Components of Skeletal Muscle Fibers

Muscle fibers are long and narrow when relaxed. They are cylindrical, running parallel to one another through the entire length of the muscle.

Many of the components of muscle fibers are similar to those of other cells. For instance, muscle fibers have a plasma membrane known as the *sarcolemma* and a cytoplasm known as the *sarcoplasm*. As noted earlier, they may have many nuclei and mitochondria. Large numbers of myoglobin molecules, which store the oxygen used by the mitochondria, are found in the sarcoplasm. The endoplasmic reticulum of a muscle cell is called the *sarcoplasmic reticulum* and is used to store calcium ions that are released during contraction. Attached to the sarcoplasmic reticulum are inward extensions of the sarcolemma known as *T tubules* (transverse tubules). Familiarity with these terms will clarify the discussion of muscle physiology that comes later in this chapter.

Skeletal muscle fibers are filled with smaller fibers, called *myofibrils,* that extend lengthwise across the cell. Myofilaments are microscopic threads that make up the myofibrils. There are two types: thick and thin. Thick myofilaments are made from the chemical myosin, and thin myofilaments are made from a contractile protein called actin. According to the sliding-filament theory, these thick and thin threads slide past each other during muscle contraction. The areas of the fiber that consist solely of thin myofilaments are called I bands. They look like a band of light under the microscope. Areas of the myofilament that consist of both thick and thin myofilaments superimposed on each other are called A bands. These appear dark under the microscope. These alternating light and dark bands cause the striated appearance of skeletal muscle tissue.

The Structure of Myosin and Actin

Each thick myosin filament is composed of smaller molecules shaped like golf clubs. The shafts of the "clubs" are bundled together into a thick cord, leaving the heads sticking out in all directions along the length of the myofilament. Greene (1995) describes the myosin filament as appearing like a long braid of garlic heads (Figure 2-3).

Six actin filaments surround each myosin filament. Each is composed of two long chains of bead-shaped molecules (see Fig. 2-3). The two chains twist around each other like the wires of a cable.

Sarcomeres

Sarcomeres are the contracting units of a muscle fiber. The thick (myosin) and thin (actin) myofilaments are arranged in a series of sarcomeres that repeat down the entire muscle fiber.

The sliding-filament theory maintains that in a relaxed muscle, one sarcomere is spaced as far away from the next

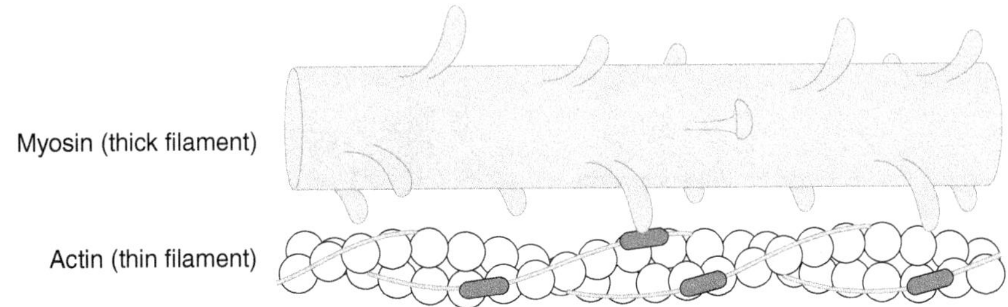

FIGURE 2-3 **Myosin and actin.** Thick myofilaments resemble braids of garlic. Each is surrounded by six thin myofilaments, which look like twisted strands of beads. Together these make up the sarcomere.

sarcomere as it can be. When the muscle fiber contracts, the sarcomeres slide closer together because the thin myofilaments move past the thick ones (Figure 2-4). (This process is described in more detail shortly.)

Muscle Tissue Physiology

An electromyogram (EMG) can measure the phases of muscle movement. Four phases have been documented by EMGs: the latent period, contraction period, relaxation period, and refractory period.

- The **latent** period is the short period of time that elapses after the initial nerve impulse and before the muscle begins to shorten. This includes time for the impulse to travel down the nerve, as well as all actions that take place within the sarcoplasm before the sliding-filament mechanism begins.
- The **contraction** phase is the period when the myosin heads bind to active sites of the actin (thin filament). Binding causes the thick and thin myofilaments to slide past one other, causing the sarcomere to shorten from both ends. The duration of a muscle contraction produced by a single nerve impulse varies according to location and function. For example, whereas eye muscles twitch for about 10 ms, the soleus may sustain a single contraction for 100 ms (Premkumar, 2004).
- During the **relaxation** period, the myofilaments slip back to their separated state.
- The **refractory** period occurs after these other phases. During this brief time, a new nerve impulse cannot cause the muscle to contract again. The refractory period in skeletal muscle is about 5 ms (Premkumar, 2004). Because the refractory period is so short, a second

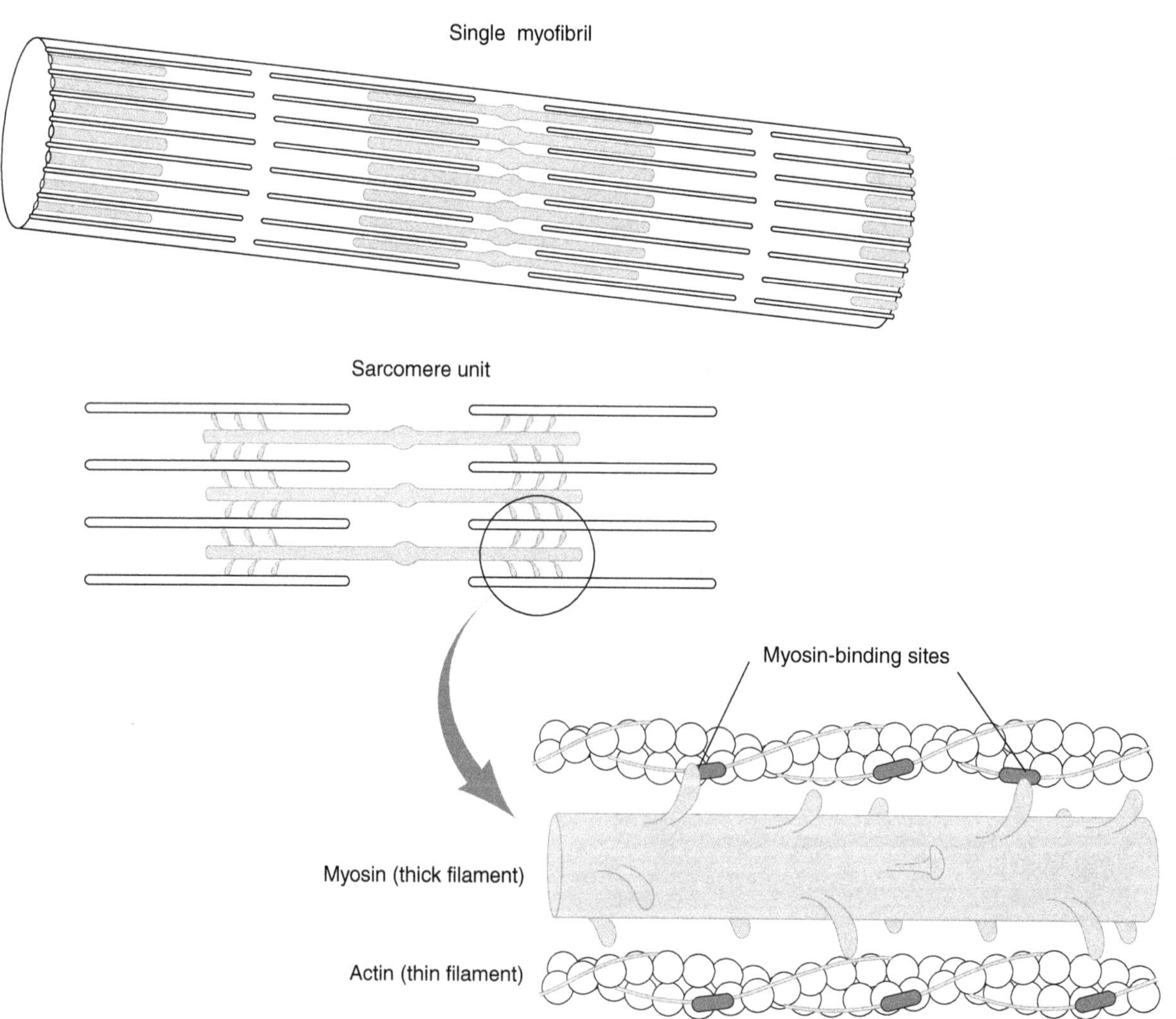

FIGURE 2-4 Sarcomere unit in sliding-filament theory. Notice how the myosin and actin myofilaments overlap when they slide past each other.

impulse can fuse with a first impulse to produce a sustained contraction (Premkumar, 2004).

THE SLIDING-FILAMENT THEORY OF CONTRACTION

Now that we have delineated the four phases of muscle movement, it is time to explore the contraction phase in more detail. Skeletal muscle contraction results from a chain of physical and chemical reactions that begin with an intention to move. Usually the impulse originates with conscious thought in the brain (e.g., "I will pick a tomato"). In the case of many reflexes (e.g., withdrawing your hand from a hot stove), however, the nerve impulse may originate lower down, in the spinal cord, to allow a faster reaction. (The spinal cord is a little closer to the muscle that is reacting.) The nerve impulse travels to a nerve ending that almost touches the edge of one or more muscle fibers. The place where the electrical impulse is transformed into kinetic energy (action) is called the **neuromuscular** (or *myoneural*) **junction**.

The nerve impulse's electrical charge causes the nerve ending to release chemicals called *neurotransmitters* into the gap (or *synaptic cleft*) between the nerve ending and the muscle cell. (This process is described in more detail in Chapter 4.) The neurotransmitters adhere to receptors on the surface of the muscle cell. When the neurotransmitter acetylcholine (ACh) binds to a muscle cell receptor, the receptor changes shape. This sets off a chain reaction that releases an electrically charged flow of sodium atoms into the muscle through the T tubules.

The electrical charge stimulates the release of calcium ions from the sarcoplasmic reticulum. The calcium ions bind to molecules that ordinarily block myosin-binding sites on the actin, leaving them exposed for myosin binding. This process also causes a release of energy, which is required to pull the thick and thin myofilaments past each other. Myosin then binds with actin and the sarcomere shortens. In relaxation, this process is reversed.

To summarize, the following stages occur during muscle cell contraction:

1. An impulse crosses the neuromuscular junction. A nerve impulse reaches the nerve ending and causes the release of the neurotransmitter ACh. ACh molecules cross the synaptic cleft and attach to receptor proteins on the surface of the sarcolemma of nearby muscle fibers.
2. The impulse enters into the body of the muscle fiber. Under the influence of ACh, an electrical charge passes over the sarcolemma and down the T tubules.
3. Calcium ions are released. The electrical charge in the T tubules causes the associated sarcoplasmic reticulum to release stored calcium ions.
4. The myofilament is activated. The calcium ions diffuse into the sarcoplasm and attach to the thin myofilaments (actin). The thin myofilaments connect to the thick myofilaments (myosin), and the thick and thin myofilaments pull past each other. This is contraction.

RELAXATION

A two-step reaction stops the contraction cycle and allows the muscle fiber to relax. First, the enzyme acetylcholinesterase breaks down the neurotransmitter ACh that was secreted across the neuromuscular junction. This stops the nerve impulse from activating muscle contraction.

Second, the calcium that has already been released into the muscle cell is removed. This occurs through two mechanisms. First, calcium is actively pumped out of the cell. Second, a special protein binds with the calcium that remains in the cell. When calcium levels decrease, the myosin–actin bond is released and the myofilaments slip back to their relaxed state.

THE RATCHET MODEL OF MYOSIN–ACTIN BINDING

The sliding-filament theory asserts that the filaments slide past each other but does not specify precisely how. Thus, a supplementary model of myosin–actin binding was developed (Greene, 1995). Called the **ratchet model** of myosin–actin binding, it proposes that myosin has a swiveling head that acts like a ratchet to pull the sarcomere together. Specifically, when actin's binding sites are exposed, the nearby myosin heads bind to them (Figure 2-5). This binding causes the myosin to swivel where the head attaches to the shaft. Recall that myosin shafts are bundled together to form thick myosin filaments. Thus, the myosin head's swiveling "power stroke" pulls on the actin, shortening the entire sarcomere unit and causing the muscle to contract.

The chemical breakdown of adenosine triphosphate (ATP) provides energy for the myosin head to swivel back to its original position, only now it is across from the next actin down the filament chain. The cycle is ready to begin again. This whole process takes less than 1 second and is somewhat similar to the gears of a bicycle as they catch and fit together to propel the bike forward.

ENERGY USE IN MUSCLE CONTRACTION

The energy that we use in muscle contraction is mostly stored in the chemical bonds that hold the three phosphates together in the ATP molecule. ATP is the universal energy carrier in all animal cells. It is manufactured by the cell's mitochondria. Muscle fibers store enough ATP to

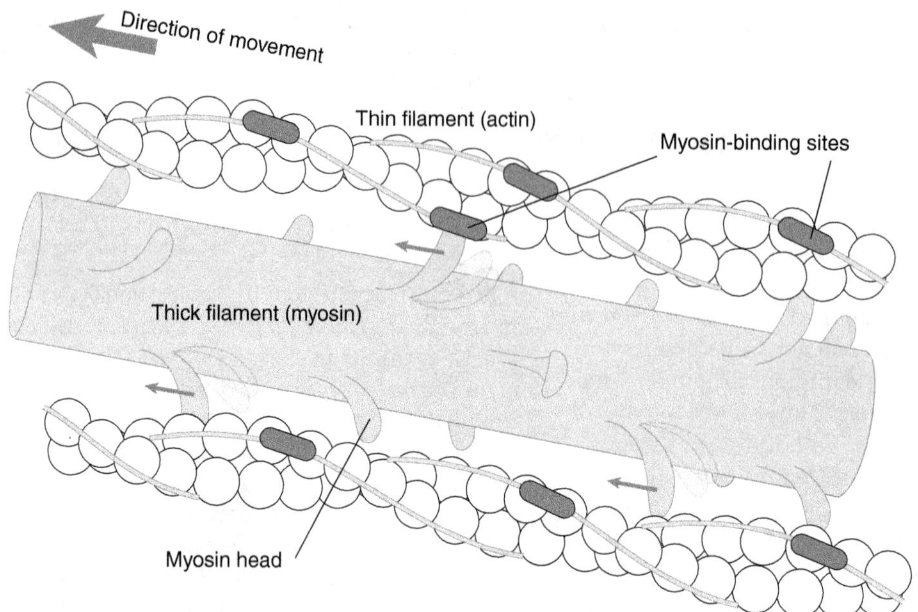

FIGURE 2-5 **The ratchet model of myosin-actin binding.** Myosin heads at both ends of the sarcomere act like ratchets, pulling the sarcomere together.

contract continuously for only about 3 seconds (Thompson and Manore, 2005).

Muscle fibers also contain phosphocreatine, a high-energy storage molecule that can be broken down into ATP. This provides an additional 15 seconds of contraction for muscle fibers (Tortora and Grabowski, 2003).

Further energy can be provided by the breakdown of carbohydrates into glucose. Muscle fibers, as well as the liver, store glucose in the form of glycogen. When needed, the glycogen is converted back into glucose and ATP. Oxygen needed to generate ATP is stored in myoglobin and hemoglobin. Myoglobin is found in muscle fibers and hemoglobin is part of red blood cells.

The muscles have only a limited supply of glycogen, so fats are another source of energy when the body is at rest and are a major source during physical activity. When fat is needed, it is released from the adipose cells and travels in the blood attached to a protein (as a *lipoprotein*) to muscle tissue. There it enters the mitochondria and uses oxygen to produce ATP.

THE ROLE OF NERVES IN MUSCLE CONTRACTION

As noted earlier, skeletal muscle fibers are stimulated to contract by nerve cells (neurons). The junction of a motor neuron with the muscle fiber it affects, called the neuromuscular junction, has three parts: the neuron, the synaptic cleft, and the muscle fiber (Figure 2-6).

Neurons that attach to and affect the muscle fibers are known as somatic motor neurons. Somatic motor neurons meet the sarcolemma (plasma membrane) of the muscle at the motor end plate. The space between the somatic motor neuron and the sarcolemma of the muscle cell is called the synaptic cleft (or synapse).

When a nerve impulse reaches the end of the somatic motor neuron, it stimulates the release of the neurotransmitter ACh from sacs at the end of the neuron known as *synaptic vesicles*. The neurotransmitter diffuses out of the synaptic vesicle, travels across the gap, and attaches to receptors on the sarcolemma. Note that the CT matrix in the synaptic cleft contains acetylcholinesterase enzymes that can destroy ACh (Premkumar, 2004). Without ACh, the nerve impulse has nowhere to go and the muscle cannot receive the message to contract.

A motor unit is a somatic motor neuron and all of the muscle fibers it innervates. The number of fibers can vary from 10 (in muscles that are associated with precise movements) to 2,000 (in muscles that perform less precise movements).

MUSCLE TONE

Normally, parts of each muscle are in a state of tension. Muscle tone (tonus) is defined as the resting tension in a muscle. In any muscle, certain motor units are always active. Although this activity is too small to cause actual contraction, it makes the muscle firm or "toned." Muscle tone is also partly an effect of the elastic property of muscles.

Muscle tone stabilizes the bones in position and helps maintain posture. Some degree of tone ensures that muscles are not limp and flaccid. Too much tone can result in

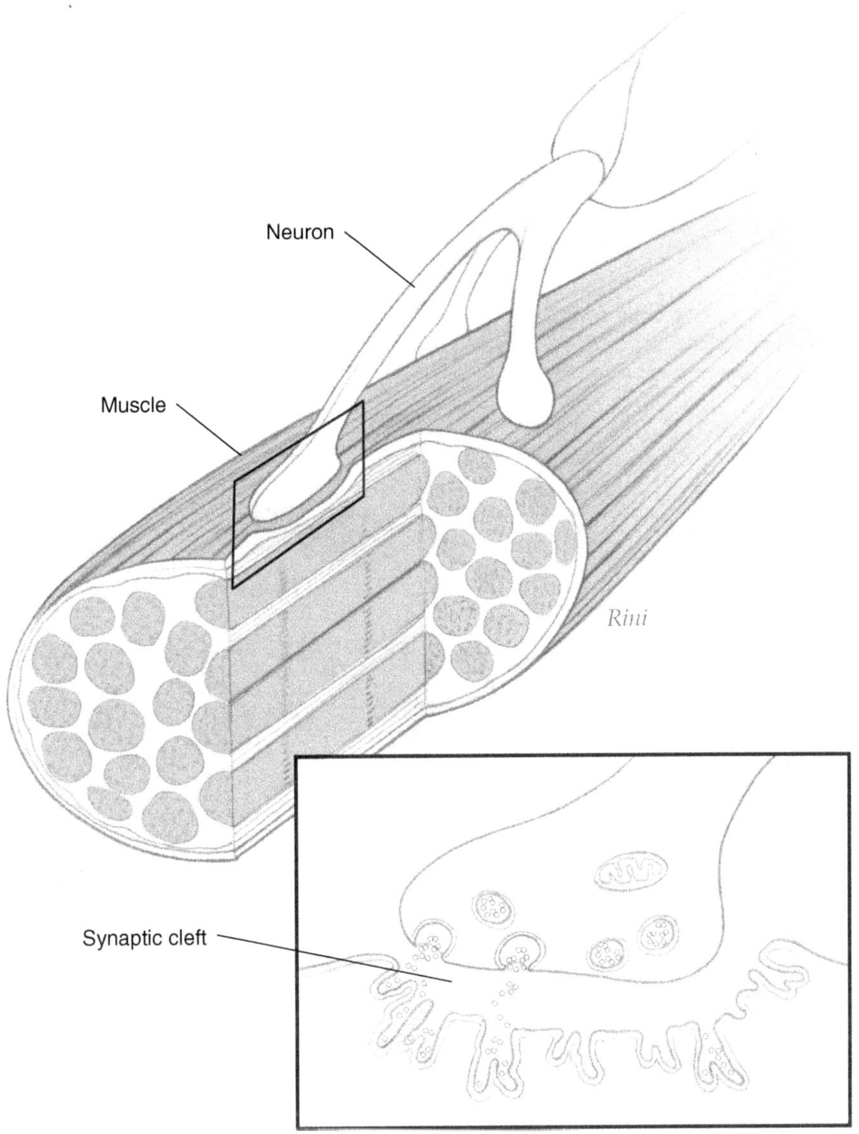

FIGURE 2-6 **The neuromuscular junction.**

hyperreactivity or rigidity in the muscles. Muscles with moderate tone feel firm and solid.

Muscle tone is maintained in part by the stimulation of *proprioceptors,* which are sensory receptors that fire in response to changes in tension, position, or acceleration of the muscles and joints. Muscle spindles are proprioceptors that are distributed throughout skeletal muscles and monitor their degree of stretch (Figure 2-7). They are composed of three to 10 modified skeletal muscle fibers innervated by sensory neurons and surrounded by a CT capsule, giving them a spindle shape. The ends of the muscle spindle capsule are attached to endomysium and perimysium. The muscle spindles are located parallel to other muscle fiber cells; their length is altered as the whole muscle lengthens or shortens. Actin and myosin within the muscle spindle are concentrated at the ends of the capsule. Special sensory nerves that surround the center of the muscle spindle generate impulses every time the length of the muscle spindle changes. These sensory nerves generate a reflex response (discussed in more depth in Chapter 4) so that the muscle contracts when stretched to prevent overstretching. Thus, muscle spindles are sometimes referred to as "stretch receptors," implying that they are nerves, although only part of the muscle spindle is actually nerve tissue.

GOLGI TENDON ORGANS

Golgi tendon organs (GTOs) are proprioceptors that monitor the degree of tension within tendons. They consist of sensory nerve endings that are wrapped around the collagen fibers of tendons (Figure 2-8). Approximately 10 to

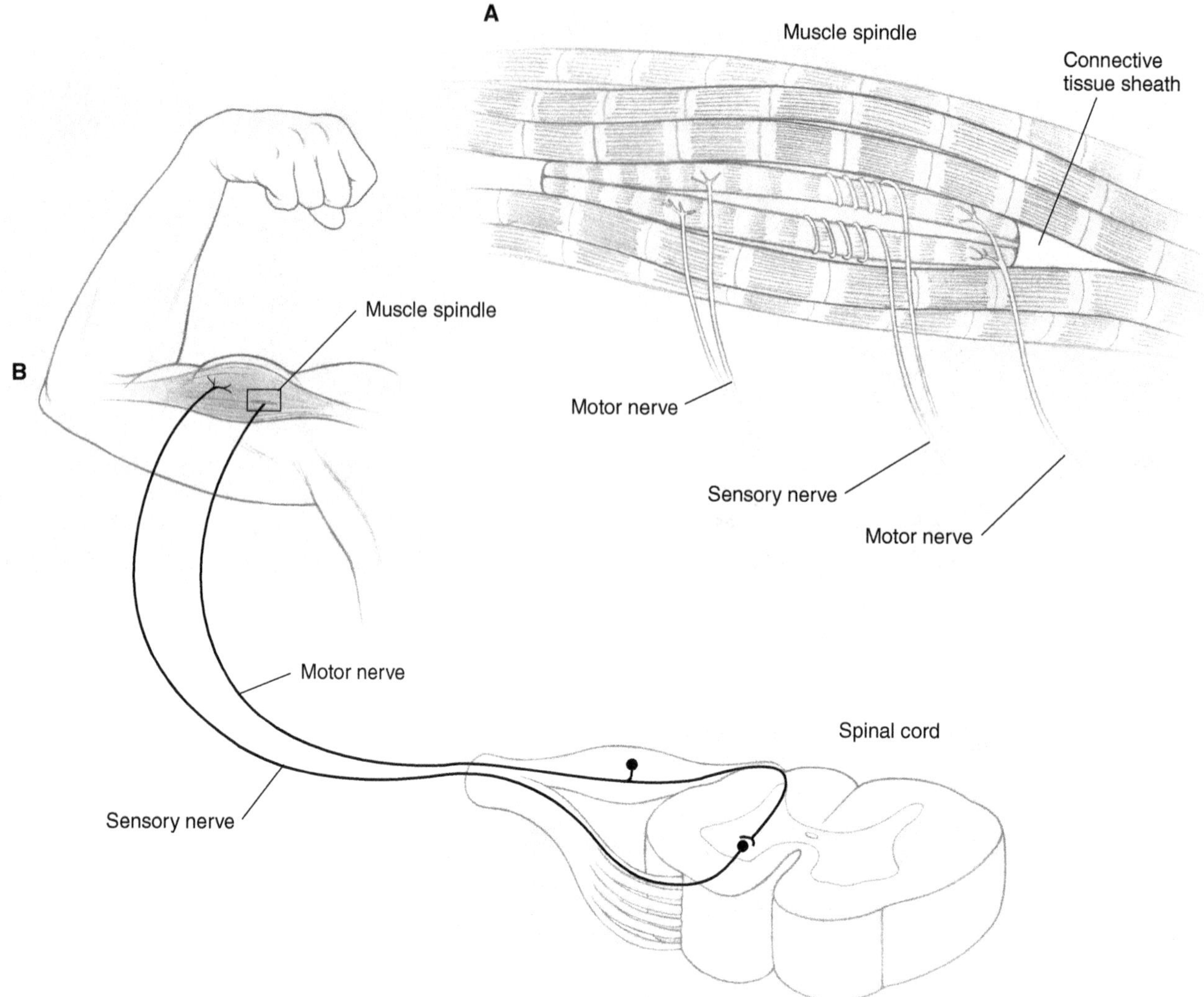

FIGURE 2-7 **Muscle spindles.** (**A**) Structure of the muscle spindle. (**B**) Location of the muscle spindle within the muscle.

15 muscle fibers are attached to each GTO. Stretch on a GTO produces reflex muscle relaxation by inhibiting the somatic motor neuron that attaches to that tendon's adjacent muscle. Thus, GTOs protect the muscle from injury caused by contracting with excessive force or speed. (Because GTOs are nerve tissue, they are discussed in more detail in Chapter 4. Other proprioceptors are also discussed in Chapter 4.)

The Implications of Myofascial Massage for Muscle Tissue

Because muscle tissue is inseparably intertwined with CT (deep fascia) and because skin is separated from muscle by more CT (superficial fascia), any bodywork that affects CT also affects the muscles within its protective wrapping. Although massage that affects muscle also affects fascia, the effects of myofascial massage may be arguably more potent than other forms of massage that do not directly address the fascia. After practicing the forms of myofascial work presented in this text (see Chapters 5 to 10), many manual therapists have reached this conclusion.

REFLEXIVE EFFECTS

Reflexive effects are caused by a nervous system response to physical manipulation of the surface or underlying tissues of the body. Usually a generalized whole-body response, reflexive effects include increased blood and lymph circulation, slowed heart rate, generalized relaxation and stress reduction, and increased immune response. Reflexive effects also include pain relief and muscle relaxation caused by alterations in the function of the motor unit and sensory receptors similar to those in muscle spindles and GTOs.

Bodywork that is intended to relax muscle tissue also has some degree of reflexive effect on the surrounding CT. Relaxation is a powerful tool that is necessary to prepare

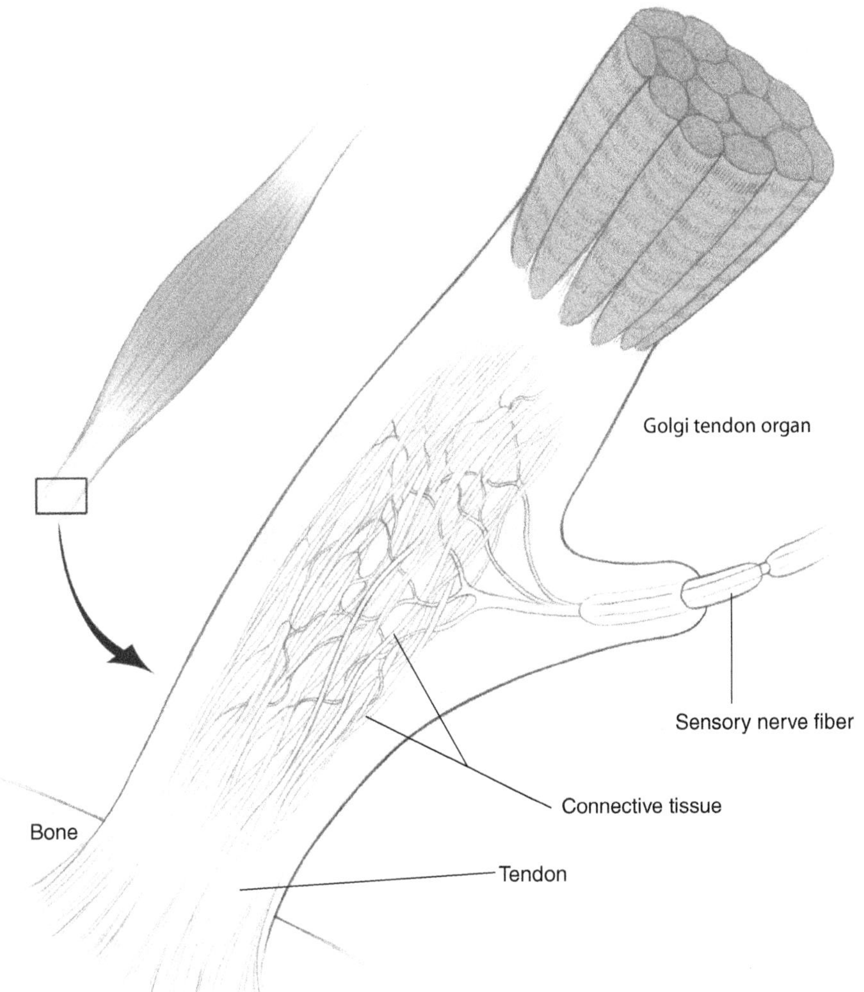

FIGURE 2-8 **Structure of a Golgi tendon organ.**

the body for more specific change. Generalized relaxation massage achieves a significant degree of change as the muscles relax their baseline tone.

Deeper forms of relaxation are possible with myofascial approaches because they directly involve the ANS. (See Chapter 4, where the connection between relaxation, the ANS, and fascia is explored.)

Massage that targets specific sensory receptors such as GTOs at a certain joint or stretch receptors within a particular muscle's muscle spindles (e.g., muscle energy techniques described in Chapter 5) may provide more specific reflexive effects such as increased range of motion at a given site.

MECHANICAL EFFECTS

Mechanical effects are effects directly caused by physical manipulation of the body tissue by the massage therapist's hands (Fritz, 1995). Mechanical effects of massage include fluid movement (e.g., circulation of blood to and from muscle and of lymph away from the muscle), heat production, compression, stretching, and broadening of the muscle fibers. Massage directed deeper than the surface of the skin (e.g., pétrissage, friction, vibration, deeper tapotement, effleurage) has some mechanical effect on muscles and at least the superficial layer of fascia.

Although the contractile (shortening) mechanism is the same for all muscles, it is important for myofascial massage practitioners to remember that the force applied is modified by the direction of the muscle fibers, the action of the muscle, and where the muscle originates and inserts on the bone. Thus, it cannot be emphasized enough that a familiarity with muscle kinesiology (i.e., fiber direction, origin, insertion, and action) helps students to accurately apply myofascial massage techniques.

Yet even with an underlying knowledge of muscle anatomy and physiology, practitioners may find that bodywork that does not specifically address CT is not as long lasting or effective as myofascial massage. When a muscle is manually relaxed but guarded by a tight and tendinous covering that will not move, it is prevented from maintaining its fully relaxed length. If the muscle is relaxed but the protective armoring remains, that muscle becomes more likely to return to a shortened, contracted state after a bodywork session.

But if muscle and fascia are so interwoven, why doesn't CT soften whenever muscle lengthens? One explanation of the need for specific fascial massage is that because CT does not contract, it does not relax. Fascia is more similar to Silly Putty, which must be molded directly to be made more soft and pliable. (See Chapter 3 for more on CT.)

Another reason why the muscle can be relaxed without an analogous pliability in the fascia is that CT is not as richly vascularized as muscle. Thus, increasing general circulatory flow is not optimally effective in getting fluids and nutrients into and releasing toxins out of the fascia. Thus, although knowledge of muscle anatomy, physiology, and kinesiology can help therapists achieve a degree of mechanical specificity over and above the broad mechanical effects of relaxation massage, the rest of the myofascial unit (connective and nerve tissues) must also be studied.

SUMMARY

The anatomy and physiology of muscle tissue determines the structure and function of the entire human body. All bodywork addresses muscles. Myofascial massage affects muscles along with the surrounding CT and innervating nerve tissue.

There are three types of muscle tissue: skeletal, cardiac, and smooth. This chapter focuses on skeletal muscles because they are the object of most myofascial massage

Each muscle is wrapped in three layers of CT: endomysium, perimysium, and epimysium.

Muscle cells are also known as muscle fibers because they are long and thin and are arranged in parallel. Some important parts of muscle fibers are the sarcolemma (plasma membrane), T tubules (inward extensions of the sarcolemma), sarcoplasmic reticulum (endoplasmic reticulum that is used to store calcium ions released during contraction), and sarcoplasm (cytoplasm).

Skeletal fibers have many mitochondria to produce energy and many nuclei. Large numbers of myoglobin molecules, which store the oxygen used by the mitochondria, are found in the sarcoplasm.

Skeletal muscle fibers are filled with smaller fibers, called myofibrils, which extend lengthwise across the cell. Myofilaments are microscopic threads that make up the myofibrils. There are two types, thick and thin. Thick myofilaments contain the chemical myosin, and thin myofilaments contain actin.

Skeletal muscles cannot move without a signal from a nerve. A motor unit includes the nerve and the collection of muscles that it causes to contract. The connection between nerve and muscle along with the gap between the two is called the neuromuscular junction. Proprioceptors include muscle spindles and GTOs.

The functioning or contractile unit of a muscle cell is the sarcomere. The sliding-filament theory describes the chain of reactions that shorten the sarcomeres, resulting in muscle contraction. The ratchet model further explains the pulling and pivoting action of the myosin heads as they bind to the thin filaments and shorten the sarcomere.

An understanding of muscle anatomy and physiology can guide the intentions of myofascial therapists. Discussions of the connective and nerve tissue components of the myofascial unit follow in Chapters 3 and 4, respectively.

Review Questions

1. The theory that explains how skeletal muscle contraction results from a chain of physical and chemical reactions is called __________.
   a. sliding-filament theory
   b. muscle fiber theory
   c. myofascial theory
   d. neuromuscular theory

2. The thick threads that make up part of the muscle fiber are composed of __________.
   a. myosin
   b. actin
   c. troponin
   d. calcium

3. The thin threads in the muscle fiber are composed of __________.
   a. myosin
   b. actin
   c. troponin
   d. calcium

4. The functional unit of a muscle fiber is a __________.
   a. sarcoplasm
   b. sarcoplasmic reticulum
   c. sarcomere
   d. myofilament

5. The ratchet model is a refinement of the sliding-filament theory that explains the movement of the __________ heads.
   a. muscle
   b. myosin
   c. actin
   d. troponin

6. Skeletal muscle tissue is __________ and __________.
   a. striated and involuntary
   b. striated and voluntary
   c. nonstriated and involuntary
   d. nonstriated and voluntary
7. Individual muscle cells are also known as muscle __________ because of their shape.
8. The middle covering of CT that bundles individual muscle fibers into muscle fascicles is called __________.
9. True or false: The three types of muscle tissue do *not* include smooth muscle tissue.
10. True or false: A motor unit is a somatic motor neuron and all of the muscle fibers to which it connects. The number of fibers can vary from 10 to 2,000.

REFERENCES

Chaitow L, DeLany JW. Clinical Application of Neuromuscular Techniques. Vol. 1: The Upper Body. Edinburgh, UK: Elsevier Science, 2002.

Fritz S. Mosby's Fundamentals of Therapeutic Massage. St. Louis: Mosby, 1995.

Greene E. Mystery of how muscles contract—solved. Massage Therapy 1995(Spring):76–80.

Premkumar K. The Massage Connection: Anatomy and Physiology. 2nd Ed. Baltimore: Lippincott Williams & Wilkins, 2004.

Thompson J, Manore MM. Nutrition and Health: An Applied Approach. San Francisco: Benjamin Cummings, 2005:430.

Tortora GJ, Grabowski SR. Principles of Anatomy and Physiology. 10th Ed. New York: HarperCollins College Publishers, 2003.

SUGGESTED READINGS

Biel A. Trail Guide to the Body. Boulder, CO: Books of Discovery, 2001.

Clay JH, Pounds DM. Basic Clinical Massage Therapy: Integrating Anatomy and Treatment. Baltimore: Lippincott Williams & Wilkins, 2003.

Juhan D. Job's Body: A Handbook for Bodywork. Barrytown, NY: Barrytown Ltd., 1998.

Moore KL, Dalley AF. Clinically Oriented Anatomy. 4th Ed. Philadelphia: Lippincott Williams & Wilkins, 1999.

Premkumar K. The Massage Connection: Anatomy and Physiology. 2nd Ed. Baltimore: Lippincott Williams & Wilkins, 2004.

Chapter 3

The Anatomy and Physiology of Connective Tissue

OBJECTIVES

- Describe the anatomy of connective tissue, focusing on structure and classification.
- Explain the physiology of connective tissue.
- Discuss how unique properties of connective tissue are affected by myofascial massage.

CHAPTER OUTLINE

KEY TERMS

Matrix: Noncellular part of connective tissue containing fibers and a solid, semisolid, or liquid ground substance.

Piezoelectricity: A property of connective tissue whereby it conducts electricity when compressed.

Thixotropy: A property of connective tissue whereby it can sometimes change form from thick and hard to more pliable and soft.

Chapter 2 addressed the muscular or "myo" component of myofascia. This chapter looks at "fascia" in its broader role as a connective tissue (CT). The first section reviews the anatomy of CT, focusing on its structure and classification. The next section reviews the physiology of CT, including its functions and unique properties.

Early in my career as a massage educator when teaching anatomy and physiology classes to massage students, I began the class on CT by saying that CT was easy to remember because "all it does is connect." Now I know how naïve that statement was. In some sense, it is true that "all that CT does is connect," but connections are the means to many ends (e.g., form, structure, safety and support, definition, entry and exit, protection, and repair). By virtue of the connections it makes, CT plays many and diverse roles in biological maintenance and healing.

Connective Tissue Anatomy

Tissues are cohesive organizations of cells that have special functions based on their specific properties. In the broadest sense, any tissue that provides structure or holds the body together can be classified as a CT. Thus, CT has many different forms. Some kinds of CT are hard (e.g., bones); some are flexible yet strong (e.g., ligaments and tendons). Blood is a fluid CT, connecting every cell in the body. These dissimilar tissues all share a distinctive function: they link one part of the body with another. All types of CT also share a distinctive structure that can be detected under a microscope. This common structure is described shortly.

To better explain what CT is, it might help to identify what it is *not*. Three types of tissue in the human body are not CT. These are epithelial, nerve, and muscle tissue.

Epithelial tissue is made of densely packed cells. It serves two functions. First, epithelial tissue covers the surface of the body and many of its organs, and lines its tubes, vessels, and cavities. Second, it forms most of the body's glands, which are structures that produce secretions such as sweat, milk, and hormones. In the human body, epithelial tissue is found joined to an underlying layer of CT called the *basement membrane.*

Nerve tissue is composed of neuroglia (which may actually be more accurately classified as CT) and neurons. Neurons produce electrical charges in response to stimuli. Characteristically of CT, neuroglia surrounds the neurons and provides them with protection and support.

As discussed in Chapter 2, muscle tissue is made up of muscle fibers, groups of fibers (called fascicles), and whole muscles, encircled by sheaths of CT. It is "excitable" because, when stimulated by an electrical charge, it contracts. Muscle tissue can also be stretched beyond its normal resting length, and upon release, return to its original length. Figure 3-1 illustrates the four basic tissue types found in the human body.

TYPES OF CONNECTIVE TISSUE

The four broad types of CT are CT proper, which is known as fascia, cartilage, bone, and blood. Figure 3-2 is a simple diagram of the relationship of these types to one another. Fascia includes two specific types of CT: superficial fascia (loose CT) and deep fascia (dense CT). CT classification is discussed in more detail later in the chapter.

Superficial fascia lies just beneath the surface of the skin. Deep fascia makes up the sheathing that surrounds and penetrates muscles as well as the tendons that link muscles to bones and the ligaments that tie bones to bones. Because fascia shares important characteristics with other kinds of CT and is continuous with them, it seems appropriate to examine the tissue that secures us into our human form as one entity.

COMPONENTS OF CONNECTIVE TISSUE

Unlike epithelial tissue, which consists mainly of cells, CT consists of only a few cells rooted in a "matrix." The matrix (meaning *mother substance*) is built of fibers and a solid, semisolid, or liquid ground substance. Compare Figures 3-1A and 3-1B to see this difference in cellular structure.

Ground Substance

Ground substance is the embedding material that holds the fibers and cells. The type of CT varies according to the degree of solidity of the surrounding ground substance. For example, whereas a liquid ground substance is characteristic of blood, a harder, denser ground substance is characteristic of bone.

Connective Tissue Cells

Connective tissue cells include fibroblasts, mast cells, plasma cells, and macrophages:

- *Fibroblasts* ("fiber makers") synthesize fibers and the ground substance. Nonactive fibroblasts are known as fibrocytes ("fiber cells").
- *Mast cells* gauge the amount of water that diffuses in and out of cells through osmosis. They also produce allergic and inflammatory symptoms (e.g., increased blood flow to the area) through the release of histamine and bradykinin.
- *Plasma cells* secrete antibodies that destroy pathogens (i.e., disease-causing microorganisms).
- *Macrophages* (literally "big eaters") are white blood cells that migrate into areas to destroy pathogens and dead cells by engulfing and eating them.

Connective Tissue Fibers

Fibers in the matrix include collagen, reticular fibers, and elastic fibers:

- *Collagen fibers* are strong and resistant to injury yet are soft and flexible. Collagen provides the extensibility and mobility in CT.
- Reticular means "like a spider's web," and indeed, *reticular fibers* intertwine and branch to form a frame that looks very similar to a web. Turchaninov and Cox (1998) consider reticular fibers to be immature collagen fibers.

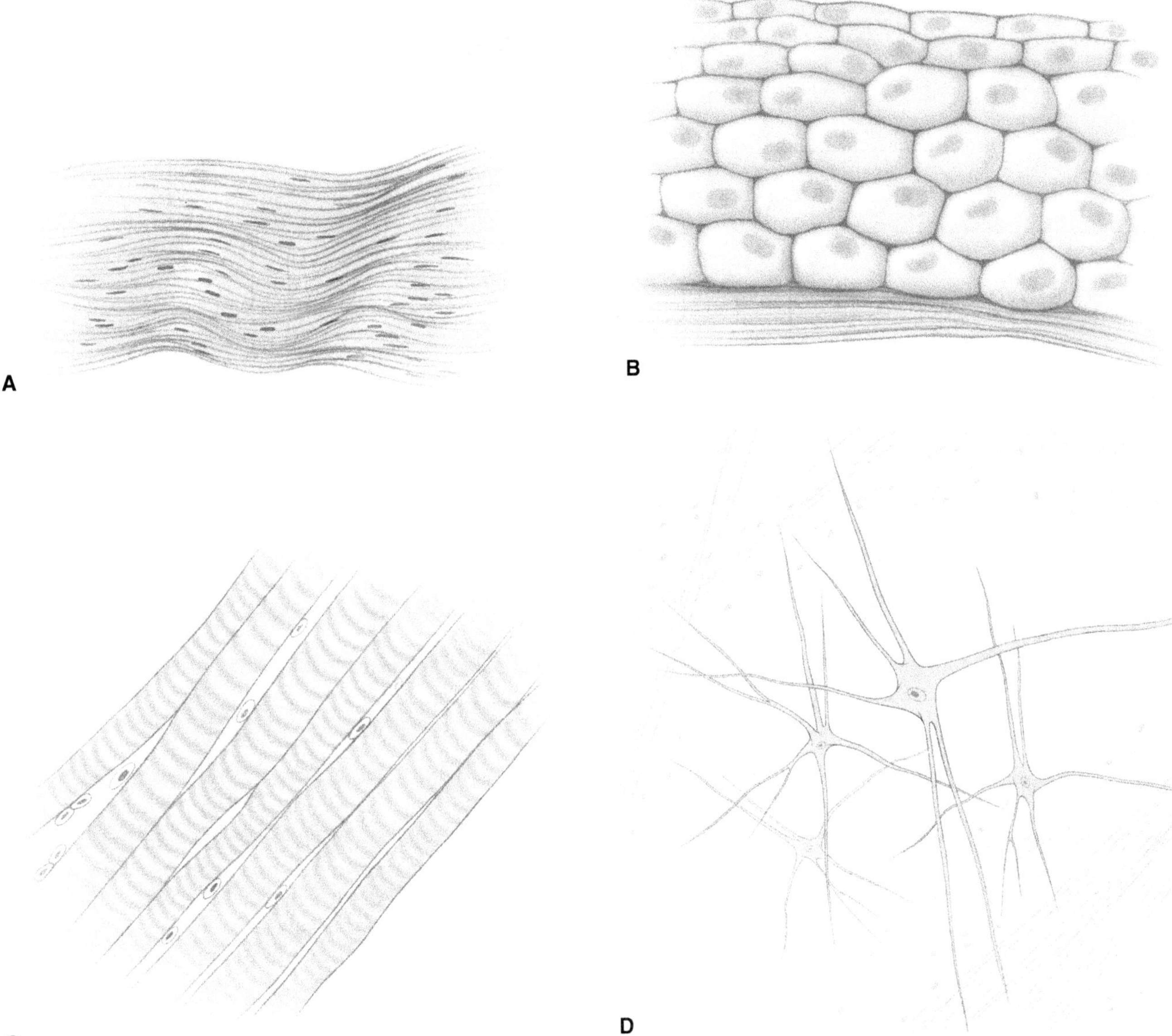

FIGURE 3-1 **Four tissues of the human body.** (**A**) Connective tissue. (**B**) Epithelial tissue. (**C**) Muscle tissue. (**D**) Nerve tissue.

Reticular CT can provide structural support (e.g., in the walls of organs and blood vessels) or perform filtering duties (e.g., in the lymph nodes and spleen).

- *Elastic fibers* are able to stretch and snap back to their original size, thereby providing the tensile strength of CT. Certain organs that require pliability (e.g., the bladder, arteries, and skin) contain an abundance of elastic fibers.

Table 3-1 summarizes the components and characteristics of CT.

A developing embryo has embryonic CT up to 2 months after conception. One important type of embryonic CT is *mesenchyme,* the original substance from which all other types of CT arise. Adults retain some mesenchyme in addition to their adult CT. This is interesting because mesenchyme has the potential for regeneration into any type of CT that is needed by the body. The ability to regenerate and renew is the model for healing.

CLASSIFICATION OF CONNECTIVE TISSUE

Postembryonic CT is classified according to the composition of its matrix. The differences in matrix consistency are based on what kinds of fibers are present (if fibers are present at all) and whether the ground substance in the matrix is solid (also called *sol*) or semisolid (also called *gel*). These properties

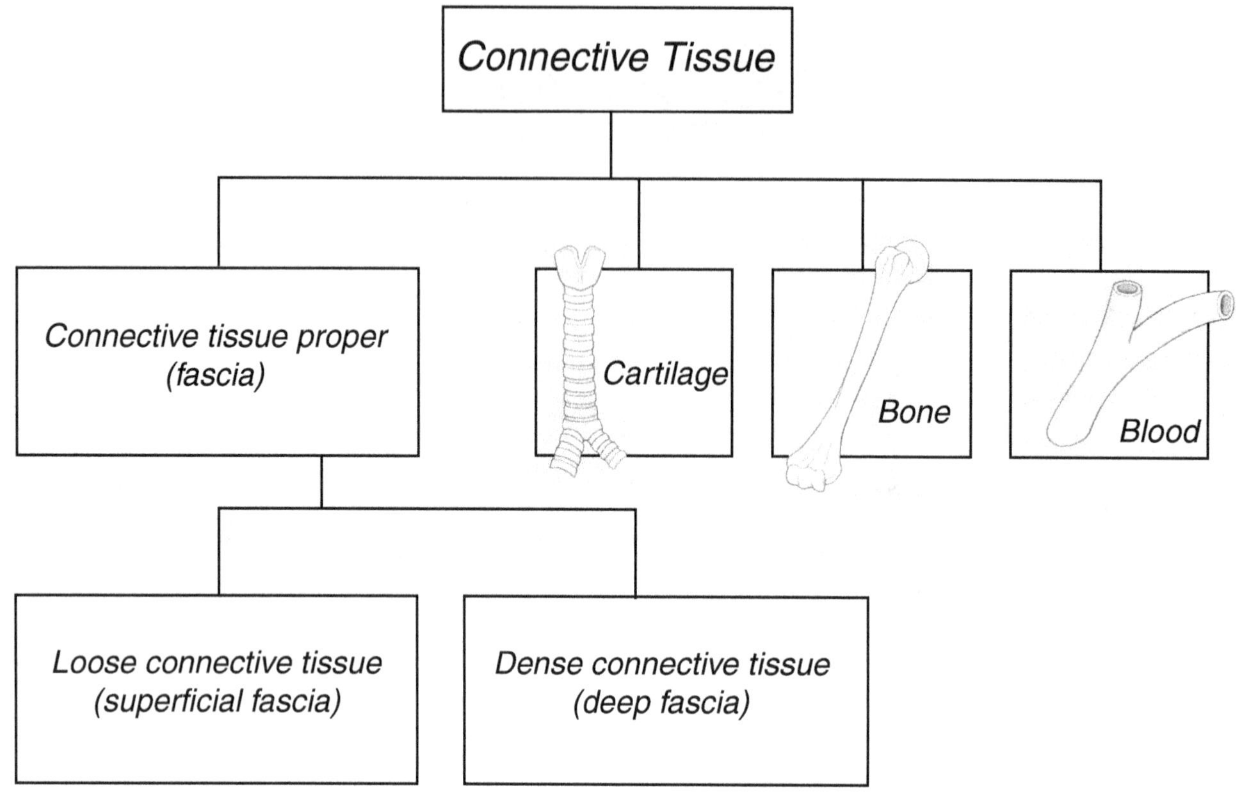

FIGURE 3-2 **Types of connective tissue present in the human body.**

cause the different types of CT to exhibit vastly different qualities. These types, their varieties, and their characteristics are discussed next and are summarized in Table 3-2.

Superficial Fascia

The three types of loose CT (superficial fascia) all contain fibers loosely interspersed among many cells. Loose areolar CT contains collagen, elastin, and reticulin fibers loosely arranged in a gel. It surrounds organs and is found between muscles and deep to the skin. Loose adipose or "fat" CT contains cells that are specialized for storing fat. It provides insulation and long-term energy reserves. Fibers interlaced in a small amount of ground substance make up loose reticular CT, which provides a protective webbing on the walls of many organs and filters foreign substances in the spleen and lymph nodes.

TABLE 3-1 Components of Connective Tissue

Component	Types	Characteristics and Examples
Fibers	Collagen	Strong yet moldable
	Reticulin	Spider-like
	Elastin	Can stretch and snap back
Cells	Fibroblasts	Make fibers
	Mast cells	Make histamines and regulate water flow
	Plasma cells	Secrete antibodies
	Macrophages	Destroy pathogens and dead cells
Ground substance	Liquid	Blood
	Semisolid	Ligaments and tendons
	Solid	Bones

TABLE 3-2 Categories of Connective Tissue

Category	Varieties	Characteristics
Loose	Areolar Adipose Reticular	Fibers loosely interspersed among many cells
Dense	Dense regular Dense irregular Dense elastic	Also called fibrous CT because it contains more numerous and thicker fibers, or collagenous CT, because the fibers are often made of collagen
Cartilage	Hyaline Fibrocartilage Elastic	Made of densely woven collagen and elastic fibers packed in a jelly (chondroitin sulfate)
Bone (osseous tissue)	Compact Cancellous (spongy)	The matrix consists of mineral salts containing calcium and phosphorus to make bones hard and collagen fibers to provide strength and flexibility
Blood (vascular CT)		Consists of a liberal watery matrix (plasma) and red and white blood cells and cell fragments (platelets) suspended in the plasma

Deep Fascia

Dense CT (deep fascia) is also called *fibrous CT* because it contains more numerous and thicker fibers, or *collagenous CT,* because the fibers are predominantly made of collagen. The fibers of dense regular CT (found in tendons and ligaments) are oriented in parallel directions. This array resists tearing and is very strong. Because the dense regular CT fibers are arranged in parallel, it has a very strong tensile strength but only in that one direction. In dense irregular CT, the collagen fibers do not have a regular pattern. This type is found in parts of the body where stresses are exerted in many directions, such as in the periosteum, liver, and capsules of the spleen. Dense elastic CT is made of mostly elastin strands suspended in a semisolid (gel) ground substance. Dense elastic fibers provide the elasticity and strength needed for the vocal cords, artery walls, and lung passageways to continually stretch and recoil.

Cartilage, Bone, and Blood

Unlike other CT, cartilage does not contain blood vessels or nerves; however, it is nourished by blood vessels in its surrounding membrane. Cartilage is made of densely woven collagen and elastic fibers packed in a jelly (chondroitin sulfate). The collagen fibers impart strength, and the jelly-like ground substance adds resiliency. Hyaline cartilage (known as *gristle* in meat products), the most common type, wraps the ends of long bones, the walls of the trachea, and the flexible part of the nose. It contains delicate collagen filaments that are difficult to spot under a microscope. Fibrocartilage contains bundles of collagen that are clearly visible. It is more rigid than hyaline cartilage and is found in the intervertebral discs. Strands in elastic cartilage form a net that maintains the shape of the ear, the top of the larynx, and the auditory tubes.

Bone (osseous tissue) can be classified as either compact (dense) or spongy (cancellous) depending on how the matrix and cells are organized. The matrix of bony matter consists of mineral salts containing calcium and phosphorus to make the bones hard and collagen fibers to provide strength and flexibility. Without collagen, bones would shatter from the impact of jumping or any type of hard contact. Compact bone forms the outer layer of the long bones, and spongy bone is found primarily in the pelvis, ribs, sternum, vertebrae, skull, and proximal ends of the femur and humerus. Spongy bone contains a gel (red bone marrow) that produces blood cells and cell fragments.

Blood (vascular CT) has a liquid matrix called plasma. Suspended in the plasma are red and white blood cells as well as cell fragments called platelets. According to Chikly (2001), lymph and cerebrospinal fluid (CSF), insofar as they are filtered from blood, are also CT.

Connective Tissue Physiology

Connective tissue is the most abundant tissue in the body, making up more of the human organism than any of the other three tissue types. This preponderance of CT directly influences myofascial functioning and indirectly influences all of the organs, tissues, and cells touched by CT. On the other hand, hormone levels, hydration, local metabolic rates, and mechanical activity can all alter the physical state of CT. These factors can all be positively affected by myofascial massage. Pressure and manipulation (i.e., assisted or resisted movement) stimulate tissues to soften, fluids to circulate, and metabolic processes to return to healthy levels.

FUNCTIONS OF CONNECTIVE TISSUE

The functions of CT are discussed next and are summarized in Table 3-3.

Connects Physical Structures

The first function of CT is to connect structures in the body. This seems simple enough, yet the connections established by CT allow a number of supplementary healing and homeostatic functions for the body. These connections give shape to the human body, provide safety and support for the organism, define areas used for cooperative roles, provide a way in and out of specific body regions, and—as blood coursing through the body—provide protection and repair.

Provides Reinforcement and Boundaries

Connective tissue provides a framework for protecting and embracing each part of the body and uniting the body as a whole. In every level of organization, from the cell to the whole human organism, connective fibers keep the unit together and functioning. CT joins cells into tissue, glues one kind of tissue to another, gathers tissues into a functioning organ, surrounds and protects organs, joins organs into organ systems, and defines organ systems and connects them to complementary systems in the body. To the degree that form follows function, the shapes outlined by CT follow the way that humans operate in the physical world. For example, CT defines and separates individual nerves, keeping them in their appropriate channels.

CONNECTIVE TISSUE WRAPS MUSCLES

As discussed in Chapter 2, CT wraps every single muscle fiber (as endomysium), fascicle (as perimysium), and muscle (as epimysium; Figure 3-3). Sheaths of deep fascia bundle muscle fibers together to keep them parallel and determine how vectors of force will pull in the endomysium, perimysium, epimysium, and tendons. Massage therapists who address CT use their bodywork to keep the fascial wrappings aligned and establish a vector of force that therapeutically influences the pull on muscles, tendons, and, by extension, bones. Some therapists do not realize the importance of the protective sheath and concentrate only on relaxing the muscles. When a muscle is manually relaxed but guarded by a tight and tendinous covering, it is prevented from maintaining its fully relaxed length. That muscle becomes more likely to return to a shortened, contracted state after a bodywork session. Manual treatments that focus only on muscles without regard to fascia take longer to effect a change and are less likely to last.

CONNECTIVE TISSUE WRAPS NERVE CELLS

In the nervous system, neurons (i.e., nerve cells that transmit electrical signals) are organized and maintained by specialized CT cells called *neuroglia*, or simply *glia*. The name, glia, literally means "glue." Glial cells do not conduct nerve impulses. Instead, they provide protection and support. In the same way that endomysial, perimysial, and epimysial CT surround individual fibers, fascicles, and entire muscles, neuroglia protect and support individual neural cells, cell bundles, and entire nerves (Figure 3-4). Glial cells can also provide the tensile strength and elasticity needed for stretching, and they can secure nerves to other structures.

Six types of glial cells are satellite cells, astrocytes, microglia, ependymocytes (ependyma), neurolemmocytes (Schwann cells), and oligodendrocytes:

- *Satellite cells* surround and protect collections of neurons in the peripheral nervous system (ganglia).
- *Astrocytes* are star-shaped cells that wrap neurons in the brain and spinal cord, binding them to one another and to blood vessels.
- *Microglia* are small "Pac-Man–like" macrophages in the brain that can move to injured areas to consume pathogens and damaged cells.

TABLE 3-3 Functions of Connective Tissue
Provides structure and form ("order out of chaos")
Transfers muscular contraction to bones
Transfers muscular contraction to internal organs, blood and lymph vessels, and nerves
Supports the skeleton so it can bear weight
Draws the boundaries around individual cells so they can perform specialized functions; provides the safe space for each cell to express its individuality
Provides defense and repair services: fibroblasts, inflammatory response
Transports nutrients into and conducts wastes out of cells

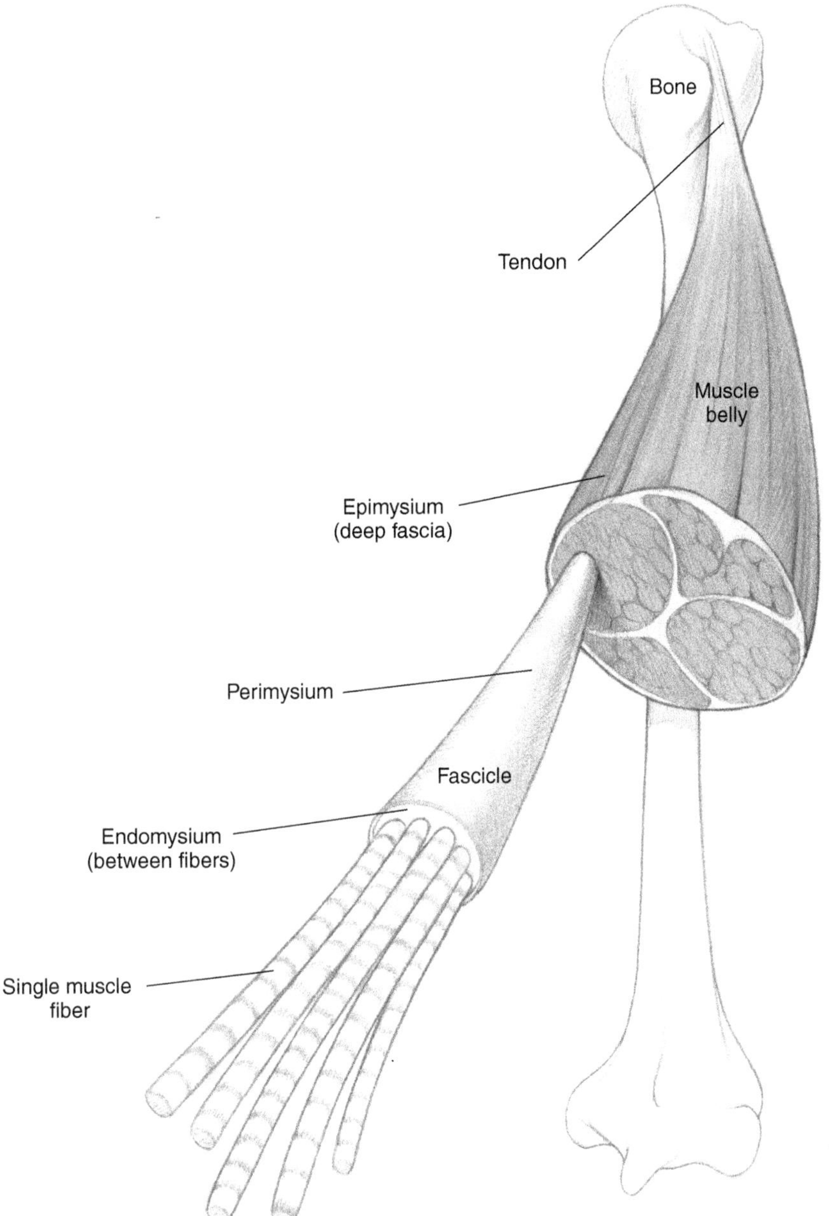

FIGURE 3-3 **Every layer of muscle is surrounded by fascia.**

- *Ependymocytes* form sheets that line the spaces in the brain (ventricles) and spinal cord. Their hair-like cilia may help to circulate the CSF that bathes the CNS.
- *Neurolemmocytes* (*Schwann cells*) produce the fatty myelin sheath that spirals around the long axons of peripheral nerves and speeds up electrical transmissions.
- *Oligodendrocytes* produce the same white myelin coating for nerve processes in the brain and spinal cord.

Nerves with a myelin coating are known as "white matter." Their color distinguishes them from uncoated grey cell bodies and axons, collectively known as "grey matter." Physical benefits from bodywork that concentrates on CT will affect the specialized CT of the nervous system (neuroglia) and in turn improve the function of the nerve cells that they support (Tortora and Grabowski, 2003).

CONNECTIVE TISSUE WRAPS ORGANS, BLOOD VESSELS, AND EACH INDIVIDUAL CELL

As previously noted, fascia wraps not only every muscle and nerve cell but also every bone, blood vessel, and organ. Around bones, CT is called *periosteum*. It is continuous from bone surface to joint capsule to ligament to tendon to muscle sac and wraps every bone, joint, and muscle in a seamless complex. CT contains every drop of

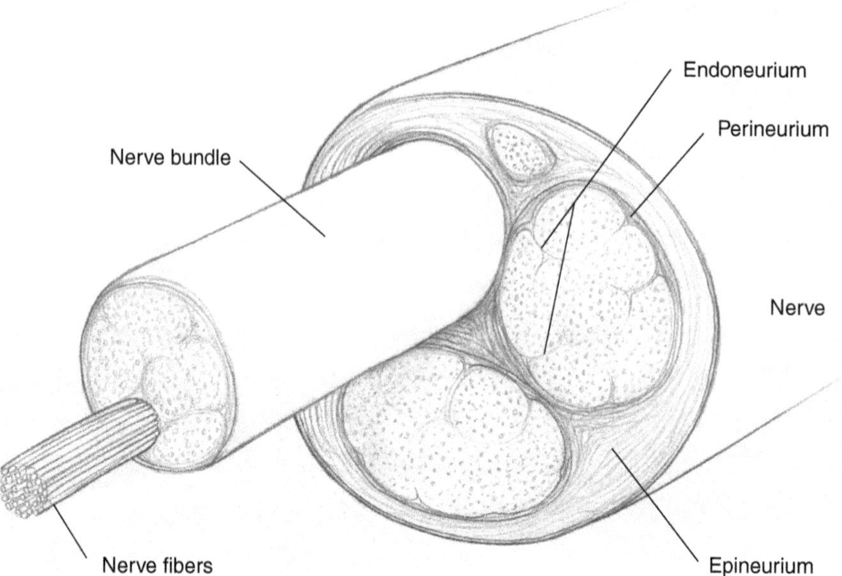

FIGURE 3-4 **Every layer of nerve is surrounded by fascia.**

fluid in our bodies, that is, it forms the fibrous bed that supports all lymph and blood vessels and keeps them in their appropriate channels. Peritoneal CT supports the richly vascularized mesentery membranes that hold the intestines in place while defining the curves of the gastrointestinal tract. The CT that forms a sheath around the heart is called pericardium. Arteries and veins are surrounded and held into place by CT. Fat cells are surrounded and held together into adipose tissue by collagen networks. Tendons, ligaments, tendon sheaths, and the retinaculum holding tendons in place are all continuous structures of CT.

Supports Bones and Other Structures

Ligaments secure bone to bone. Tendons attach muscle to bone. Without CT to hold it up, the skeleton would collapse under its own weight. CT connectors act like the rigging on a ship to provide tension to support the masts (bones) and sails (skin and musculature) of the human body (Figure 3-5).

Assists in the Transfer of Muscle Contraction

Muscles contract, but that is all that they do. Bones by themselves cannot contract. Without a direct tendinous connection and the indirect connection provided by ligaments, muscles could not exert force on the skeleton. In this sense, the ability of bones to be moved is dependent on CT. Muscles are ineffectual without the CT ropes and sheets that transfer muscular effort to the levers of the skeleton. The relative length and resilience of CT connections can make the difference between what gestures and movements we can and cannot perform.

Similarly, a dynamic balance is sustained between movements of the muscles, vessels, nerves, and viscera. Muscle action is transferred by way of CT to continually stretch and massage internal organs and promote blood flow through veins back to the heart.

Provides First-line Defense

Connective tissue mounts the first line of defense against noxious agents that invade the body by building a physical barrier to compartmentalize and isolate those agents from the system as a whole. Fibroblasts produce collagen to close wounds with new scar tissue. Fibers are manufactured and plastered over injured sites to wall off toxic substances that might otherwise encroach through a break in the skin.

Provides Secondary Defense and Repair

Connective tissue also constitutes the major repair mechanism of the body via the inflammatory response. It provides the fluid medium for substances in the blood and lymph to circulate into areas where a secondary defense against toxic invaders is needed. Blood delivers antibodies and white blood cells to fight off infection.

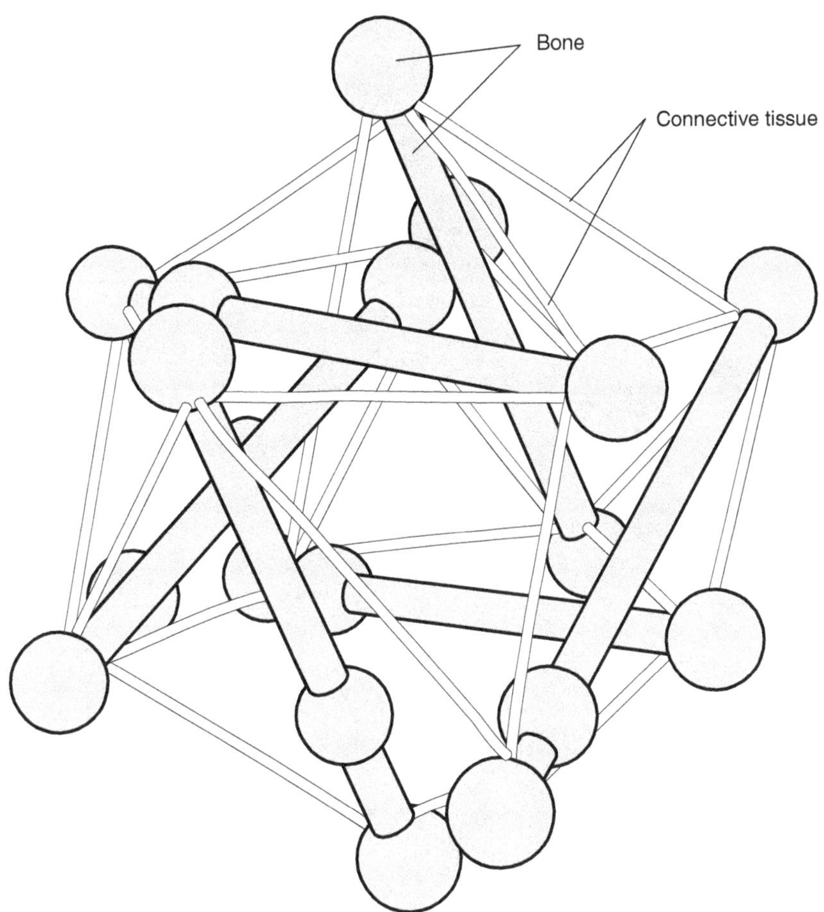

FIGURE 3-5 **Supportive function of connective tissue (CT).** CT is similar to the wires that hold the shape of the object, and bone is similar to the spacers (bars and spheres) in between. Just as in the human body, without the connective strands, the entire structure would collapse.

Assists in the Transport of Nutrients and Wastes

As blood, lymph, and CSF, CT is the medium for carrying food to and waste away from every cell.

PHYSIOLOGIC PROPERTIES OF CONNECTIVE TISSUE

Connective tissue has three physiologic properties that can be accessed and accentuated with effective manual therapy. These are:

1. **Pervasiveness:** The ever-present nature of CT
2. **Piezoelectricity:** The ability to conduct a current under pressure
3. **Thixotropy:** The ability to soften or harden as a result of warmth, manipulation, and pressure or the lack thereof

Pervasiveness

Juhan (1998) uses the metaphor of a body stocking to describe the pervasiveness of the CT web. CT is like a stretchy sweater that covers the entire body:

> Connective Tissue forms a continuous net throughout the entire body. Although it contains many specialized structures, CT is really all one piece, from scalp to soles and from skin to marrow. If all the muscle, nerve, and epithelial tissues were removed, the connective web would preserve all of the dimensions of the human form. (Juhan, 1998)

Because CT is everywhere, any place that the bodyworker touches will extend to other parts of the body (Fig. 3-6). The indirect effects are an added practical benefit of using touch to focus the client on healthy change.

The cross-section in Figure 3.6C demonstrates the lovely spiraling pattern that dense CT makes as it winds between the fascicle bundles and corkscrews from the exterior muscle into the periosteum around the bone.

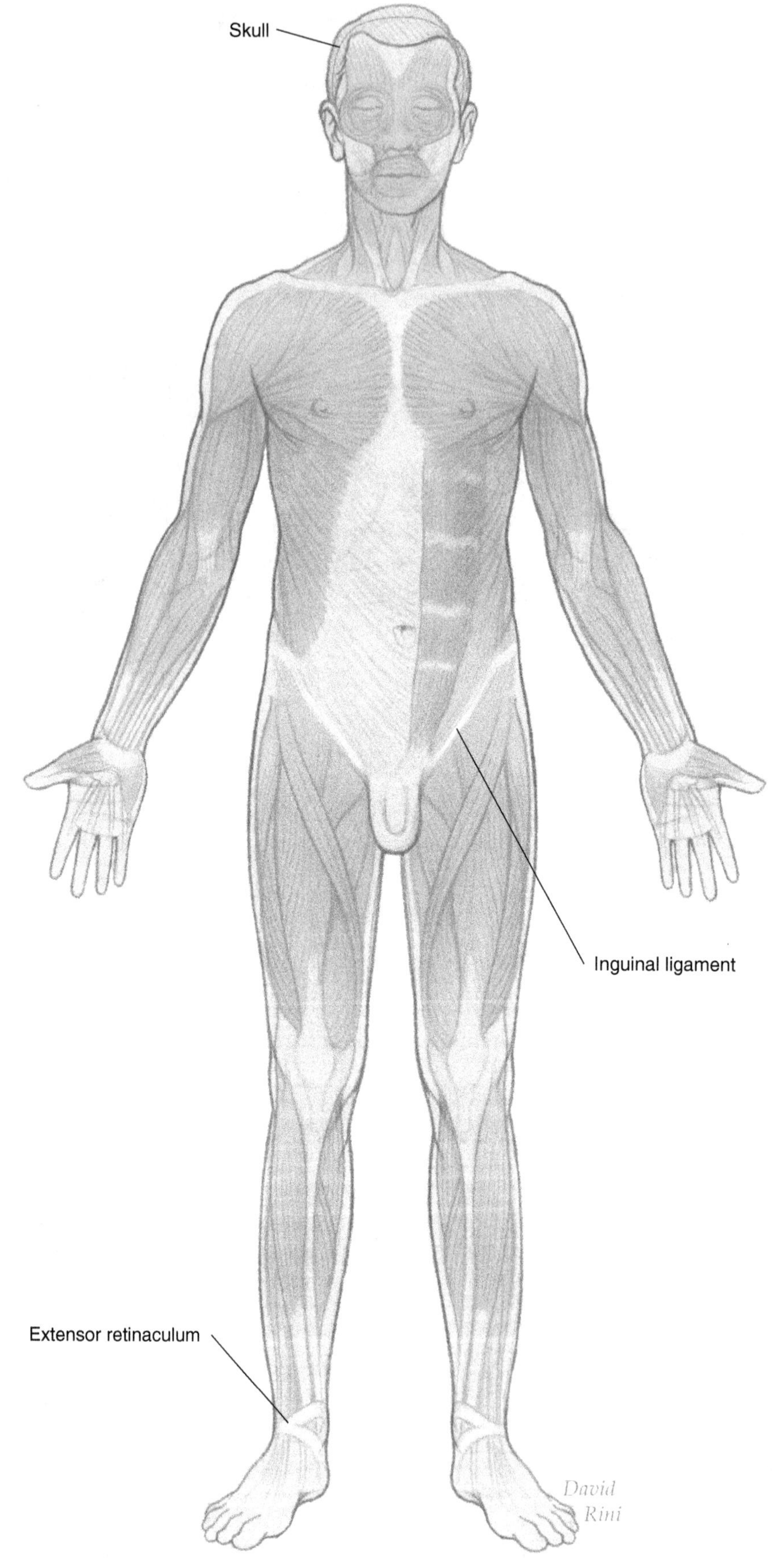

FIGURE 3-6 Location of connective tissue (CT). CT is clearly seen as the white areas of the figures. (**A**) Anterior view.

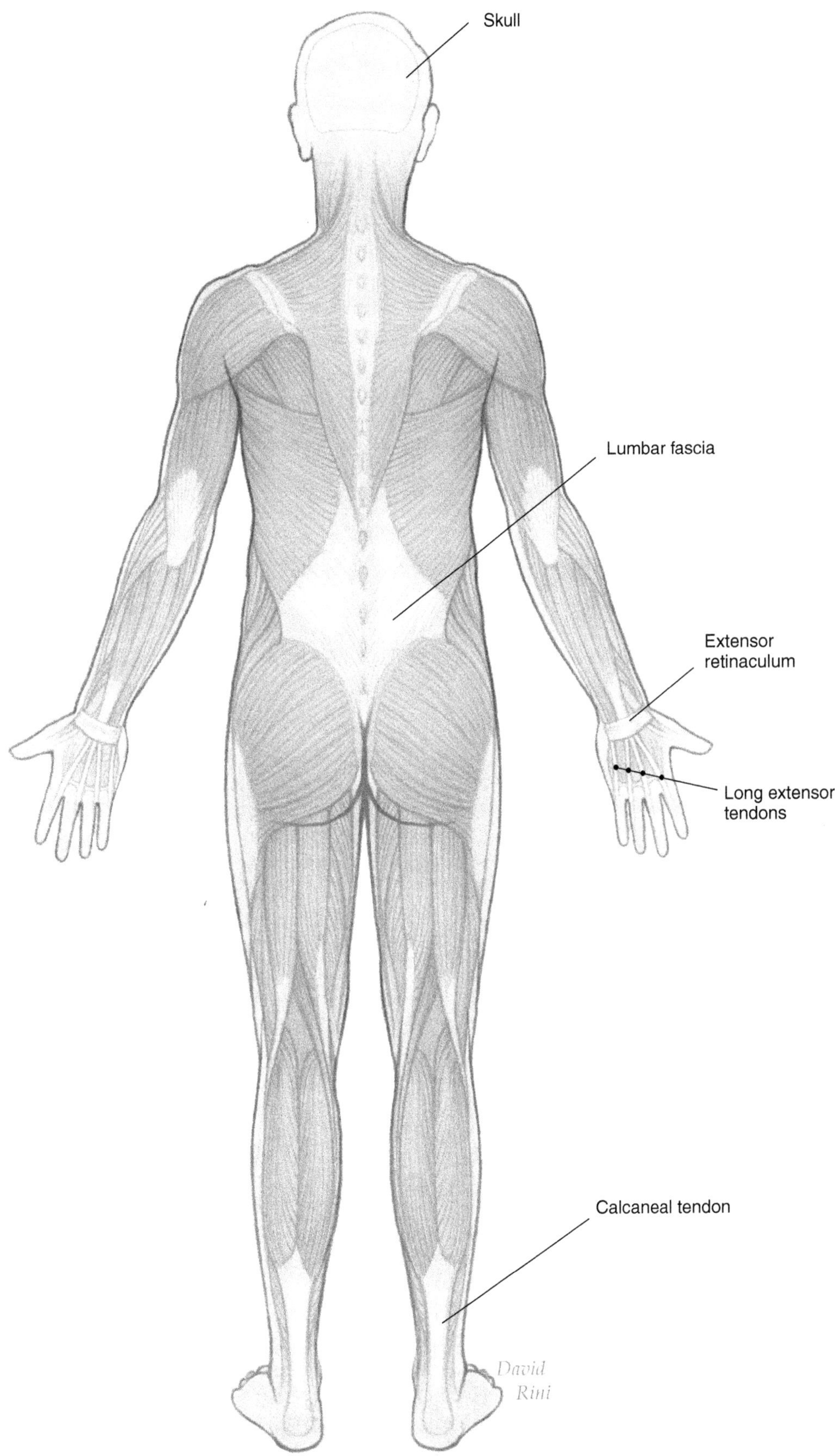

FIGURE 3-6 Location of connective tissue (continued). (**B**) Posterior view.

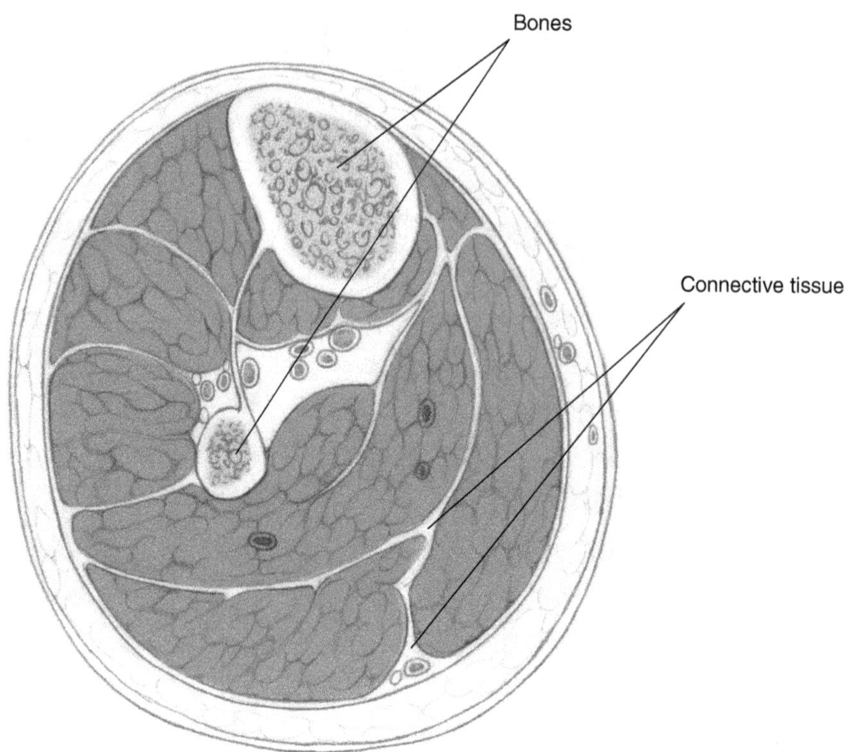

FIGURE 3-6 Location of connective tissue (continued). (C) Cross-section. Notice how the CT walls that separate muscles seem to spiral in toward the bone.

Just beneath the skin, the superficial fascia (loose CT) envelops the body in its entirety. Deep to this, the deep fascia (dense CT) organizes muscles into functional groups, wraps each individual muscle, and burrows into the muscle belly to strengthen it from the inside. Deep fascia continues from the ends of muscles as tendons. Tendons blend into periosteum, which forms a fibrous jacket over bones. Periosteum is also continuous with ligaments, as it is with *endosteum,* the inner coating of the hollow bones.

Reticular CT's spider-like webbing gives rise to its name and gives shape to the organs. It joins organs together and provides cabling to suspend them in body cavities. Reticular CT also surrounds vessels and ducts that supply the organs, as well as the muscles, bones, and nerves.

Piezoelectricity

The collagen in deep fascia is a gelatinous material with molecules arranged like those in solid crystal arrangements, such as those found in quartz crystal. All crystalline structures are piezoelectric. *Piezo* means pressure; therefore, a substance that demonstrates piezoelectricity conducts electricity when compressed. In liquid crystals, a weak electric current causes molecules to realign. This phenomenon can be observed in the liquid crystal displays (LCDs) of a calculator or watch. If the crystals in an LCD are charged (i.e., if the device is turned on), the molecules align so that all the light waves are made to vibrate in the same plane (i.e., they are polarized). A mirror in the back of the device reflects these light rays so that the numbers on the display become visible. If there is no current, the LCD is dark.

Another way to see this property in action is to press down on a quartz crystal in the dark. When you compress the rock, it sends off a spark of light that is visible to the naked eye. The same thing happens within the human CT matrix when pressure is applied to the body. Similar to the nervous system, which uses electrical impulses to send important messages throughout the body ("My finger hurts" or "I'm hungry"), CT may be a medium for transmission of electrical messages.

Thixotropy

One of the signs that a piezoelectric phenomenon has occurred is that the client's soft tissue appears to become longer, more responsive, and generally more supple under the fingers. Thixotropy describes the way a material substance can sometimes be thicker and harder and sometimes more pliable and soft. A good example of thixotropy in reverse occurs when you sit through a long movie. When the 3-hour feature is over and you try to get up out of your seat, you may notice that it is difficult to move. It is almost as if part of your body has grown into your seat and solidified its position. The "couch potato" phenomenon can be explained by the thixotropic nature of CT. Whenever we stay in one position for a very long time, CT stiffens independently and quite effectively. CT is not so good at softening by itself. That is where exercise and massage can be very helpful. Stirring it up like molasses or a thick soup helps the mixture to become thinner and less congealed.

The Implications of Myofascial Massage for Connective Tissue

Now let's examine the interrelationship of myofascial massage and these unique properties of CT.

PERVASIVENESS

Because CT is continuous throughout the human body, one body region can be adversely affected by injuries in a distal site. A snag in the shoulder area may pull on fibers from as far away as the opposite foot. One fortuitous aspect about wearing a fascial body stocking is that traumatized areas can be positively affected by manual manipulations anywhere along the client's body. Thus, the bodyworker may be able to loosen the snag at the painfully inflamed shoulder by softening fibers at the foot. This avoids aggravating a painful site with bodywork directly over a traumatized area.

PIEZOELECTRICITY

Perhaps piezoelectricity is the observable trace of impulses carried by the CT medium. Indeed, Oschmann (2000) indicates that voluntary movement generates electrical signals that spread through CT. These weak currents are said to signal cells about changes in movement, forces, or other activities occurring in the body. Theorizing an electrical impulse signaling system that runs through the connective matrix helps explain why movement and exercise maintain the skeleton and long periods of bed rest or space travel in zero gravity lead to loss of bone mass.

The writings of Juhan (1998), Oschmann (2000), and Langevin et al (2001) suggest that the CT network is responsible for the therapeutic effects of acupuncture and acupressure. Meridians are presumed to be channels of least resistance for electrical signals, and acupuncture points are described as semiconductors that process and refine the energy flow (*chi*). Understanding the CT as this kind of electronic messaging mechanism may partly explain the profound effectiveness and some unusual effects (e.g., twitching, slow arcing of the body, feeling of electricity reported by the client) of myofascial massage.

Semiconductors transform electricity into other kinds of energy and information. In the human body, semiconductors are sites where electrical information is converted to perceptions of light, sound, or touch. Oschmann (2000) states that collagen, the primary fiber found in ligaments, tendons, muscles, nerves, and blood and lymph vessel sheaths, is a piezoelectric semiconductor. Thus, not only does the CT complex transmit electrical current, but it also transforms the current into information and may increase, decrease, or change the signal.

Piezoelectricity is truly an exciting phenomenon for bodyworkers because the electricity can be felt while it is spreading. Sometimes the therapist senses only the end results of the piezoelectric response—the client's soft tissue appears to yield, lengthen, and become generally more supple under the fingers. Sometimes the client reports a sensation of tingling or electricity that does not feel like numbness or any other nerve phenomenon. The piezoelectric response may also be experienced as arising in the therapist's own body as a response to change in the client. I do not know the mechanism for this phenomenon (although I will speculate about the possible physical and energetic physiology in Chapter 11). I have sensed a softening in my own body and sometimes a palpable feeling of electricity that signals the piezoelectric effect. When I check in with my client in these moments, I find that shifts that I am feeling inside my body correspond with reported physiological or psychological changes, such as a feeling of sparking or softening or a change in attitude, sense of letting go, or memories.

THIXOTROPY

As noted earlier, CT stiffens by itself very well but needs help to soften. As we age, our CT becomes less flexible and more infused with deposits of mineral that cause crepitus. That is where exercise and massage can be very helpful. Stirring up the CT with pressure and movement helps the mixture to become thinner, more pliable, and less congealed. Thus, myofascial massage can actually help patients to become biologically (not chronologically) younger.

JING-LAO: INTERCONNECTIVITY

Jing-lao is a concept of traditional Chinese medicine that is loosely translated as structure or CT. *Jing* describes the connections between things and how relationships allow individual parts to work optimally as well as contribute to the system as a whole. Practitioners who work on the Jing level have an intellectual and often a kinesthetic idea of connection. This understanding shapes the massage session so that, for example, the practitioner is aware of the motion of the client's head that is caused by rocking the foot. This may lead to an alteration from preconceived patterns of bodywork and exploration of new areas in the client's body.

The notion of Jing well expresses my respect and reverence for touching CT. Because CT connects, it supports. Because it supports, it allows the organism to be safe. Because it is safe, it can more fully express its potentiality for being all that it can be. To touch and free these qualities in my clients is an honor and a joy.

SUMMARY

Connective tissue has a unique anatomy and physiology with profound effects on the structure and function of the whole human body. Myofascial massage addresses this important tissue to attain lasting therapeutic effects.

The components of CT are cells that are embedded in a matrix of ground substance, and fibers. Depending on the nature and arrangement of the cells, fibers, and ground substance, CT can be liquid or solid, dense or loose, fibrous or elastic, or regular or irregular. Types of CT include superficial fascia, deep fascia, cartilage, bones, and blood.

Because of the connections that CT establishes within and between entities, it performs seven important functions in the human body. These are:

1. Providing structure and form
2. Allowing bones to move by transferring the effects of muscular contractions to the bones
3. Massaging internal organs and vessels of blood and lymph by transferring the effects of muscular contractions to these structures
4. Supporting the skeletal system so that it will not collapse under its own weight
5. Providing the boundaries between cells, tissues, organs, and organ systems so that they can maintain their individual functions
6. Repairing injuries (manufacturing fibers to wall off wounds) and fighting invaders (as the blood delivering white blood cells and antibodies to fight off infections in the inflammatory response)
7. Delivering nutrients to the spaces where they are needed and transporting wastes out of the body through the blood (which is a CT)

The physiology of CT is unique because of its prevalence in all types of human organ systems and in all parts of the body. CT also has a tendency to act as if it were a liquid crystal, conducting electricity when pressure is applied (piezoelectricity). CT tends to become more liquid when it is manipulated and more solid when it is left alone (thixotropy). Piezoelectricity and thixotropy can be directed with myofascial therapies.

Review Questions

1. All of the following are CT cells except __________.
   a. fibroblasts
   b. mast cells
   c. hammer cells
   d. plasma cells
2. The __________ of CT is the bed in which the CT cells are found. It is made up of ground substance and fibers.
   a. fibroblast
   b. matrix
   c. fibrous bed
   d. ground
3. The fibers in CT can determine whether a structure is more like a spider's web, more or less elastic, or more or less resistant to injury. Fibers that are moldable but strong are probably made of __________.
   a. collagen
   b. fats
   c. minerals
   d. water
4. __________ is a type of embryonic CT that has the potential to regenerate into any type of CT that is needed by the body.
   a. Ground substance
   b. Macrophages
   c. Mesenchyme
   d. Collagen
5. Which of the following is NOT a function of CT?
   a. transfers muscular contractions to bones, organs, and vessels
   b. keeps the skeletal system from collapsing under its own weight
   c. makes blood
   d. repairs injuries and fights pathogenic invaders
6. True or false: Fascia refers to two specific types of CT, which are superficial and loose.
7. True or false: Any tissue that provides structure or holds the body together can be classified as CT.
8. True or false: Bone is *not* a type of CT.
9. __________ is the capacity to conduct electrical impulses when compressed.
10. __________ refers to the capacity of CT to become more similar to a solid or a fluid.

REFERENCES

Chikly B. Silent Waves—Theory and Practice of Lymph Drainage Therapy. Scottsdale, AZ: IHH Publishing, 2001.

Juhan D. Job's Body: A Handbook for Bodywork. Barrytown, NY: Barrytown, Ltd., 1998.

Langevin HM, Churchilk DL, Cipolla MJ. Mechanical Signaling through Connective Tissue: A Mechanism for the Therapeutic Effect of Acupuncture. Burlington, VT: Department of Neurology, University of Vermont, 2001.

Oschmann JL. Energy Medicine—The Scientific Basis. London: Churchill Livingstone, 2000.

Tortora GJ, Grabowski SR. Principles of Anatomy and Physiology. 10th Ed. New York: HarperCollins College Publishers, 2003.

Turchaninov R, Cox C. Medical Massage. Scottsdale, AZ: Stress Less Publishing, Inc, 1998.

SUGGESTED READINGS

Juhan D. Job's Body: A Handbook for Bodywork. Barrytown, NY: Barrytown, Ltd, 1998.

Myers TW. Anatomy Trains—Myofascial Meridians for Manual and Movement Therapists. London: Churchill Livingstone, 2002.

Rolf IP. Rolfing—Reestablishing the Natural Alignment and Structural Integration of the Human Body for Vitality and Well-Being. Rochester, VT: Healing Arts Press, 1989.

Schultz RL, Feitis R. The Endless Web—Fascial Anatomy and Physical Reality. Berkeley, CA: North Atlantic Books, 1996.

Chapter 4

The Anatomy and Physiology of Nerve Tissue

OBJECTIVES

- **Describe the anatomy of nerve tissue and discuss the neuroglia as distinct from neurons.**
- **Provide an overview of the physiology of the nervous system.**
- **Discuss how neural responses are affected by myofascial massage.**

CHAPTER OUTLINE

KEY TERMS

Nerve impulse (action potential): Electrical message transmitted by nerves.

Neurons: Nerve cells that send and receive electrical impulses.

Cell body: Part of the neuron that contains the nucleus and the organelles needed to sustain cell metabolism.

Axon: Long extension of the neuron that carries information away from the cell body to another neuron, a muscle, or a gland.

Dendrites: Neuron projections that receive signals from the outside environment, inside the body, or from another neuron.

Neuroglia (glia): Cells in the nervous system with a connective function; they insulate, bind, support, and protect the neurons and help the neurons transmit their messages more efficiently.

Myelin: Lipid-insulating coat of neuroglia that surrounds some axons.

Central nervous system (CNS): The brain and spinal cord.

Brain: Largest and most complex organ of the nervous system. It is made up of approximately 100 billion neurons and neuroglia that together interpret, regulate, and coordinate information.

Spinal cord: The part of the central nervous system that extends from the base of the occiput to the low back.

Peripheral nervous system (PNS): The cranial and spinal nerves.

Sensory fibers: Nerves that transmit information from the external or internal environment to the brain or spinal cord.

Motor fibers: Nerves that transmit information from the brain or spinal cord to effect responses in muscles, glands, or other nerves.

Autonomic nervous system (ANS): Functional division of the nervous system through which automatic motor responses are sent primarily to organs via their smooth muscles and glands; these responses may be either sympathetic (fight or flight) or parasympathetic (rest and repose).

Endoneurium: Thin connective tissue sheath that wraps each individual axon or dendrite.

Perineurium: Connective tissue sheath that wraps groups of axons or dendrites.

Epineurium: Connective tissue sheath that wraps the entire nerve.

Meninges: Three connective tissue layers that together form a sac that surrounds and protects the brain and spinal cord.

Spinal cord reflexes: Automatic reactions to a stimulus that involve at least three neurons: a sensory neuron, an interneuron, and a motor neuron.

The nervous system is the primary communications network for the human body. Bundles of specialized cells, called nerves, allow us to feel sensations such as pressure, cold, and pain; to initiate action; and to interpret information about the world.

When a nerve is triggered by a sensation, it sends off a message in the form of an electrical wave called a nerve impulse (action potential). This impulse travels to the spinal cord and then up to the brain. Without the brain to make sense of the impulse, you would not recognize that an old carrot in your refrigerator is foul smelling or that it hurts to touch a hot stove.

It is important for myofascial therapists to understand how the nervous system can interact with the manipulation of soft tissue, especially through myofascial massage. (Chapter 2 discusses the relationship of nerve and muscle tissue.) The first section of this chapter reviews the anatomy of the nervous system, focusing on nerve cells—the building blocks of nerve tissue—and the structure and basic roles of the various parts of the nerve system. The next section reviews the physiology of the nervous system, and the chapter closes with a discussion of the implications of myofascial massage for nerve tissue.

This chapter discusses nerve tissue and the nervous system insofar as they relate to CT. It is not intended to teach the entire nervous system. Much of the information is presented in summary form, with some specific topics (e.g., meninges, neuroglia, and neurological principles) receiving a fuller discussion because of the significance they have in respect to myofascial massage. Whole sections relating to nerve location, brain function, and other important topics are omitted from the discussion here. Please consult an anatomy and physiology text for complete discussion of the nervous system.

Nervous System Anatomy

The structure of nerve tissue and its organization into an information-distribution network establish conditions that influence the transfer of messages to and from the myofascia.

COMPONENTS OF NERVE TISSUE

Two distinct kinds of cells are found in what is collectively called nerve tissue. True nerve cells (neurons) conduct electrical impulses. Neuroglia are cells that support and protect neurons but do not send or receive impulses themselves.

Neurons

Neurons are nerve cells (also called *nerve fibers*) that receive and send electrical impulses. Neurons receive information from the external environment (e.g., light, pressure, sound, odor, taste) or from other neurons in the body. They transmit this information in the form of electrical signals to muscles, glands, or other neurons. Neurons consist of a cell body and two types of projections, an axon and many dendrites (Figure 4-1).

CELL BODY

The cell body contains the nucleus and the organelles (tiny organs) that carry out the functions of the cell. Some

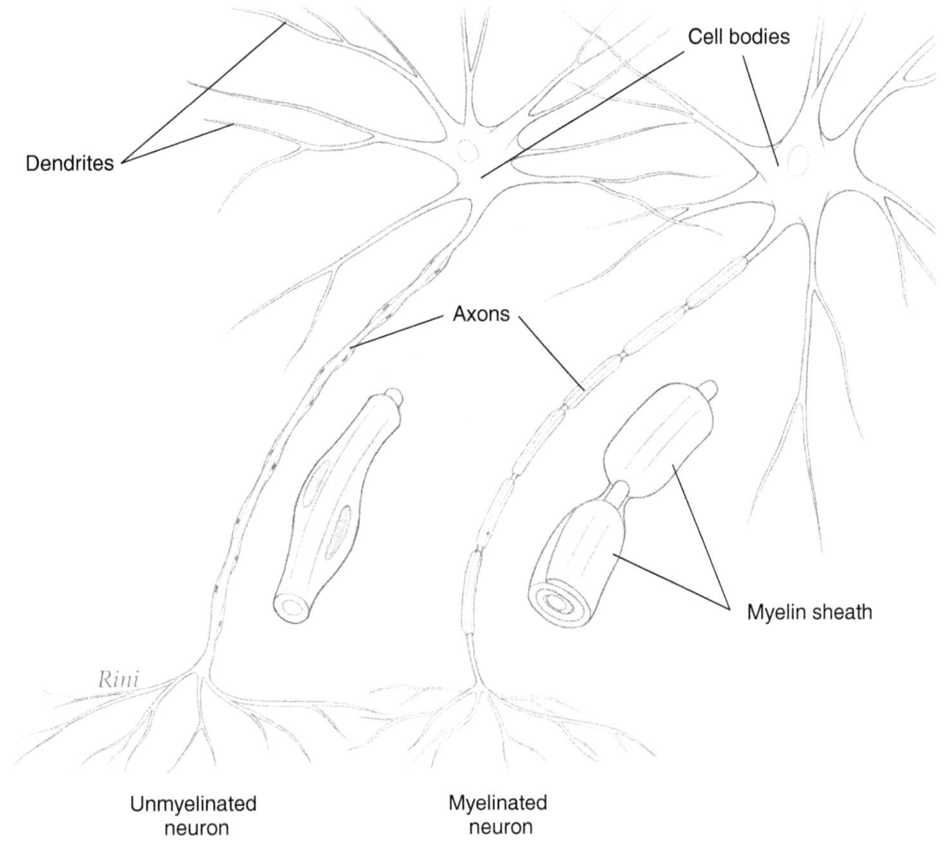

FIGURE 4-1 **Structure of a typical neuron.** Both unmyelinated and myelinated neurons contain a cell body, axon (or axons), and many dendrites.

organelles found in neurons but not in other types of cells include *neurofibrils* (for transporting substances and structural support) and *Nissl bodies* (to produce proteins used in the chemical transmission of messages from neuron to neuron).

AXON

An axon is a fiber-like process that conducts electrical impulses away from the cell body. Axons vary in length from a few millimeters to more than 1 meter long (e.g., in the vagus nerve). Axons have an *axoplasm* (cytoplasm), *axolemma* (plasma membrane), *axon terminals* (branches off the axon), and *synaptic vesicles* or *sacs* at the end of the axon terminals.

DENDRITES

Dendrites look like small hairs that branch out from the cell's cytoplasm. They receive impulses and direct them to the cell body.

Neuroglia

Specialized CT cells or neuroglia (glia) are five times as prevalent as neurons in nerve tissue (Moore and Dalley, 1999). As discussed in Chapter 3, the primary functions of neuroglia are to bind, support, and protect neurons. For example, glia form sheaths of a lipoprotein called myelin that insulates some axons. Table 4-1 provides a review of the major types and functions of glia.

Glial cells differ from neurons in a number of ways:

- Neurons have two types of processes (axon and dendrites). Glial cells have only one type.
- Neurons generate electrical impulses. Glial cells do not.
- There are many more glial cells than neurons. In the brain, the ratio is as much as 50:1. In other nerve tissue, the ratio is about 5:1.

CENTRAL NERVOUS SYSTEM

Because they are in the center of the neural network, the brain and the spinal cord are called the central nervous system (CNS) (Figure 4-2).

Brain

Contained within the protective skull, the brain is the largest and most complex organ of the nervous system. It

TABLE 4-1 Major Types and Functions of Neuroglia

Glial Cell	Function
Astrocyte (astroglia)	Star-shaped cells that provide physical and nutritional support for neurons in the CNS Clean up brain debris Transport nutrients to neurons Hold neurons in place Digest parts of dead neurons Regulate content of spaces between cells (interstitial)
Ependymocytes	Line spaces in the brain (ventricles) and spinal cord Hair-like cilia may help circulate cerebrospinal fluid in the CNS
Microglia	Digest parts of dead neurons and invading microorganisms in the CNS; immunity
Oligodendrocytes	Provide insulation (myelin) to neurons in the CNS
Satellite cells	Provide physical support to spinal ganglia in the PNS
Neurolemmocytes (Schwann cells)	Provide insulation (myelin) to neurons in the PNS

CNS = central nervous system; PNS = peripheral nervous system.

is made up of approximately 100 billion neurons bundled together with supporting neuroglia inside the skull (Fritz, 2000). Most people know that we use our brains to think, but the brain's long list of duties also includes regulating movement, behavior, and bodily functions; developing speech and personality; and coordinating the four special senses—seeing, hearing, tasting, and smelling. The brain plays an integral role in the way we think, feel, and act, and determines the way we interpret, regulate, and coordinate information. The brain weighs an average of 3 pounds, making up more than 97% of the nervous system by weight (Fritz, 2000). More than half of this weight comes from the neuroglia. The brain contains a higher percentage of fluid than blood.

Spinal Cord

Stretching from the base of the brain to the lower back, the spinal cord resembles a long, white worm covered with blood vessels. Anatomically, it is a continuation of the brain stem, beginning just below the foramen magnum ("big hole") at the base of the occiput. A lengthwise view shows that the spinal cord gradually decreases in thickness from the foramen magnum (with the exception of the cervical and lumbar enlargements) to its pointed end at the second lumbar vertebra. Similar to the trunk of a tree, the spinal cord branches off into thousands of miles of tiny nerves that reach all parts of the body. When these distant nerves transmit impulses, they travel first to the spinal cord, then up into the brain. This all happens in less than a second.

An integral part of the nervous system, the spinal cord is protected within the bony vertebral column. Nevertheless, a severe injury to or disease of the spinal cord can cut off the communication of impulses between the nerve branches and the brain. In such cases, the individual experiences varying degrees of paralysis according to the level and extent of the damage.

PERIPHERAL NERVOUS SYSTEM

The peripheral nervous system (PNS) consists of all the nerve tissue that is not part of the brain or spinal cord (see Figure 4-2). It includes the nerves that emerge from the spinal cord (*spinal nerves*) and those that emerge from the brain (*cranial nerves*). Whereas the CNS functions to integrate information, the job of the PNS is to send information to and receive information from the periphery of the body.

The PNS has three types of sensory fibers and two types of motor fibers:

- *General sensory fibers* from the skin and organs convey data about temperature, touch, deep or light pressure, and pain.
- *Special sensory fibers* carry signals from the eyes, ears, tongue, and nose about vision, hearing, taste, and smell.
- *Proprioceptive sensory fibers* carry signals about skeletal muscle contraction and the position and movement of joints and the head.
- *Somatic motor fibers* carry signals from the CNS to the skeletal muscles.
- *Autonomic (visceral) motor fibers* carry signals from the CNS to glands, smooth muscles, and cardiac muscles.

These fibers are discussed in more detail in the Physiology section of this chapter.

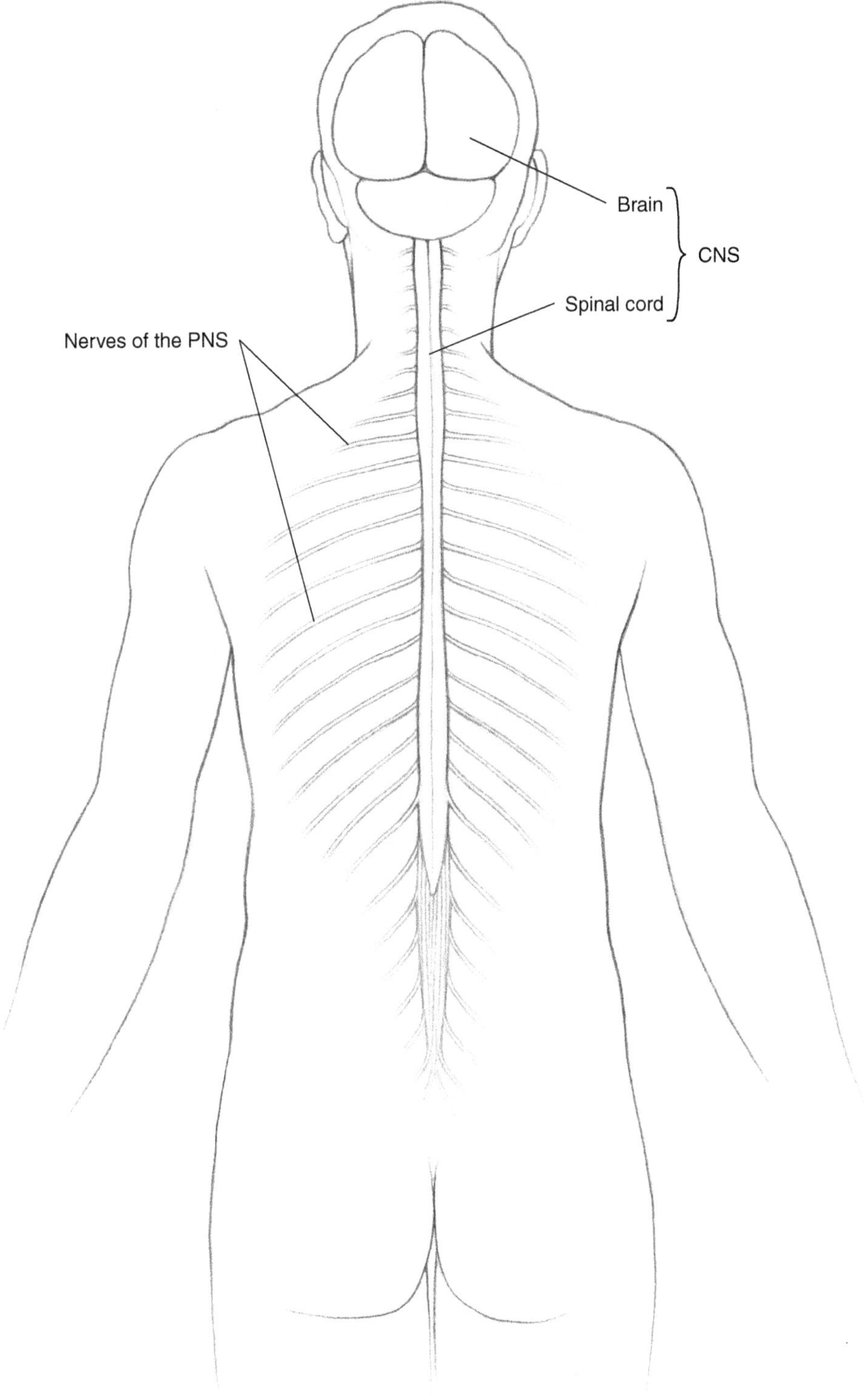

FIGURE 4-2 Central nervous system (CNS) and peripheral nervous system (PNS). The CNS is composed of the brain and spinal cord. The PNS is made up of the cranial and spinal nerves.

AUTONOMIC NERVOUS SYSTEM

As we have seen, the nervous system can be divided structurally into the CNS (brain and spinal cord) and the PNS (everything else). But it can also be divided functionally into the somatic nervous system (which innervates skeletal muscles) and the autonomic nervous system (ANS), which innervates smooth and cardiac muscle and glands). The ANS is an important physiological link between the myofascia and reflex responses and the myofascia and the stress response (Figure 4-3).

Autonomic motor nerves regulate pupil and blood vessel size, movements of the digestive tract, the size of respiratory passageways, and the rate and force of the heartbeat, as well as the secretion of hormones and other chemicals. ANS effects are immediate but short lived. Because the ANS originates in either the brainstem or spinal cord, it does not involve conscious input or thought.

The ANS consists of two divisions, the sympathetic (thoracolumbar) division and the parasympathetic (craniosacral) division. Nearly every organ is innervated by a sympathetic nerve fiber and a parasympathetic fiber. These two nerve tracts have complementary and opposing effects.

Sympathetic Nervous System

Sympathetic stimulation activates a series of events that supply skeletal muscles with oxygenated, nutrient-rich blood. Its actions are commonly summarized as "fight or flight" responses. Associated physiological changes include an increase in the force of the heart muscle contractions, vasodilation of arteries that supply working muscles, vasoconstriction of arteries that lead to nonworking muscles, dilation of pupils and bronchial tubes, increased heart and breathing rate, reduced digestive activity, and release of blood sugar from the liver. Because cell bodies of sympathetic neurons are found in the thoracic and lumbar regions of the spinal cord, the sympathetic division is often called the *thoracolumbar outflow*.

Parasympathetic Nervous System

Parasympathetic activity is responsible for energy conservation and relaxation, allowing body cells to regenerate and healing to occur. Its actions, commonly summarized as "resting and digesting," include reduced heart rate, slowed breathing rate, decreased muscle tension, and increased digestion. Because cell bodies of parasympathetic neurons are found in the brain stem (cranium) and in the sacral spinal cord segments, the parasympathetic division is often called the *craniosacral outflow*.

Dual Innervation

The parasympathetic and sympathetic systems are exclusive in that they cannot dominate organ and muscle activity simultaneously. Sympathetic arousal, similar to a gas pedal in a car, becomes the dominant driver during stress, whereas parasympathetic activity promotes homeostasis at all other times. Therefore, it is impossible to be physically aroused and relaxed at the same time (Figure 4-4).

There are some exceptions to the sympathetic equals "go," parasympathetic equals "rest" model. For example, both sympathetic and parasympathetic nerves stimulate the secretion of saliva. And although blood vessels generally dilate under sympathetic dominance, during sexual arousal, parasympathetic fibers tell the vasculature of the penis and clitoris to dilate. Also, digestion is activated under the influence of parasympathetic, not sympathetic nerves. These last two examples make a kind of intuitive sense in that it does not make sense to take energy away from "fight or flight" to digest a big meal or to procreate the species.

ANATOMICAL RELATIONSHIPS BETWEEN NERVE AND CONNECTIVE TISSUE

Nerves, like muscles (as shown in Chapter 2), are inseparable from CT. CT is woven throughout nerve tissue itself. As you will see below, the interweaving of connective and nerve structures is even more extensive than that found in the myofascia.

Predominance of Glial Cells in Nerve Tissue

It is somewhat confusing that true nerve cells (neurons) are physically entangled with cells that have a connective function (neuroglia) and the whole bundle is referred to as nerve tissue. *Webster's Dictionary* of 1913 defined neuroglia as "the delicate CT framework which supports the nervous matter and blood vessels of the brain and spinal cord." Currently, it is somewhat controversial to say that more than half the cells in nerve tissue are really CT. A modern biology dictionary (Anderson, 1997) defines neuroglia as "*nerve tissue* of the CNS other than the signal transmitting neurons." An electronic source, word.net, defines neuroglia as "*sustenacular* tissue that surrounds and supports neurons." I believe that neuroglia function as CT but are best categorized as nerve tissue. Bodywork that focuses on the CT web affects these specialized CT cells and thus improves the function of the neurons that they support (Tortora and Grabowski, 2003).

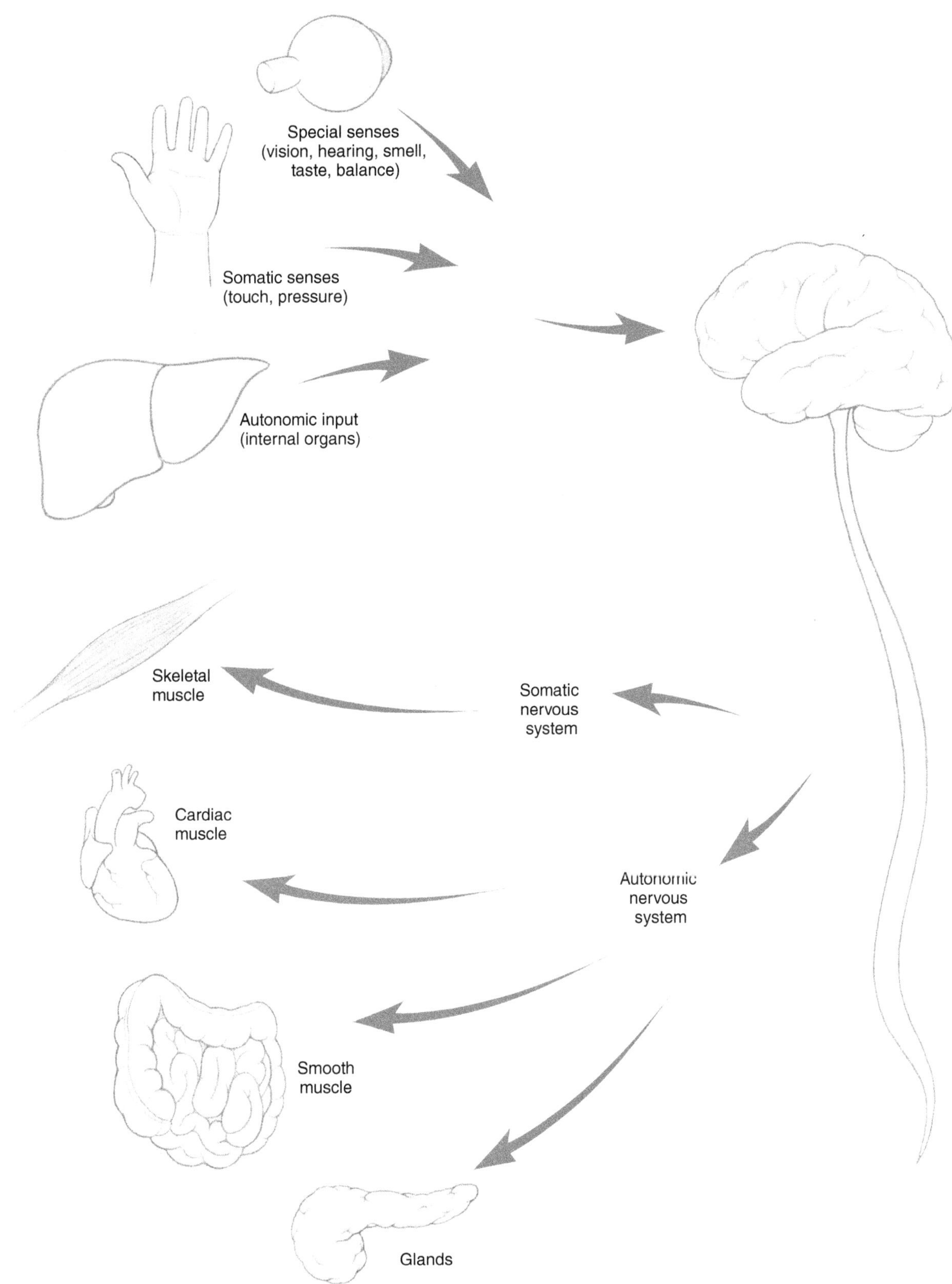

FIGURE 4-3 **Autonomic and sensory nervous systems.**

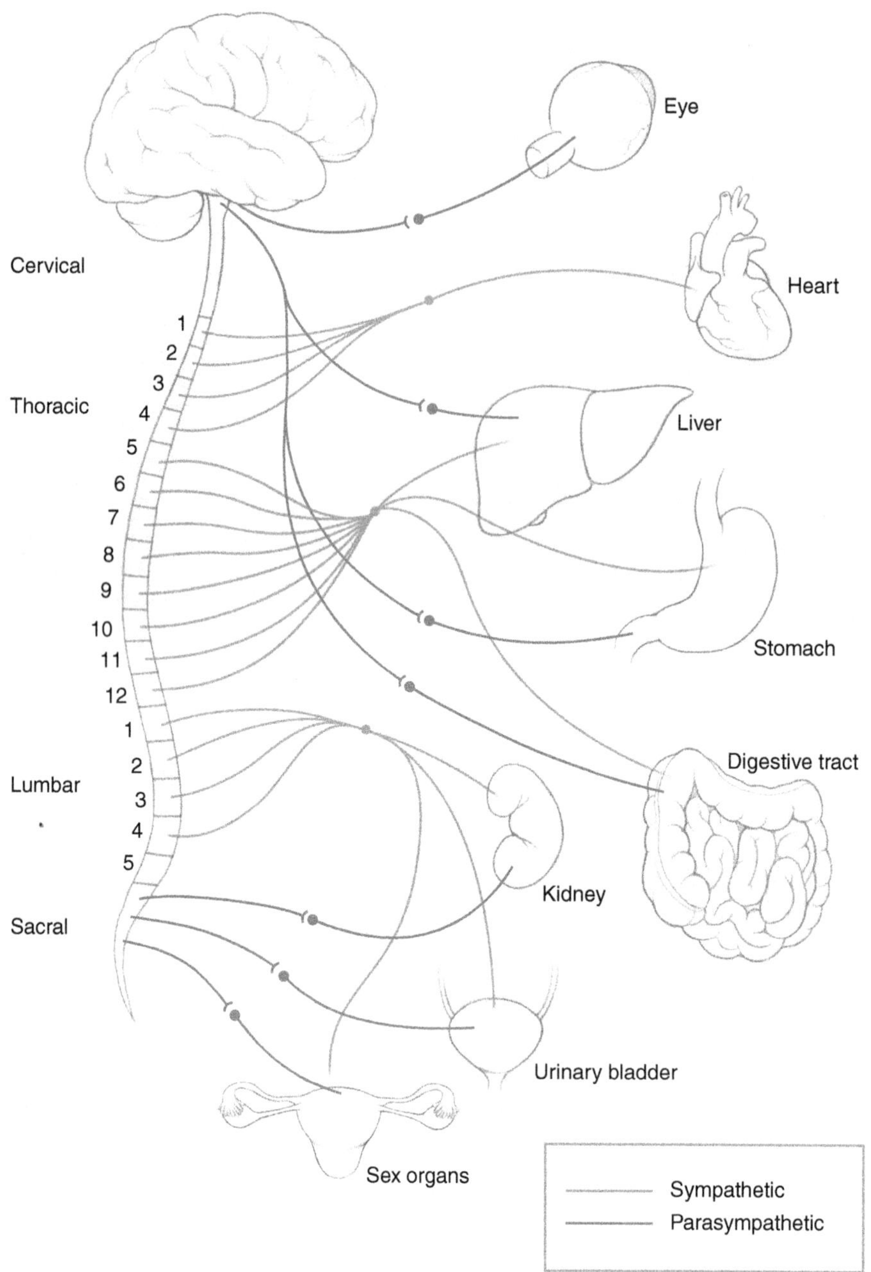

FIGURE 4-4 Dual innervation in the autonomic nervous system.

Glial cells provide tensile strength and elasticity needed for stretching. They also secure nerves to other structures, such as the periosteum around bones. Moreover, Barres (1997) showed that without glia, the neuronal transfer of messages is inefficient and often fails. With glia around, the connections rarely fail and neurons pass on more and stronger signals. As mentioned earlier, glia wrap around some neuronal axons and insulate them with a lipoprotein called myelin. Glia at synapses act as a physical barrier to dispose of extra neurotransmitters released by neurons and prevent the confusing chaos of signals that would otherwise result.

In the brain and spinal cord (CNS), types of glia include astrocytes, microglia, ependymocytes, and oligodendrocytes. In the PNS, types of neuroglia include satellite cells and neurolemmocytes. Recall that the types and functions of neuroglia are identified in Table 4-1.

Connective Tissue Wraps Nerve Cells, Fascicles, and Nerves

Connective tissue wraps individual neural cells, cell bundles, and entire nerves. Individual axons and dendrites are wrapped with a thin sheath of endoneurium. Nerve fascicles are wrapped in perineurium, and the entire nerve is covered in a CT sheath known as epineurium.

Because myelin is white, CNS nerves with a myelin coating are known as "white matter" (Figure 4-5A). Their color distinguishes them from the grey cell bodies and axons that are not protected by myelin. Uncoated brain tissue is called "grey matter."

Myelin also insulates neurons in the PNS (Figure 4-5B). The PNS myelin sheath has an outer membrane known as the neurolemma. Small gaps between the segments of the myelin sheath are called *nodes of Ranvier.* These gaps enable "saltatory" conduction of impulses, that is, they cause impulses to leap (or literally, "dance") from one node to another without having to travel the portion of the axon between them.

Neurons can be grouped according to the size of their CT coating. "A" fibers have a large diameter because of their thick coating of myelin. They conduct impulses quickly because of their increased saltatory conduction. "A" fibers typically carry messages associated with danger. "B" fibers are also myelinated, but less so. They are smaller in diameter and send impulses at an intermediate speed. "B" fibers generally transmit sensory information that is not associated with danger. "C" fibers are small, unmyelinated fibers that conduct impulses slowly. They typically carry pain sensations or motor impulses to the eyes, heart, and bladder.

Meninges Protect the Brain and Spinal Cord

The meninges are three CT layers that together form a sac that surrounds and protects the brain and spinal cord (Figure 4-6). The outermost layer is a tough fibrous connective lining that attaches to the inner surface of the skull and folds down into the fissure between the lobes of the brain. Its name, *dura mater,* means "tough matrix (mother)." The middle layer, called the *arachnoid mater,* means "spider matrix (mother)" and looks like a web. The inner layer, the *pia mater,* is delicate, transparent, and richly supplied with

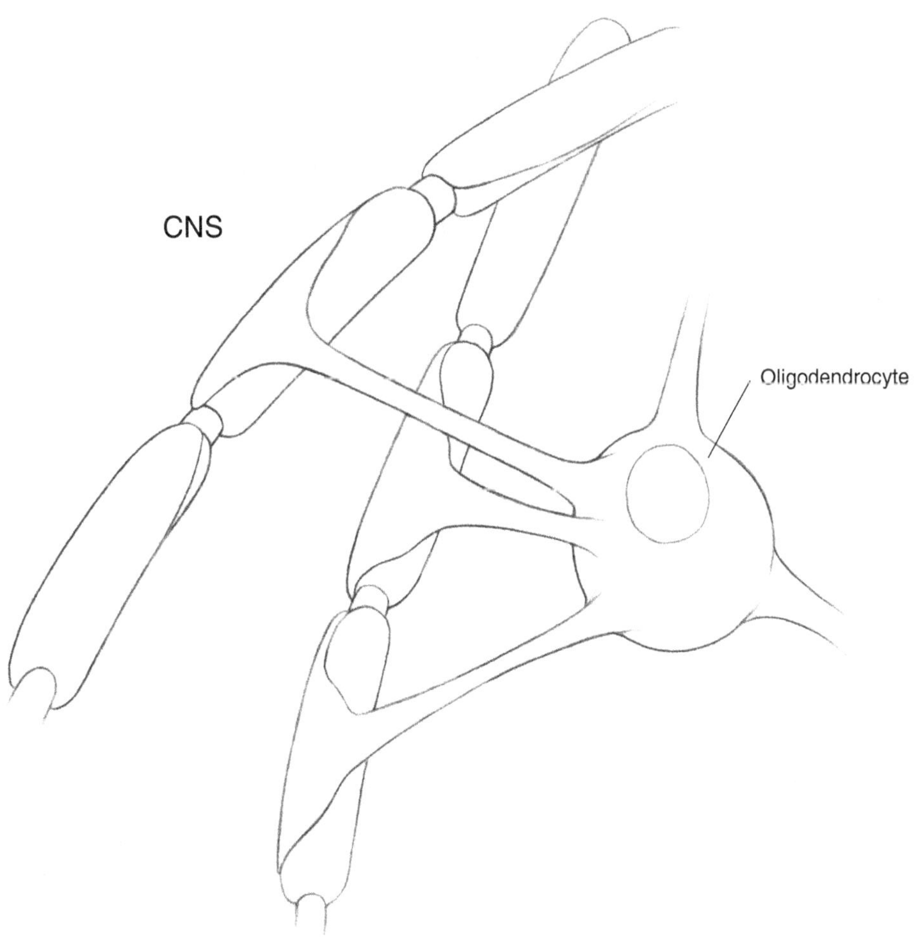

FIGURE 4-5 Myelin sheaths. (**A**) In the central nervous system, myelin sheaths are formed by oligodendrocytes.

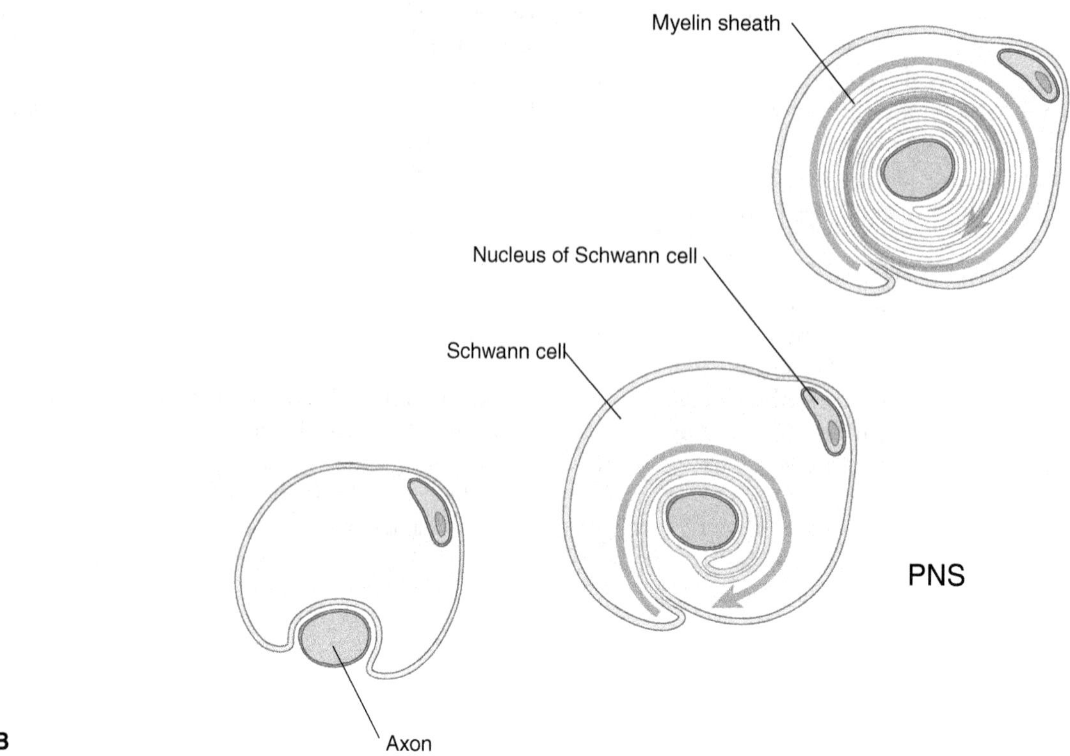

FIGURE 4-5 **Myelin sheaths (continued).** (**B**) In the peripheral nervous system, myelin sheaths are formed by Schwann cells.

blood vessels. Pia mater adheres directly to the surface of the brain (see Figure 4-6A).

Meninges also protect the spinal cord from trauma, extending downward from the cranium in a continuous sac. Dura mater hangs freely within most of the vertebral canal, attaching only at the sacrum and at cervical vertebrae 2 and 3. The epidural space between the dura and the vertebra contains adipose and loose CT that provides a shock-absorbing pad around the spinal cord. Deep to the spinal arachnoid mater is a large channel called the subarachnoid space, which contains cerebrospinal fluid. The delicate innermost layer, pia mater, is attached to the surface of the spinal cord (see Figure 4-6B).

Other Interrelationships

Neural receptors within fascia inform the brain and spinal cord about changes in the speed or direction of movement. Muscles, tendons, and ligaments contain specialized neural structures (muscle spindles and Golgi tendon organs [GTOs], discussed in Chapter 2) that send additional information about body position to the brain. These proprioceptive sensory receptors are discussed further in the Physiology section of this chapter.

Nervous System Physiology

Despite the prevalence of neuroglia, the neuron remains the functional unit of nerve tissue. Neurons have a single function, which is the transmission of nerve impulses. Therefore, it is essential to comprehend nerve impulse transmission to understand how the nervous system works.

NERVE IMPULSE TRANSMISSION

A neuron's cell membrane is selectively permeable, which means that it allows some chemicals, but not others, to move into and out of the cell. Neurons retain selective permeability because of the presence of ion channels, proteins in the cell membrane that allow some ions through, depending on their size and charge. Some ion channels, known as leakage or nongated channels, are always open. Other channels, called gated channels, require a stimulus to make them open. Stimuli that cause gated channels to open include changes in voltage (e.g., when an electrical charge travels from one part of a neuron to another), chemicals (e.g., release of a neurotransmitter or hormone), mechanical stimuli (e.g., pressure or vibration applied by a massage therapist), and light (e.g., stepping outside into bright sunlight).

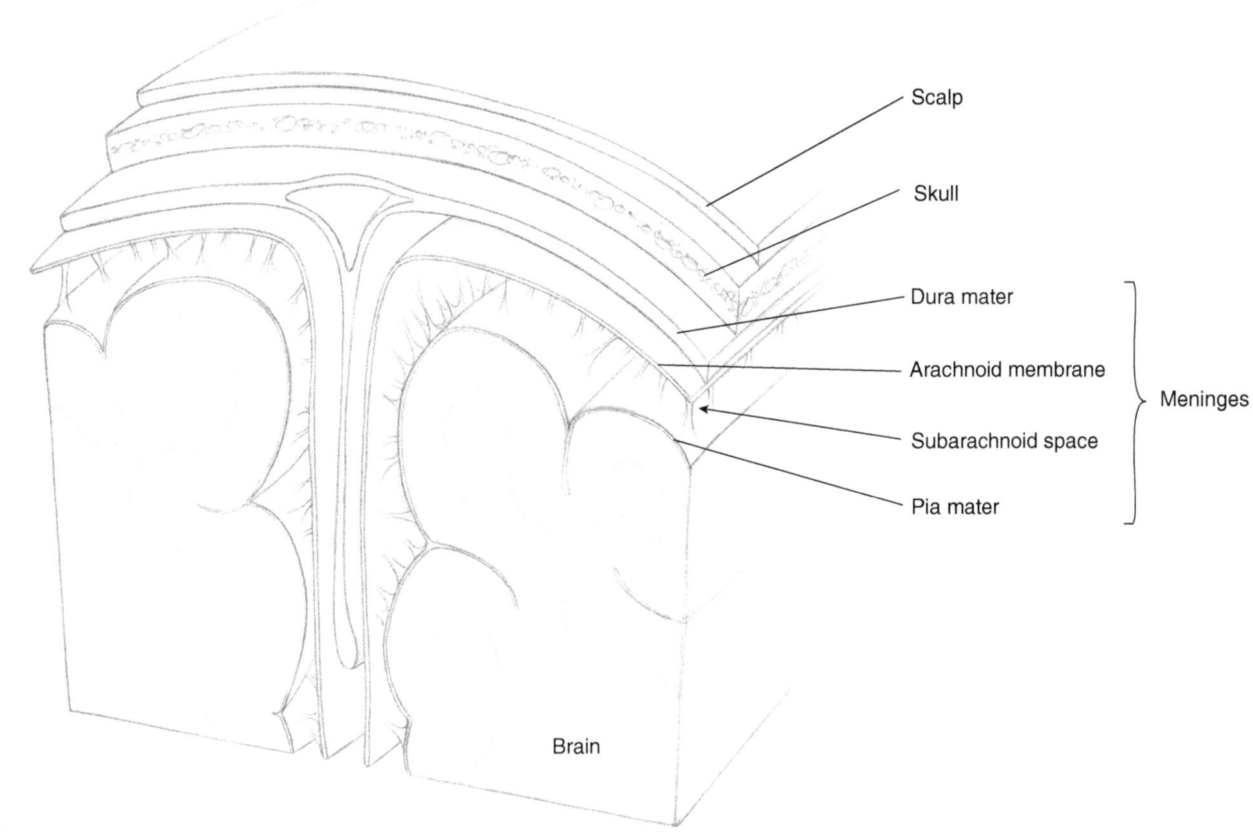

FIGURE 4-6 **Meninges.** (A) The cerebral meninges protect the brain.

The ions outside a neuron are different from the ions inside. This difference helps maintain an electrical charge (potential difference). Inside a resting (unstimulated) neuron, there is a high concentration of potassium (K+) ions. These carry a positive charge. There are also many phosphate (PO_4^-) and protein ions that carry a negative charge. Outside a resting neuron, there is a high concentration of positive sodium (Na+) ions and negative chloride (Cl^-) ions.

In a resting neuron, the neuron's plasma membrane is not permeable to the negatively charged ions inside the cell. It is, however, permeable to the positively charged potassium ions inside. Because there is such a high concentration of potassium inside the neuron, the ions easily leave the neuron through the potassium leakage channels, leaving a negative charge inside the cell membrane. This is the potential difference or *resting membrane potential*. Therefore, the membrane is charged or polarized just like a battery.

Depolarization

A stimulus such as pressure, light, temperature, or the release of a neurotransmitter results in a very brief change in one segment of the neuron. Sodium-ion gated channels open, and positively charged sodium ions (Na+) rush into the neuron. This reduces the negative charge inside the membrane. This change is called *depolarization* because the cell membrane briefly reduces its difference in charge between inside and outside the cell.

Propagation of an Action Potential

If a stimulus is strong enough, the polarity inside and outside of the cell reverses completely, triggering an action potential (or nerve impulse). Voltage-gated channels open on either side of the original stimulus, the process spreads in both directions, and the nerve impulse moves down the axon. This movement is called *conduction*.

In an unmyelinated neuron, depolarization continues through each and every point on the neurolemma; this is continuous conduction. In a myelinated neuron, the charge leaps from gap to gap in the myelin sheath because CT is a poor conductor of electricity. This saltatory conduction is faster and uses much less energy than continuous conduction.

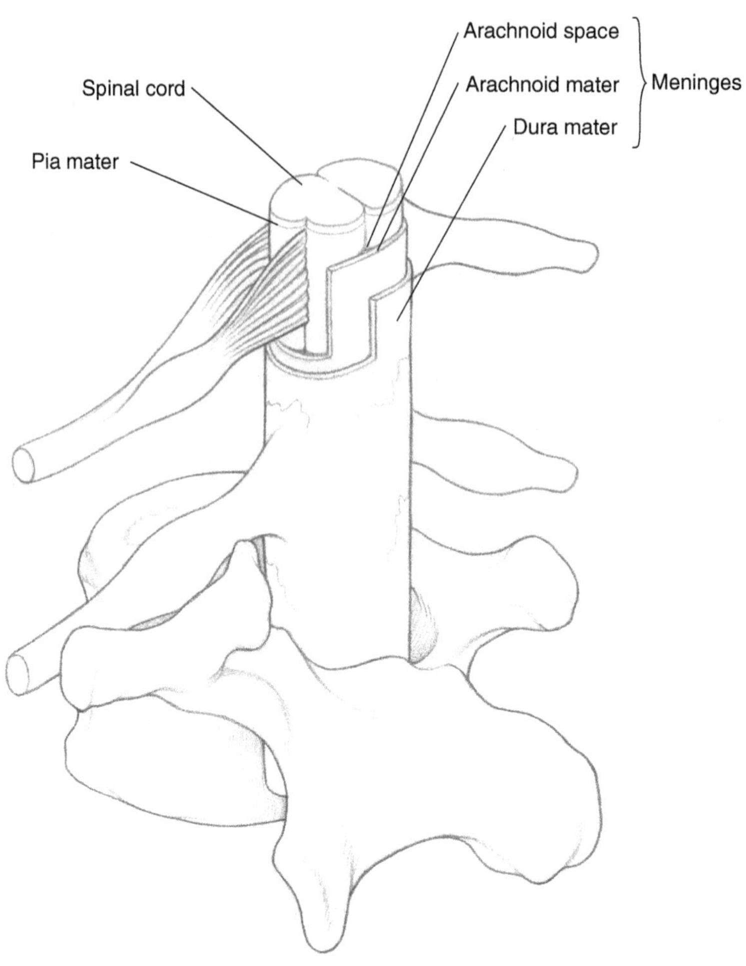

FIGURE 4-6 Meninges (continued). (**B**) The spinal meninges protect the spinal cord.

Transmission Across the Synapse

When a nerve impulse reaches the end of the axon, the charge stimulates the release of chemical neurotransmitters stored in the synaptic vesicles. The neurotransmitter diffuses out of the axon terminal, travels across the synaptic cleft, and attaches to receptors on the cell membrane of the effector. Some common neurotransmitters are acetylcholine (ACh), norepinephrine (noradrenalin), dopamine, and serotonin. ACh is the only neurotransmitter released at the neuromuscular junction.

Reception and Response

The effector (i.e., cell that is stimulated to do something) can be another neuron, a gland (epithelial cell), or a muscle cell. If the effector is another neuron, it is stimulated to carry the impulse farther. The gland is stimulated to increase or decrease the production and secretion of hormones or fluids (e.g., perspiration). The muscle cell (which can be smooth muscle, such as that found in the bladder, or skeletal muscle, such as that in the biceps brachii) is stimulated to contract.

The junction of a motor neuron with the effector is called the neuroeffector junction. Each junction has three parts, the presynaptic neuron, the synaptic cleft, and the effector. Chapter 2 describes and provides an illustration of a neuromuscular junction.

PATHWAYS INVOLVING THE BRAIN

One of the most important functions of the brain is the integration of all sensory and motor information. The result of this integration may be voluntary motor activity; vision or hearing; or other complex functions such as remembering, communicating, thinking, or worrying. These functions require the involvement of neurons in the cerebral cortex, the thin layer (about 1/8 inch) of gray matter that is the seat of human consciousness.

REFLEXES

Some human activity does not require the participation of neurons in the brain. Sometimes the spinal cord independently integrates sensory and motor information through spinal cord reflexes. Reflex actions can occur even if spinal cord connections with the brain have been completely severed. Reflexes usually protect the body from danger, such as when you pull your finger away from a burning flame. They can also regulate the activities of organs. A reflex (illustrated in Figure 4-7) can be described in five steps.

1. A receptor is stimulated.
2. A sensory impulse travels to the spinal cord.
3. The spinal cord transfers the message from the back (sensory) area of the cord to the front (motor) area.
4. A motor response is sent.
5. A muscle moves or a gland secretes.

SENSORY RECEPTION

Information about the external environment is fed into the nervous system from sensory receptors in the skin, muscles, and CT, and from the eyes, ears, nose, and tongue (Table 4-2). Internal sensors also transmit data on muscle tone and the position and movement of every body part.

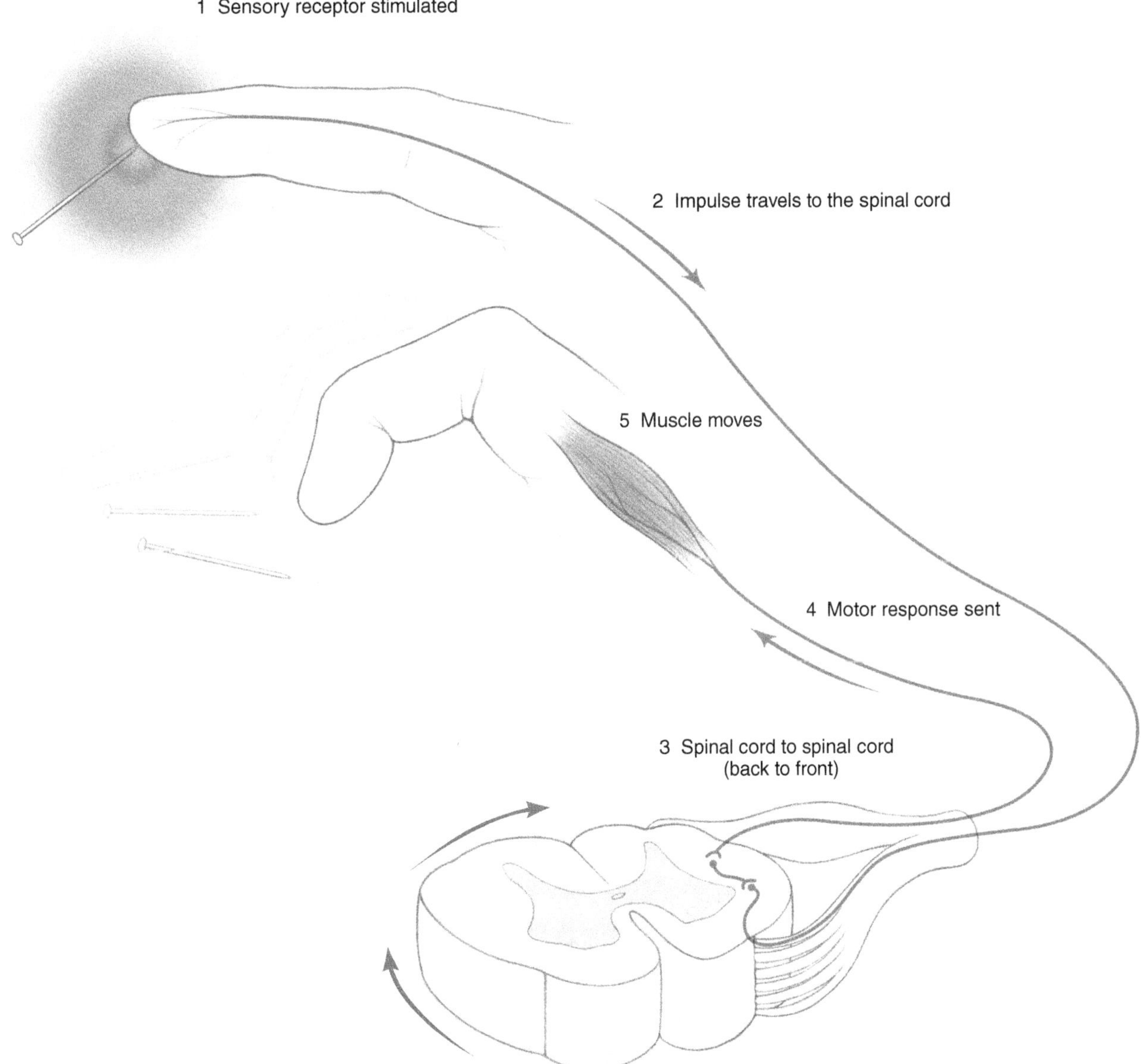

FIGURE 4-7 The reflex arc. (**1**) Sensory receptor stimulated. (**2**) Impulse travels to spinal cord. (**3**) Spinal cord to spinal cord (back to front). (**4**) Motor response sent. (**5**) Muscle moves.

TABLE 4-2 Sense Organs, Locations, and Sensations

Sense Organ	Location	Sensation
Rods and cones Hair cells Olfactory neurons (hairs) Taste buds	Eye Ear Nose Tongue	Vision Hearing Smell Taste
Vestibular apparatus	Ear	Acceleration
Pacinian (lamellated) corpuscles Meissner's corpuscles (corpuscles of touch)	Connective tissue around the joints, subcutaneous fascia Dermal papillae, enclosed in a connective tissue capsule	Touch, pressure, vibration
Thermoreceptors (free nerve endings)	Skin	Warmth Cold
Merkel's (tactile) discs	Skin	Light touch
Root hair plexuses	Skin	Movement on the skin (air or object moving on the skin)
Proprioceptors	Neck	Balance and position of head in space
Nocioceptors (free nerve endings and any cutaneous receptor that is overstimulated)	Skin	Pain
Golgi end organs Ruffini end organs	Ligaments Within the joint capsule, around joints, and in the dermis of the skin	Joint position and movement
Muscle spindle	Muscle belly	Muscle length
Golgi tendon organs	Muscle belly and junction between muscle and tendon	Muscle tension

Myofascial massage is concerned with the general sensations of touch, body position, and movement (Table 4-3). These sensations are detected by cutaneous and proprioceptive receptors.

Cutaneous Sensory Reception

Cutaneous sensations include light and heavy touch, pressure and vibration, sensations of heat and cold, and pain. Cutaneous receptors are found in the skin, CT, and ends of the gastrointestinal tract. In some parts of the body, such as the fingertips, these receptors are densely packed. In contrast, the back has few cutaneous receptors, making it much less sensitive to specific touch.

Cutaneous receptors are mechanoreceptors, excited by stimuli that deform them. They are constructed simply, consisting of dendrites that may or may not be enclosed in capsules of epithelial or CT (Kinnaird, 1993). They function to detect touch, pressure, vibration, heat and cold, and pain. Cutaneous receptors include the following (Figure 4-8):

- *Root hair plexuses* are dendrites wrapped around the roots of hairs. They are sensitive to movement on the body surface (e.g., sensation of wind or an insect moving over the skin).
- *Free nerve endings* can detect pain and register pressure, heat, and cold. These receptors are found in many layers of the skin and other tissues.
- *Merkel's (tactile) discs* are disc-shaped dendrites attached to deeper layers of epidermal cells, making them sensitive to light touch.
- *Meissner's corpuscles (corpuscles of touch)* are egg shaped and contain a mass of dendrites enclosed in a CT capsule. They are found in the skin's dermal papillae and are abundant in the more sensitive areas of the body (e.g., fingertips).
- *Ruffini end organs (type II cutaneous mechanoreceptors)* are devoted to cutaneous sensations and lie deep within the dermis of the skin. At this level, they detect heavy and continuous touch and pressure. Ruffini end organs are also found within the joint capsule around the joints, where they serve as proprioceptors (see next section).

TABLE 4-3 Sensory Receptors and Their Specialized Functions

Type of Receptor	Function
Mechanoreceptors	Detect deformation of adjacent tissues
Chemoreceptors	Report on taste, smell, carbon dioxide, and oxygen levels
Thermoreceptors	Detect change in temperature (most prevalent on hands, forearms, and tongue)
Photoreceptors (electromagnetic receptors)	Respond to light entering the retina
Nocioceptors	Register pain

- *Pacinian (lamellated) corpuscles* have an oval-shaped capsule with layers of CT similar to an onion, between which is a sodium ion–rich solution of interstitial fluid. Located in the subcutaneous fascia, in serous membranes, around joints and tendons, and in the perimysium of muscles, they respond to deep pressure.

Proprioception

Proprioception is information about the position and motion of the body. This information comes from sensory receptors in the muscles, skin, CT, and joints. Schafer (1987) more broadly defines proprioception as *kinesthetic*

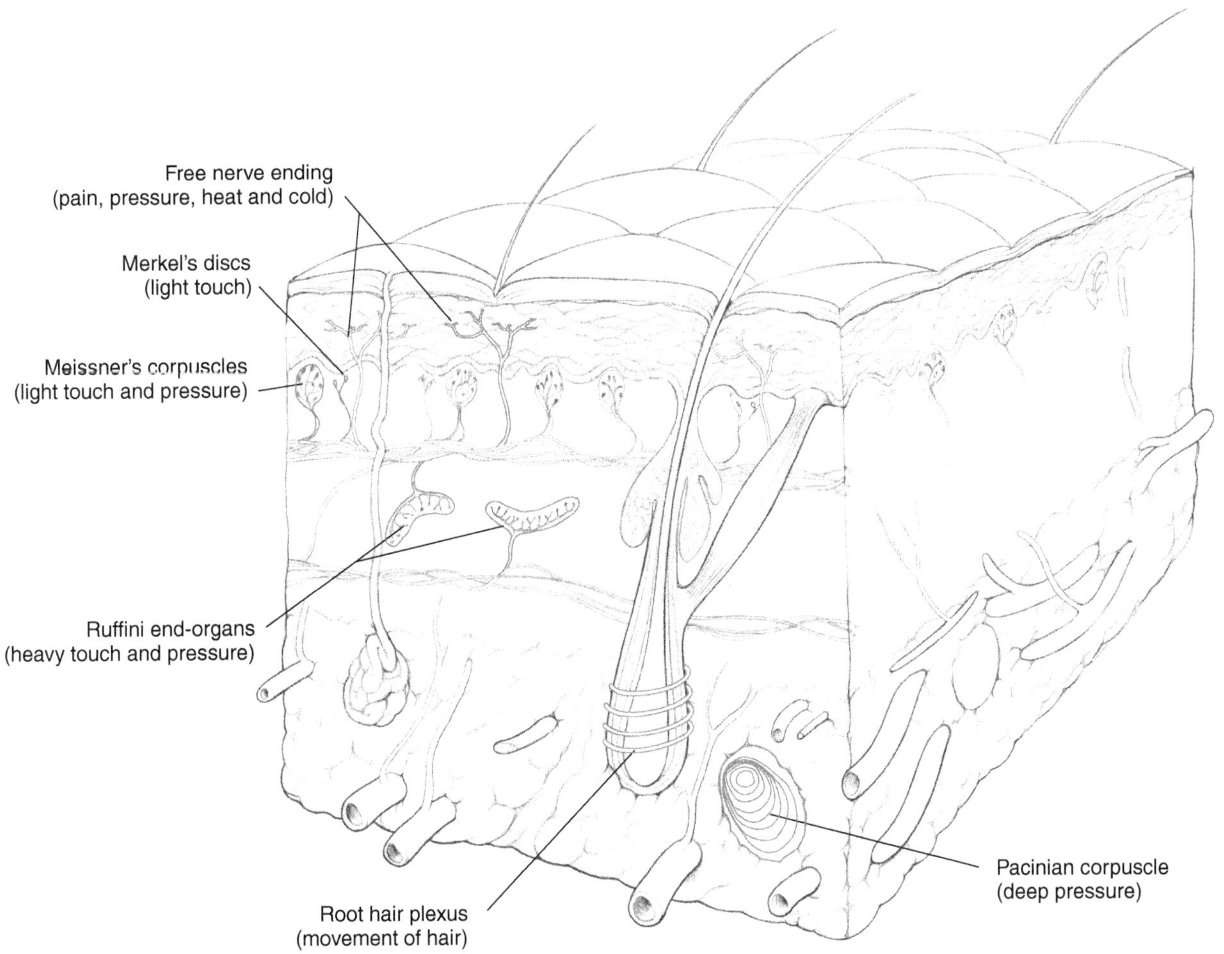

FIGURE 4-8 **Sensory receptors of the skin.**

awareness and includes data about body posture, position, movement, weight, pressure, tension, changes in equilibrium, resistance of external objects, and associated habitual patterns.

Proprioceptors provide information on muscle contraction, tendon tension, joint position, and the orientation of the head. These data can inform us about the location of a body part in space and in relation to the rest of the body and can provide a sense of how much muscular force is needed to move an object. Proprioceptors relevant to myofascial massage include muscle spindles and GTOs (discussed in Chapter 2), Ruffini end organs, Golgi end organs, Pacinian corpuscles, and cervical receptors (Kinnaird, 1993). We discuss their role in proprioception here:

- *Muscle spindles* are tiny bundles of muscle tissue embedded within skeletal muscle fibers; however, nerve receptors are wrapped around them. Muscle spindles are found attached to the belly of muscle or to the musculotendinous junction parallel to the muscle fibers. Nerve receptors in muscle spindles detect, evaluate, report, and adjust the length of the muscle, thus setting its tone. Central muscle spindle receptors fire in response to small changes in muscle length; receptors on each side of the center fire in response to bigger changes. Receptors in muscle spindles are sometimes called *stretch receptors* because they respond to a muscle that has been stretched too quickly or too far. They may discharge for long periods at a time, registering information about how long the muscle is, how fast it is contracting, and changes in contraction speed.
- *GTOs* are found in the tendons, as mentioned in Chapter 2. Because they register the tension on the attachment, they indicate how hard the muscle is working. If the GTO detects excessive tension, a message is sent to inhibitory motor neurons that come back to the same muscle. This relaxes the muscle by stopping muscle contraction and in turn decreases tension on the tendon.
- *Ruffini end organs* can also be found within the joint capsule, where they respond to gentle, active muscular contraction that alters joint tension. Ruffini end organs adapt slowly, are not easily fatigued, and are progressively recruited as the joint moves, inducing continuous smooth movement and preventing movement from being "disjointed" and jerky. Ruffini end organs are affected by the first 15 degrees of movement and report on steady position and to a lesser degree on direction of movement.
- *Golgi end organs* are stimulated by gentle, passive joint movement. They adapt slowly and continue to fire over a long time. Because they are found in ligaments, they deliver information that is not dependent on muscular contraction. This helps the body to keep track of where the joint is at any given moment, irrespective of muscle activity.
- *Pacinian (lamellated) corpuscles* are found in CT around the joints. Under deep pressure, they discharge and cease firing in a short period. They are sometimes called *acceleration receptors* because they respond to changes in the direction or speed of movement.
- *Cervical receptors* interact with equilibrium receptors inside the ear to maintain balance and an appropriate position of the head in space.

Myofascial massage techniques stimulate these proprioceptors below the pain threshold but at a level high enough to elicit self-healing and regeneration of soft tissues.

The Implications of Myofascial Massage for Nerve Tissue

This section outlines myofascial discoveries and neurological principles or theories that reveal how myofascial massage may affect the nervous system.

Cathie (1983) notes that many trigger points are found in sites where nerves pierce the fascia. He infers that sustained pulls on the fascia may lead to entrapment of neural structures at these sites and subsequent dysfunction and pain.

Staubesand (in Chaitow and DeLany, 2002a, 2002b) shows that fascia is regularly perforated by nerve and blood vessels. Heine (1995) previously showed an 82% correspondence of fascial perforation sites with acupuncture points. Looking at these data, Schleip (1998) concludes that intervention in the fascial system (e.g., myofascial massage) may affect the ANS. Shea (1993) claims that myofascial massage lowers sympathetic dominance to alter the supply of blood to all the cells in the body.

Shea (1993) argues that the sympathetic division modulates organ functioning to respond to the needs of the skeletal muscles. As discussed in Chapter 2, the skeletal muscles are the largest consumer of energy in the body. They produce heat, oxygen, and waste more rapidly and more than any other part of the body. Shea claims that when an individual starts a new exercise regimen or undergoes a lot of stress, the nerves shut down nonessential organ functions because of the additional energy requirements of the skeletal muscles.

Stimulating the sympathetic fibers results in a measurable increase in muscle energy activity within 5 to 15 minutes (Shea, 1993). With myofascial massage, a rapid decrease in the client's sympathetic tone becomes apparent as dizziness, sweating, or flushing. Other signs of a rapid ANS shift can include tremoring in the muscles, shaking, jerking, skin color changes, sweating, clamminess, laughing, crying, and talking a lot during a session.

It is important to remember that these kinds of energy discharge are not inherently bad because the ultimate goal is to reduce stress. It is possible, however, to reduce sympathetic dominance in a way that reduces or does not induce unpleasant side effects. To "gentle" out myofascial sessions, slow down your strokes when you first notice some of these signs. If you slow down and the reactions still continue, stop to allow nerve impulses to reach the client's consciousness before any more physical sensations are inputted.

THE IMPLICATIONS OF NEURAL RESPONSE THEORIES FOR MASSAGE

Spinal cord reflexes can be influenced by conscious signals from the cerebral cortex, but when a reflex starts, it always occurs automatically, in a specific, predictable fashion. Many laws and theories have been formulated to explain the nature of these reflexes. Others attempt to explain the predictable responses of cutaneous receptors, including those that transmit data related to pain. Thus, these laws and theories provide a rationale for many principles of myofascial massage. They include the following:

- **Law of specificity** (Thomas, 1997): *Excitation of a receptor always gives rise to the same sensation regardless of the nature of the stimulus.* When a sensory receptor is activated, it will respond in a specific way, no matter whether you use vibration, deep pressure, stretching, or some other massage technique.
- **Hooke's law** (Thomas, 1997): *The stress used to stretch or compress tissue is proportional to the strain experienced, as long as the elastic limits of the body have not been exceeded.* Myofascial methods should precisely meet and match the resistance found in the soft tissue without excessive or inadequate pressure or pull.
- **All or none (Bowditch's) law** (Anderson, 1997): *The weakest stimulus capable of producing a response produces the maximum response contraction in cardiac and skeletal muscles and nerves.* Techniques do not have to be extremely intense to produce a healing response.
- **Bell's law** (Thomas, 1997): *Anterior spinal nerve roots are motor, and posterior spinal nerve roots are sensory.* Massage applied along the spine can have a powerful effect, and very light pressure applied in that area is strong enough to effect a therapeutic change.
- **Arndt-Shultz law** (St. John, 1990): *Weak stimuli activate physiological processes, and strong stimuli inhibit them.* This law describes the positive effect of steady low levels of pressure used in many myofascial approaches. It also explains how higher intensities of pressure can be counterproductive and actually shut off a response.
- **Weber's law** (Thomas, 1997): *The increase in stimulus necessary to produce the smallest perceptible increase in sensation bears a constant ratio to the strength of the stimulus already existing.* To change a sensory perception, the intensity of the massage method must exceed the existing sensation. Thus, although indirect myofascial therapies may effectively reduce pain and discomfort, the client can more easily perceive the change in sensation (deep pressure) from direct therapies.
- **Law of facilitation** (St. John, 1990): *After a nerve impulse has traversed a pathway through a certain set of neurons, it will tend to travel on that same path.* This explains the tendency to have an old pain pattern return even when there is no current injury in the area. It also describes the phenomenon of trigger points, a subject of interest in the neuromuscular approach.
- **Pflugger's law of unilaterality** (Nimmo, 1957): *If a mild stimulus is applied to a sensory nerve (or nerves), the nerve impulses will usually take place on one side only, the side of the stimulus.* Mild injuries tend to manifest only on one side of the body, and light massage stimulation affects only the side of the body on which it is applied.
- **Pflugger's law of symmetry** (Nimmo, 1957): *If the stimulation is increased sufficiently, reflex responses occur on the opposite side of the body as well as on the affected side.* So if a client has more severe pain, it may manifest on both sides. To treat, massage the unaffected side to avoid pain; such actions will have a therapeutic effect on the injured side.
- **Pflugger's law of radiation** (Nimmo, 1957): *If stimulation continues to increase, the signals will be propagated up the spinal cord and elicit reflex reactions at these higher segments.* In severe injuries, pain and guarding can manifest more superiorly than the actual injury.
- **Pflugger's law of intensity** (Nimmo, 1957): *Reflex movements are usually more intense on the side of the irritation.* At times, the movements of the opposite side equal them in intensity, but they are usually less pronounced.
- **Pflugger's law of generalization** (Nimmo, 1957): *When stimulation becomes very intense, the reticular activating system (RAS) radiates impulses to all parts of the spinal cord, causing a general contraction of all skeletal muscles.* Ongoing chronic pain or intense acute pain can make the whole body hurt or lead to the development of hyper sensitive areas that refer pain to other areas. When choosing massage techniques, avoid the generalization response by keeping aggressive or invasive techniques to a minimum.
- **Cannon's law of denervation** (Canon and Rosenblueth, 1949): *When autonomic effectors are partially or completely separated from normal nerve connections, they become more sensitive to noxious stimuli.* For example, if a person is not getting any sleep or is chronically stressed, a small stimulus may reactivate an old injury.
- **Hilton's law** (Thomas, 1997): *A nerve that supplies a joint also supplies the muscle of the joint and the skin over the insertions of these muscles.* If a joint is injured, the reflex response is to tighten the muscles to hold the joint immobile.

- **Gate-control theory** (Melzack and Wall, 1965): *A hypothetical "gate" in the spinal cord allows pain impulses through to reach the area in the brain that perceives pain signals.* Stimulation of large-diameter fibers blocks the gate and prevents pain sensations from getting through. The sensations of massage (which are transmitted by large-diameter fibers) thereby help to suppress pain sensations (which are transmitted by small-diameter fibers). Students should note that gate-control is a theory and has its detractors. It is not a law.

MANIPULATING NEURAL RESPONSES WITH MYOFASCIAL MASSAGE

Neural responses to trauma and pain can be manipulated by changing the input to sensory receptors with touch, pressure, or stretch. This is what bodywork does. Rubbing or pressing techniques affect mechanoreceptors. Conscious input (e.g., guided voluntary breathing, imagery, movement, or direct questions that require a verbal response) can also override neural responses to a degree.

Direct pressure on an area alters the amount of stretch or tension perceived by the muscle spindles or the GTOs. This increased sense of stretch stimulates the transmission of data instructing motor neurons to effect relaxation. Thus, a muscle in spasm may be helped to relax by applying direct pressure to the GTOs at the tendinous attachments or to the muscle spindle in the belly of the muscle. A muscle can be temporarily toned or strengthened by reversing the direction of pressure to pull away from muscle spindles or the GTOs.

Isometric contractions temporarily increase perceived tension on the tendons and stimulate the GTOs to initiate a reduction in tension and subsequent relaxation in the muscle. Active movements stimulate mechanoreceptors to shift the perception of touch, pressure, and pain. Voluntary movements can also help the client's brain to override habitual reflex patterns that are maladaptive. Easy movement reduces the stretch and tension on a muscle and resets the stretch receptors in the muscle spindle, allowing the muscles to relax. Passive movements activate mechanoreceptors.

CREATING NEW NEURAL PATHWAYS

Bodywork that engages the client's conscious mind affects the brain. Kinesthetic learning in a myofascial session develops new neural pathways in the brain, similar to building roads to new places. When conscious understanding or activity is coupled with bodywork, these new pathways reinforce physiological changes.

It is even possible for massage to recreate the sequence of the synaptic pathways that lead to a certain memory. Clients often report memories during massage. Massage can also provide an opportunity to reexperience pain in a safe environment and integrate that sensation in a healthier way. For example, pressure on a painful trigger point can at first be scary. When the client recognizes that her myofascial therapist will not push past her pain threshold and that she is in control, the client can relax and breathe out the experience of pain. Without a sensitive myofascial therapist, bringing up painful sensations can be harmful.

SUMMARY

Nerve tissue has a unique anatomy and physiology with profound effects on the structure and function of the whole human body. Bodywork must address this important tissue to attain lasting therapeutic effects.

Two types of cells are found in nerve tissue: neurons and neuroglia. Neurons conduct impulses (electrical charges) that carry information to and from the brain or spinal cord. The important parts of neurons are the cell body, axons, and dendrites. Dendrites carry information to the cell body, and axons carry data away from the cell body to the next connection. Neuroglia are supportive cells that have a connective function.

Nerve tissue is organized into a nervous system. The two divisions of the nervous system are the CNS, which includes the brain and spinal cord and has integrative and interpretive functions, and the PNS, which includes the cranial and spinal nerves and distributes information to and from the periphery of the body.

The function of a neuron is to conduct electrical impulses. The steps to nerve impulse transmission include depolarization, propagation of an action potential, transmission across the synapse, and reception and response.

The peripheral nerves can have a sensory or motor function. Cutaneous sensory receptors deliver information about touch, pressure, pain, and other tactile stimuli. Proprioceptors deliver information to the CNS about the position and motion of the internal parts of the body. Two proprioceptors (i.e., muscle spindles and GTOs) are reviewed in light of their significance for myofascial massage.

The motor aspect of the nervous system itself can be separated into two categories. One is the somatic nervous system, which delivers information to and from skeletal muscles. This is the division that causes muscles to move. The ANS affects the organs. Because it originates in either the brainstem or spinal cord, the ANS is said to be automatic, or below the level of conscious thought.

The ANS is an important link to the "stress response." Touch can activate the parasympathetic division of the ANS, so that self-regeneration and healing can occur.

All voluntary activity, including cognition, communication, perception, and conscious movement, involves the brain. In contrast, spinal cord reflexes always occur automatically, without voluntary control. Once activated, reflexes ensue in a specific, predictable way. Laws explaining predictable neural responses provide an important rationale for the effectiveness of myofascial massage therapy. In addition to manipulating neural responses, myofascial massage can help clients create new, more healthful neural pathways.

Review Questions

1. Nerve tissue refers to two specific types of cells, __________ and __________.
   a. neurons and nerves
   b. nervous and nerve
   c. neurons and neuroglia
   d. connective and supporting
2. The middle covering of CT that bundles individual nerve fibers into nerve fascicles is called __________.
   a. epineurium
   b. perineurium
   c. endoneurium
   d. synoneurium
3. __________ neurons conduct impulses to the spinal cord and brain.
   a. Autonomic
   b. Reflex
   c. Sensory
   d. Motor
4. True or false: Somatic motor neurons conduct impulses to the skeletal muscles.
5. True or false: GTOs are also called acceleration receptors.
6. True or false: Proprioceptors provide information about the body in space at any moment.
7. __________ are receptors that respond to pain.
8. __________ theory states that a special mechanism in the spinal cord modifies pain sensations with other sensations entering at that segment.
9. __________ forms thin sheaths around the axon of PNS neurons to aid in saltatory conduction.
10. Define and describe the "fight or flight" response.

REFERENCES

Anderson KN. Mosby's Medical, Nursing and Allied Health Dictionary. 6th Ed. St. Louis: Mosby Year-Book, 1997.

Barres B. Lowly glia strengthen brain connections. Available at: http://faculty.washington.edu/chudler/glia.html. Accessed September 12, 1997.

Canon WB, Rosenblueth A. The Supersensitivity of Denervated Substances. New York: MacMillan, 1949.

Cathie A. Selected writings. Academy of Applied Osteopathy 1974 Yearbook. Indianapolis, IN: American Academy of Osteopathy, 1983.

Chaitow L, DeLany JW. Clinical Application of Neuromuscular Techniques. Vol. 1: The Upper Body. Edinburgh, UK: Elsevier Science, 2002a.

Chaitow L, DeLany JW. Clinical Application of Neuromuscular Techniques. Vol. 2: The Lower Body. Edinburgh, UK: Elsevier Science, 2002b.

Fritz S. Mosby's Basic Science for Soft Tissue and Movement Therapies. St. Louis: Mosby, 2000.

Heine H. Functional anatomy of traditional Chinese acupuncture points. Acta Anatomica 1995;152:293.

Kinnaird DW. Neuro-Humoral Massage. Unpublished manuscript. Notes for Neuro-Humoral Workshop, Portland, OR, 1993.

Melzack R, Wall P. Pain mechanisms: a new theory. Science, 1965;150:971–979.

Moore KL, Dalley AF. Clinically Oriented Anatomy. 4th Ed. Philadelphia: Lippincott Williams & Wilkins, 1999.

Nimmo R. Receptors, affectors and tonus. J Am Chiropract Assoc 1957;27:21.

Schleip R. Interview with Prof. Dr. Med. J. Staubesand. In: Rolf Lines. Boulder, CO: Rolf Institute, 1998.

Schafer R. Clinical Biomechanics. 2nd Ed. Baltimore: Williams and Wilkins, 1987.

Shea MJ. A Manual for the Spine and Extremities with Intra-oral Supplement. Juno Beach, FL: Shea Educational Group, 1993.

St. John P. Workshop Seminar Notes (Seminar I). St. John Neuromuscular Therapy Seminars, Largo, FL, 1990.

Thomas CL, ed. Taber's Encyclopedic Medical Dictionary. 18th Ed. Philadelphia: FA Davis, 1997.

Tortora GJ, Grabowski SR. Principles of Anatomy and Physiology. 10th Ed. New York: HarperCollins College Publishers, 2003.

SUGGESTED READINGS

Juhan D. Job's Body: A Handbook for Bodywork. Barrytown, NY: Barrytown Ltd., 1998.

Premkumar K. The Massage Connection: Anatomy and Physiology. 2nd Ed. Baltimore: Lippincott Williams & Wilkins, 2004.

Tortora GJ, Grabowski SR. Principles of Anatomy and Physiology. 10th Ed. New York: HarperCollins College Publishers, 2003.

Part

II

Direct Methods Used in Myofascial Massage

Chapter

5

Neuromuscular Approach

OBJECTIVES

- Describe the neuromuscular approach, including myofascial trigger point massage, other manual neuromuscular techniques, and muscle energy techniques.
- Describe trigger points and the basic procedure for trigger point release.
- List other manual neuromuscular techniques that release pressure on nerves from soft tissue and alleviate discomfort from trigger points.
- Describe neuromuscular techniques using stretch with resistance.
- Discuss positioning, draping, and support.
- Discuss treatment planning and decision making.

CHAPTER OUTLINE

KEY TERMS

Trigger point (trigger zone, trigger spot, trigger area, TrP): Hyperirritable area that is locally tender and may refer pain, tenderness, other autonomic phenomena, or proprioceptive changes when pressed. Trigger points produce weakness and prevent complete lengthening in the muscle and may elicit a local twitch response upon compression.

Active trigger points: Hypersensitive areas that are painful without stimulation. Active trigger points are very tender and produce referred pain upon palpation

Latent trigger points: Hypersensitive areas that are not ordinarily painful but upon palpation are tender and may produce referred pain.

Tender points: Hypersensitive areas that do not cause increased tightness or radiating pain in surrounding areas. Release of a tender point does not cause a release in other areas.

Acupuncture points: Precise points (tsubos) along meridians as specified by traditional Chinese medicine.

Neuromuscular Therapy (neuromuscular techniques; NMT): Trademarked style that focuses on local dysfunctions, including trigger points, ischemia, inflammation, muscle hypertonia, and nerve impingement.

Deep pressure (ischemic compression): Sustained pressure on a trigger point (8 to 10 sec up to 1 min).

Vibration: Neuromuscular technique in which the therapist presses into the trigger point and then adds an up-and-down trembling motion.

Stripping: Neuromuscular technique that is a type of deep effleurage that travels down the length of the muscle fiber while maintaining depth.

Ice friction (intermittent cold): Slow application of ice over soft tissue with unidirectional parallel strokes.

Muscle energy techniques (METs): Set of procedures requiring client to voluntarily contract a specific muscle in a specific direction against (or with) a specific force applied by the therapist.

Post-isometric relaxation (PIR): Principle in MET by which the therapist lengthens the target muscle up to a point of mild resistance. Holding that position, the therapist coaches the client to voluntarily resist for 8 to 10 seconds. As the client relaxes, the therapist takes the muscle into a greater stretch and repeats the process two more times, ending on a stretch/relax.

Contract relax (CR): Muscle energy technique identical to post-isometric relaxation, except that the muscle is *not* taken into greater lengthening after the first resistance barrier.

Reciprocal inhibition (RI; antagonist contract): Principle in MET by which the therapist inhibits the reciprocal (or antagonist) muscle to the one he or she wants to target.

Contract relax antagonist contract (CRAC): Muscle energy technique in which the therapist alternates performing post-isometric relaxation and then reciprocal inhibition.

The direct method of myofascial massage (e.g., including both the neuromuscular approach and direct connective tissue [CT] approach) has the distinct advantage of enabling bodyworkers to meet resistances in the client's body directly. This chapter introduces the neuromuscular approach to myofascial massage. As the name implies, the neuromuscular approach uses applications based on neurologic principles governing the reflex arc, proprioceptors, sensory receptors, and other aspects of the nervous system. This approach encompasses a variety of treatments, including trigger point (TrP) massage, muscle energy techniques (METs), and manual techniques. These treatments are sometimes referred to collectively or in part under the umbrella term neuromuscular therapy.

The first section of this chapter describes the various types of TrPs and distinguishes them from tender points and acupuncture points. It also describes the basic procedure for TrP release.

The second section introduces several additional manual neuromuscular techniques, such as deep effleurage, vibration, percussion with stretch, and ice friction. Similar to the deep pressure used in basic TrP release, such techniques seek to release pressure on nerves caused by soft tissue and alleviate discomfort and pain from myofascial TrPs.

The third section describes neuromuscular techniques that stress movement, collectively known as MET. METs emphasize voluntary contraction of specific muscles by the client coupled with specific directional stretches or movements applied by the therapist. MET procedures incorporate additional therapeutic objectives such as increased range of motion (ROM), relaxation of hypertonic muscles, assessment of muscle pain or weakness, and increased sensory awareness.

The chapter also discusses positioning, propping, and draping for the neuromuscular approach to enhance the process of soft tissue release. Decision making about where and when to use the various techniques is discussed and suggestions are made for adapting the approach to specific conditions and client needs, including acute, subacute, and chronic complaints.

Myofascial Trigger Point Massage

Trigger points are intense knots of tension that refer pain to other parts of the body (Rubik, 1992). Froriep identified tight and tender bands within muscle in the 1800s. Then in 1938, Kellgren published a study indicating that many muscles in the body exhibit a characteristic referral pattern for pain when injected with a salt solution. In 1940, the term *myofascial pain* was first used in medical journals to describe trigger areas in the lumbar spine; in 1952, Travell reported the pain referral pattern of the infraspinatus muscle during a muscle biopsy. Travell and her colleague, Simons (1999a, 1999b), also a physician, went on to establish recognized diagnostic and assessment criteria and treatment procedures for myofascial TrP dysfunction.

TERMINOLOGY

According to Travell and Simons (1999a, 1999b):

> a **trigger point** (also called a **trigger zone**, **trigger spot**, or **trigger area** and often called by its abbreviation, **TrP**) is a focus of hyperirritability in a tissue that, when compressed, is locally tender and, if sufficiently hypersensitive, gives rise to referred pain and tenderness, and sometimes to referred autonomic phenomena and distortion of proprioception.

Trigger points can be found in scar tissue, tendons, ligaments, skin, fat pads, joint capsules, and periosteum, as well as in the muscle and junction of muscle with these tissues (Manheim, 2001).

According to Travell and Simons (1999a, 1999b), "distortion of proprioception" is a change in awareness about where and how the body takes up and moves in space. "Referred autonomic phenomena" may consist of pain, tenderness, and other kinds of sensations, as well as physiological processes such as increased motor unit activity (spasm), vasoconstriction, vasodilation, and hypersecretion, which occur at a distance from the TrP. Practitioners may recognize twitching, heat, cold, itching, and goosebumps as referred sensations often reported by their clients.

Myofascial TrPs are sometimes associated with fibrous nodules, palpation of which often invokes general involuntary pain responses, such as crying out, twitching, or other signs of withdrawal, known as "jump signs." Because TrPs are areas of hyperexcitability, over time, increasingly smaller stimuli activate them. Thus, clients who complain of increasing pain are reporting a real phenomenon and not simply becoming chronic complainers. No anatomic structure that corresponds with the actual TrP, however, has ever been identified (Manheim, 2001).

Active trigger points are hypersensitive areas that are painful even without stimulation. Active TrPs are very tender upon palpation and produce a characteristic referral pattern for each muscle (Kostopoulos and Rizopoulos, 2001). They produce weakness in the muscle, prevent full lengthening of the muscle, and may elicit a local twitch response upon compression.

Latent trigger points are usually quiet and not a source of spontaneous pain. They are tender upon palpation and may produce the characteristic referred pain pattern with the application of pressure. Similar to active TrPs, latent TrPs produce weakness in the muscle, interfere with flexibility, and mediate a local twitch response when adequately stimulated. Practitioners believe that an active TrP that was not properly treated may become latent and that latent TrPs may exist in the myofascia for years after recovery from an injury. These latent TrPs may become active if reinjury occurs.

Satellite TrPs may develop in the same muscle where the primary TrP exists, in other muscles within the referred pain pattern, or in other muscles altogether (Kostopoulos and Rizopoulos, 2001). Satellite TrPs seem to resolve when the "primary" TrP is resolved.

Travell and Simons (1999a, 1999b) distinguish between central myofascial TrPs, which are located near the center of muscle fibers, and attachment TrPs, which are located at musculotendinous (MTJ) or tenoperiosteal (TPJ) points between muscle, tendons, and bones. The MTJ and TPJ are inherently weak areas because they consist of a joining between two distinct anatomical structures with conflicting tensions and pulls (Figure 5-1). Therefore, proprioceptors such as muscle spindles and Golgi tendon organs are grouped in greater numbers at these junctions to protect the areas from damage caused by overstretching.

DIFFERENCES BETWEEN TRIGGER POINTS AND TENDER POINTS

Clients often complain of tenderness upon compression. It is important to distinguish whether this tenderness is attributable to a TrP or a tender point because the application of TrP release may not be appropriate for tender points. A **tender point** differs from a TrP in tightness and reported

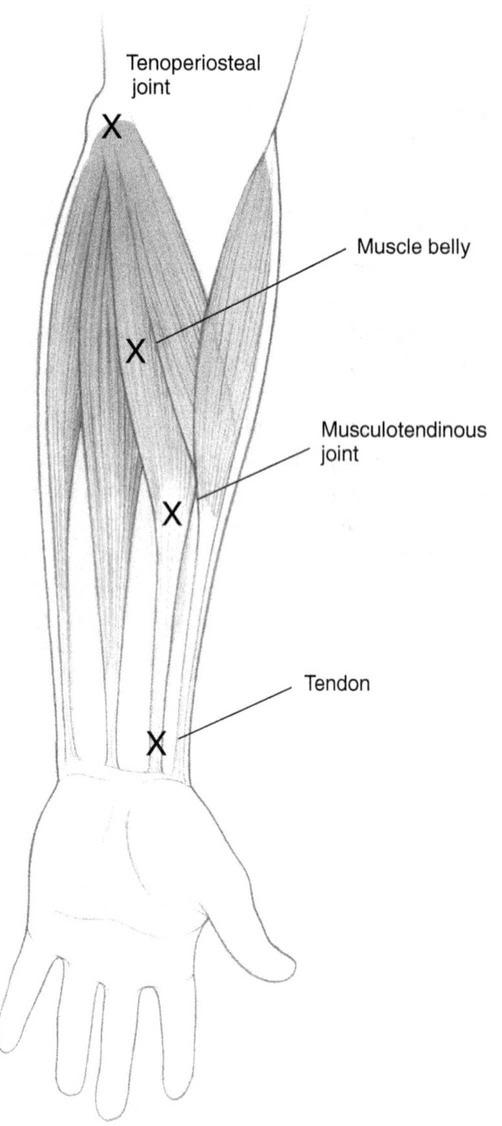

FIGURE 5-1 Common sites for trigger points in the pronator teres muscle. These include the belly of the muscle, tendon, tenoperiosteal joint, and musculotendinous joint. The sites are marked with Xs.

pain responses to pressure. Direct pressure on a tender point does not cause increased tightness in surrounding areas as it does for TrPs. Pressure on a tender point does not cause radiating pain and does not cause the therapist's finger to be drawn into a spiral path but rather, to travel a straight path down. Another difference is that release of a tender point does not cause releases in other areas, as it may for TrPs (Manheim, 2001).

DIFFERENCES BETWEEN TRIGGER POINTS AND ACUPUNCTURE POINTS

Similarly, it is important to distinguish whether this tenderness is attributable to a TrP or an acupuncture point because the application of TrP release may not be appropriate for acupuncture points. Theoretical and physiological discrepancies exist between TrPs and acupuncture points. As specified by traditional Chinese medicine (TCM), classical acu points are precise points (called *tsubos*) along meridians. Extrameridian and achi points are exceptions that lie outside of the meridian lines. In contrast, myofascial TrPs may be found anywhere within a muscle belly and are believed to originate in the vicinity of "dysfunctional endplates" (Travell and Simons, 1999a, 1999b). With acupuncture treatment, diagnosis is made according to TCM principles that have no apparent correlation with Western anatomical, kinesiology, or biomechanics principles. In contrast, such principles guide the insertion of dry needles into TrPs, when administered by physical therapists and physicians. Also, in Western medical TrP treatment, only one needle is inserted, causing a local twitch response; with acupuncture, more than one needle is usually necessary.

IDENTIFYING TRIGGER POINTS BY THEIR REFERRAL PATTERNS

Travell and Simons (1999a, 1999b) have identified specific pain patterns that can be used to identify exact TrPs. Detailed charts can be found in their definitive work, *Myofascial Pain and Dysfunction: The Trigger Point Manual, Vols. 1 and 2,* an example of which is shown in Figure 5-2.

The scope of this book does not allow for a complete discussion of all identified TrP locations and possible pain referral patterns. To give the student an idea of the information that is available, Table 5-1 presents TrP locations for selected muscles, along with some of the common referral patterns. This brief and incomplete sketch can in no way replace the detailed and unparalleled work of Travell and Simons (1999a, 1999b).

Trigger point release (and bodywork that incorporates TrP release) can focus on any region or segment of the body. It is not necessary to memorize pain referral patterns to release TrPs. Charts that show a visual representation of the patterns are available, or the therapist can simply ask the client for feedback and follow the pain as it is reported with subsequent TrP releases. Rather than rote memorization of possible pain patterns, it is more important to know the anatomical structures that lie beneath the hands. To acquire a deeper conceptual understanding of structure, review anatomy texts and practice palpating the soft tissues enough to build an experiential understanding of the muscles and CT, where the muscles attach to tendons, and where the tendons attach to bones.

A tendon feels like a cord sliding under your hand when the client's muscle contracts. As you palpate along the tendon and get closer to the muscle belly, the sensation of sliding decreases. The MTJ region is palpable; it does not feel cordlike like a tendon, and it does not feel like a softer muscle belly. The TPJ is where the tendon attaches to the bone.

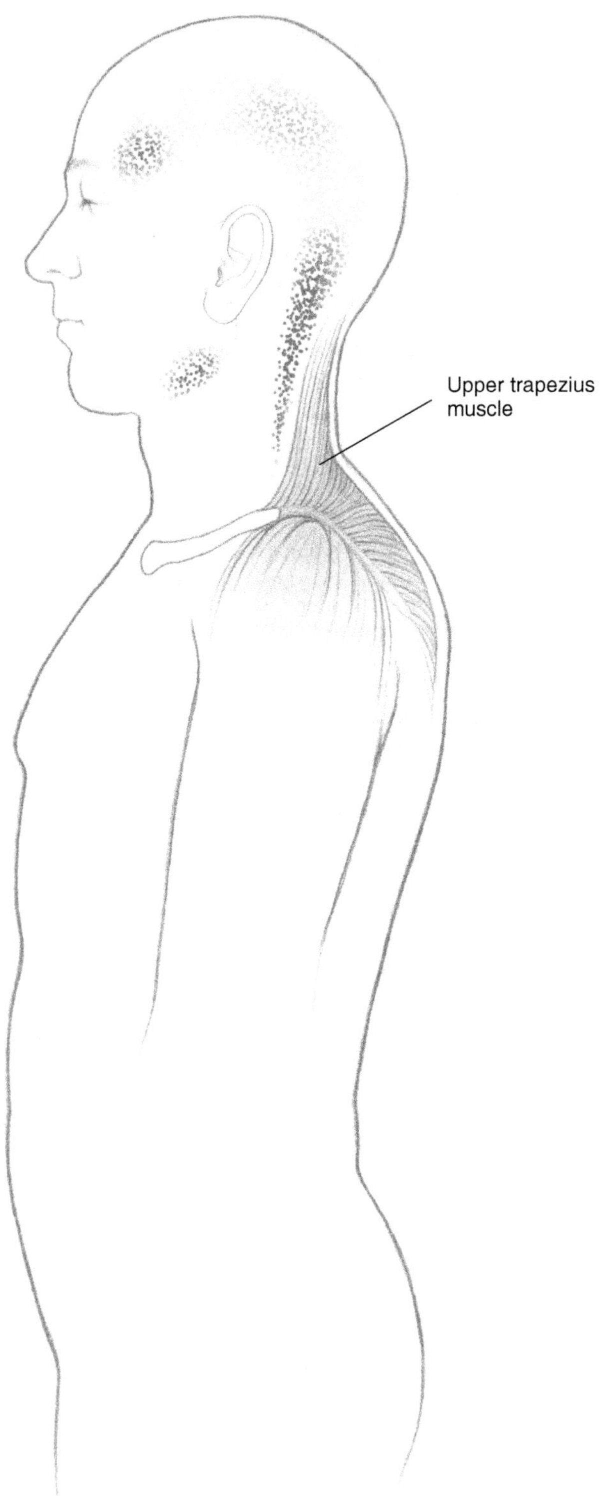

FIGURE 5-2 **Example of a common referral pattern.** *Dots* mark the trigger point referral pattern for the upper trapezius muscle. *Solid areas* (where the dots overlap) mark the primary referral pain zones (adapted from Travell and Simons, 1999a).

RELEASE OF PAIN AND EMOTION IN TRIGGER POINT MASSAGE

Some massage students may think that they must impose a certain amount of pain to affect a TrP release. Inflicting pain on clients is neither desirable nor necessary. There are many ways to perform TrP release that do not require strong pressure or discomfort.

It also is ill advised to deliberately try to evoke an emotional response from the client. Although emotional releases do sometimes occur during TrP work, they are not necessary to the work. When an emotional response does present itself, it is best to respond simply as a caring human being, rather than violating scope of practice by simulating the skills of a mental health therapist. Referrals to mental health experts are appropriate at the end of any session. During an emotional experience, it may be helpful to remind the client to tangibly experience his body and physical reality with simple sensory cues. Sensory cues could include suggestions such as "Feel your breath moving in and out of your nose" or "Feel the weight of your body supported by the massage table." Further discussion of the psychological aspects of myofascial massage can be found in Chapter 11. Psychological aspects of massage are also addressed in my previous book, *Body Mechanics and Self-Care Manual* (2001).

Practitioners who deliberately provoke intense pain to prompt their clients' emotions to surface indulge in a type of agenda setting that is potentially harmful. As bodyworkers, our area of expertise is the *body,* and a presumption of what the client "should do emotionally" to heal is never warranted. It is also a credo of this book that pain itself is considered a sign for caution and should not be confused with therapy.

For the purpose of clarity in this text, we will establish the following guideline/communication scale of 1 to 10 to describe pain:

1. No discomfort at all; very light sensation of touch, pressure
2. No discomfort at all; mild sensation of touch, pressure
3. Firm, comfortable pressure but without pain
4. Strong, stable pressure but without pain
5. Strong sensation of pressure at the threshold of pain; "that just feels good"
6. Soreness that "hurts so good"; mild release of pain
7. Soreness that feels bad, does not give satisfaction or relief
8. Sharp, stabbing pain; client trying to decide if she should complain; "I wonder if I should say that hurts?"
9. Intense pain that is barely controlled pain; flinching and twitching
10. Intense, unbearable pain

It is not necessary to memorize this scale, just to understand the relative progression. When working with clients, a good guideline is to focus on applying pressure levels

TABLE 5-1 Selected Muscles, Trigger Point Locations, and Referral Patterns

Muscle	Location of Trigger Points	Pain Referral Patterns
Pectoralis major	Clavicular: Along the lateral border of pec major, underneath the edge of the anterior deltoid Sternal: Between ribs 3, 4, and 5, near the insertion of pectoralis minor	Clavicular: Along the anterior deltoid and into the region of the TrP Sternal: Into the front of the chest and down the arm
Biceps brachii	Lower third may contain a TrP in each head	May refer pain throughout the biceps and upward into the anterior deltoid
Hand and finger extensors	Pain lodges in the portion of the muscles near the elbow	Pain is referred to the lateral epicondyle and down the forearm to the wrist and hand area
Erector spinae	Longissimus and iliocostalis are the most likely sites	Upper: Tend to refer along scapular border and between shoulder blades Lower: Down into the lumbar and hip region and into abdomen
Trapezius	Upper: Slightly above lateral portion of the clavicle Middle: Superior edge of the spine of the scapula Lower: Lateral border of middle and lower traps	Upper: Up the posterior neck to the mastoid process Middle: Shoots pain to the top of the shoulder Lower: Not reported
Rhomboids	Medial to the vertebral border of the scapula	Pain pattern is local, along the edge of the scapula
Lattisimus dorsi	Axillary fold, near the posterior deltoid	Superior: Deep under the upper portion of the scapula; may extend over posterior deltoid and down triceps Inferior: Through muscle itself and over the lowest ribs
Hamstrings	TrPs tend to cluster in the distal portion of all three hamstrings above the knee and at the borders of the muscles	Up to the gluteal area, around the ischial tuberosity, and around the back of the knee

TrP = trigger point.

that are described by the client as strong but good," level 4 or 5 on the 10-point scale. Never work deeper than a level 6, even when locating a TrP.

BASIC TRIGGER POINT RELEASE

Before a massage that will use TrP release, trim your fingernails short and rounded on the edges, so that you do not scratch the client. It will also be easier to perform TrP release techniques when the client's skin is dry and free of oil and lotion.

Let your hands (or other contact point, such as the forearm or elbow) sink into the skin at the site of the TrP until you meet a resistance (Figure 5-3). Hold that level of pressure and wait for the tissue to soften in a release. This amount of pressure may initially increase the client's pain level (slightly) at the site of the TrP and in its radiation pattern. After the initial release, the tissue may seem to draw your finger deeper in a spiral (Manheim, 2001). Continue to exert downward pressure without increasing the pressure and wait for the release again. *Note: Do not exceed the client's pain tolerance!*

Resistance in the soft tissue determines depth of pressure. By only sinking until you feel resistance, you have another safeguard that your work will not hurt your client. Sinking is most effective when you face and align your whole body with the direction of the pressure. Alignment is maintained all the way from the sole of the foot through the ankle, knee, hip, shoulder, nose, and top of the head. Scan your client for nonverbal clues of discomfort (scowl, shudder, scrunched-up face) or release (sigh, deep breath, stomach rumbling, faint smile) while holding your head in line with the rest of your spine.

Remaining at ease in the body and hands helps you to effectively use TrP release. You cannot feel very tiny releases in the TrP unless your body stays soft and relaxed throughout the process. When you let go of your own tensions, you consciously and unconsciously guide the client into letting go of her tensions as well.

When the tissue softens, reposition yourself for the next release. Repositioning means moving into your next position and letting go of any accumulated tension. It may mean taking a relaxing breath, shifting to a different part of your body as the main tool, or stepping to the other side of the table to get a better angle.

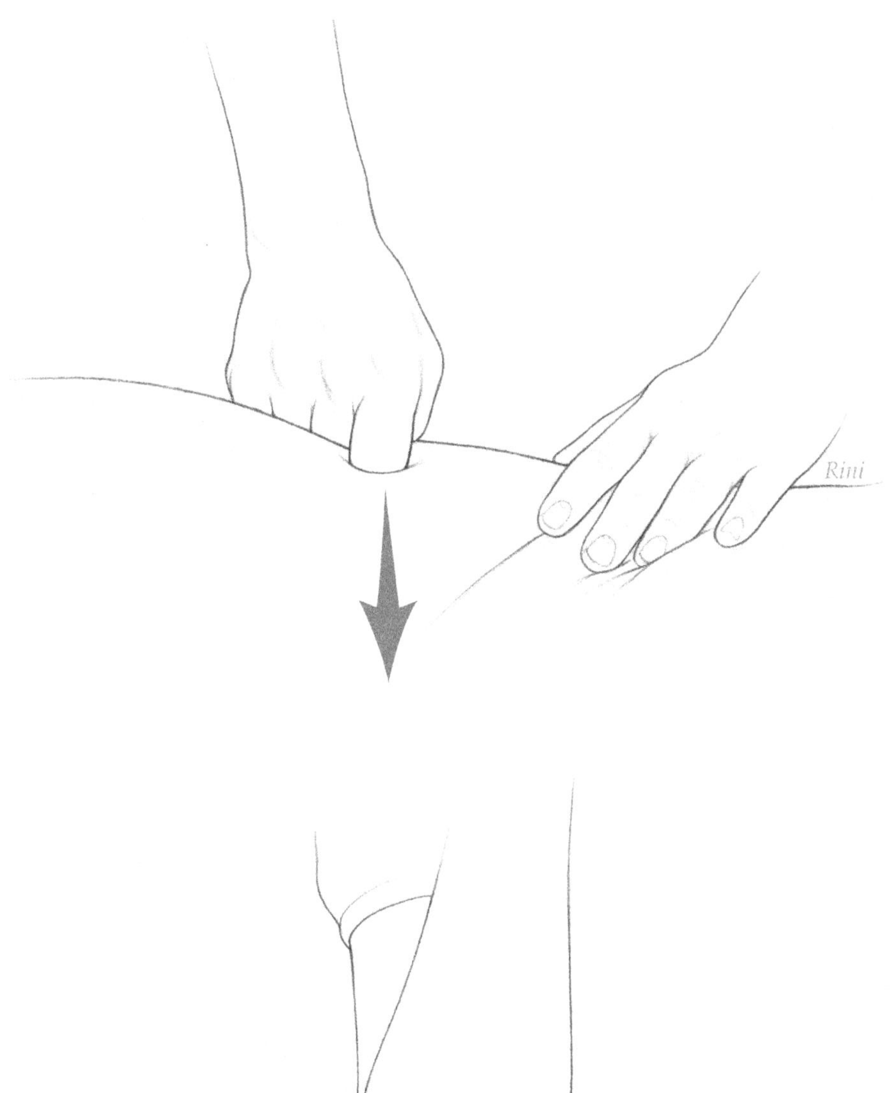

A

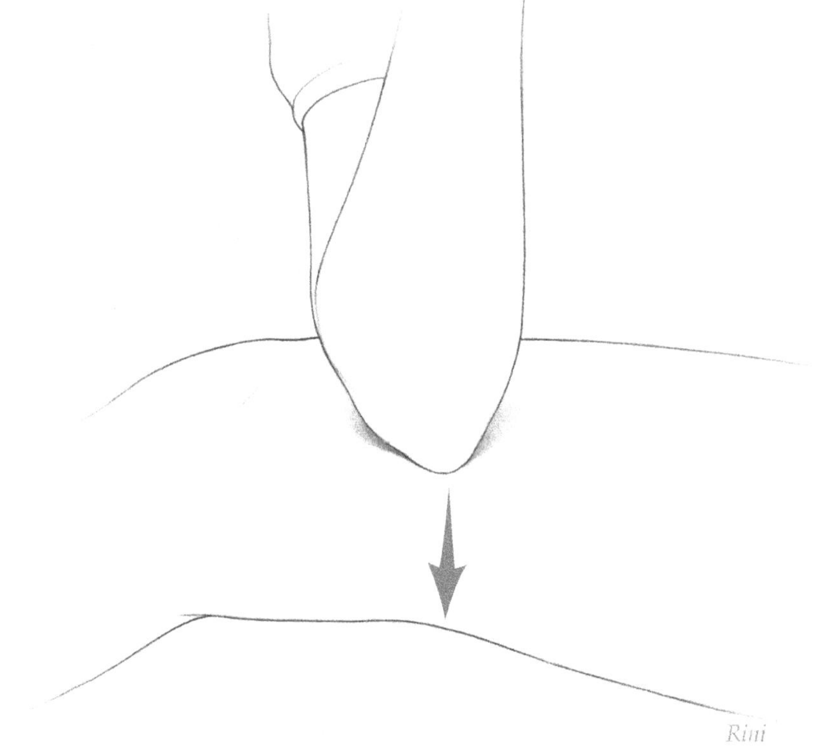

B

FIGURE 5-3 **Deep pressure or ischemic compression over a trigger point.** (**A**) Use of a knuckle. (**B**) Use of an elbow for a larger area or greater force.

RECOMMENDATIONS FOR OPTIMAL USE OF TRIGGER POINT RELEASE

The following are recommendations for the optimal use of deep pressure for TrP release. They are also pertinent when applying other manual neuromuscular techniques, which are described in the next section of this chapter.

1. Take time to position your body comfortably before compressing the soft tissues. Align your pelvis, shoulder girdle, wrists, and hands. This will allow your body efforts to work in unison rather than fighting against yourself.
2. Do *not* poke, push, or shove the tissue. Instead, allow the time to sink into the tissue and feel your way into the line that leads out of the restriction.
3. Sink into the tissue past the surface of the skin. Sink straight down toward the bone until you feel that you have accessed the TrP. *Note: This may differ widely for different people. Some clients only let you in to the superficial layer, just beneath the surface of the skin. Others let you in much deeper.*
4. Do NOT spend more than 8 to 10 seconds in each placement. You can rework a TrP site two or three times if you do not get a release the first time. But if the TrP does not release after two or three tries, leave that area and work someplace else. Do not spend more than 1 minute in total time on the TrP.
5. Good places to find TrPs are in muscle bellies, MTJs, TPJs, and tendons.
6. Know the anatomical structures that you are palpating (i.e., muscles, ligaments, tendons, vessels, bones) and use that knowledge to guide pressure and movement as you free the TrP.
7. Release in the TrP can be signaled by a softening, lengthening, or a spiralling or twitching in the area where you are working, as well as communication with the client that indicates the pain level has decreased.
8. As you press the TrP, ask the client to breathe and relax the area directly underneath your hands. Breath cues (i.e., telling your client to breathe in and out deeply in conjunction with your pressure) will increase your patient's awareness and decrease his pain level.
9. End with a stretch of the area. This can be a passive stretch performed entirely by the therapist or it can involve the active resistance (MET) techniques described later in this chapter.

Other Manual Neuromuscular Techniques

Travell and Simons (1999a, 1999b) describe four manual techniques for reducing pain and discomfort from myofascial TrPs. These manual myofascial massage techniques include deep pressure (ischemic compression, described at length in the previous section), deep effleurage (stripping), percussion with stretch, and ice massage (intermittent cold). These authors also recommend a procedure called relaxation upon exhalation to enhance the manual techniques. I include vibration directly over a TrP as a therapeutic tool when more aggressive release techniques do not seem to be appropriate. These techniques provide the foundation for a style of bodywork called Neuromuscular Therapy (Ezzo, 1994).

DEEP PRESSURE (ISCHEMIC COMPRESSION)

Deep pressure (ischemic compression) is described as sustained digital pressure on a TrP for 8 to 10 seconds (Travell and Simons recommend sustaining pressure from 20 seconds to 1 minute.) According to Travell and Simons (1999a, 1999b), pressure on the site can be gradually increased as the patient's pain sensitivity decreases. Others (Alexander, 2003; Hart, 1999) do not see a need for increasing pressure in the course of the procedure. Pressure is released when the tension subsides or when the TrP is no longer tender.

VIBRATION

Use vibration directly over the TrP to help release areas that do not soften in response to direct pressure. The mechanism for action is unknown, but it is hypothesized that vibration may help to shift the muscle or joint pain perception by stimulating the surrounding nerves. Vibration for TrP release begins with a light compression and adds an up-and-down trembling motion (Figure 5-4).

STRIPPING

Stripping is a type of deep effleurage that follows the length of the muscle fiber (Figure 5-5). (If the effleurage is deep enough, it actually no longer glides on the surface of the skin but moves the underlying tissue. Then it is more properly termed *longitudinal friction.*) Stripping is applied along the length of the taut band, through the entire region of the TrP. Danneskiold-Samsoe et al (1983, 1986) claim that 10 massage sessions of stripping may help relieve signs and symptoms of fibrositis or myofascial pain.

PERCUSSION AND STRETCH

Percussion and stretch starts with a passive stretch on the affected muscle to the first signs of resistance (Figure 5-6).

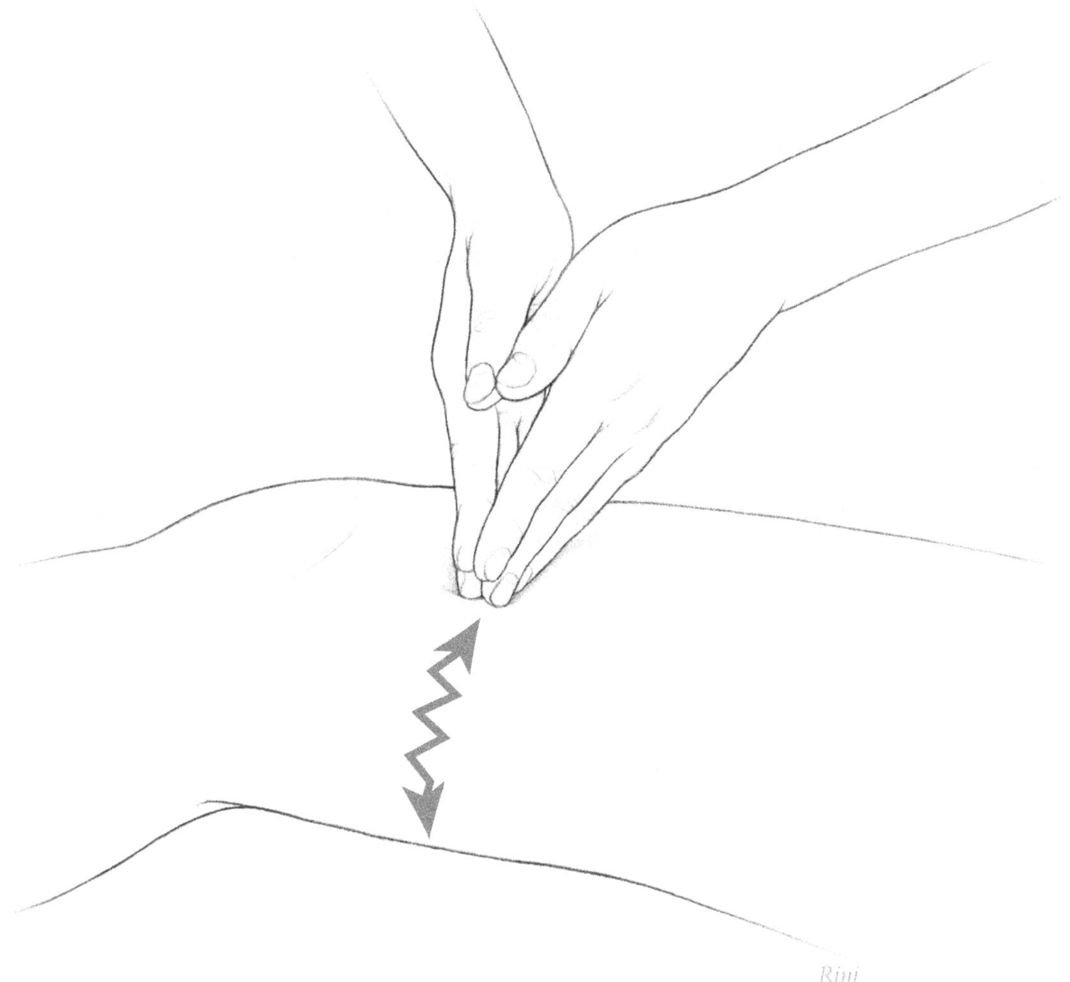

FIGURE 5-4 **Vibration begins with pressure into the TrP and then adds an up-and-down trembling motion.** It may help to soften a trigger point that does not respond to deep pressure.

Then percussion is performed on the TrP 10 times (at a rate less than 1 per second and greater than 1 every 5 seconds). When taught as a self-help technique, percussion on a stretched muscle is particularly recommended for the quadratus lumborum (QL) and also recommended for the brachioradialis, finger extensors, and peroneus muscles (Travell and Simons, 1999a, 1999b). Travell and Simons caution against applying this procedure to anterior or posterior leg compartment muscles because of the risk of aggravating anterior compartment syndrome.

ICE FRICTION MASSAGE (INTERMITTENT COLD)

Ice friction massage is the application of ice to the TrP to help it release. One of the easiest ways to use ice friction (intermittent cold) is to freeze water in a paper cup with a stick inserted like a popsicle (Figure 5-7). When you are ready to apply the intermittent cold, tear back the cup and cover the popsicle with plastic wrap to keep the skin dry. Use unidirectional parallel strokes and a slow speed of application.

RELAXATION DURING EXHALATION

Relaxation during exhalation is not really a separate procedure but can be incorporated into techniques that use pressure and movement. To include this procedure in a massage, first lengthen the muscle with a passive or active stretch. Coach your patient to breathe slowly and deeply while concentrating on relaxing the site of the TrP during exhalation. This breathing technique can be used in conjunction with deep pressure or stretching (MET), or it can stand alone as a self-help tool.

Table 5-2 provides a quick reference for the manual neuromuscular techniques we have discussed.

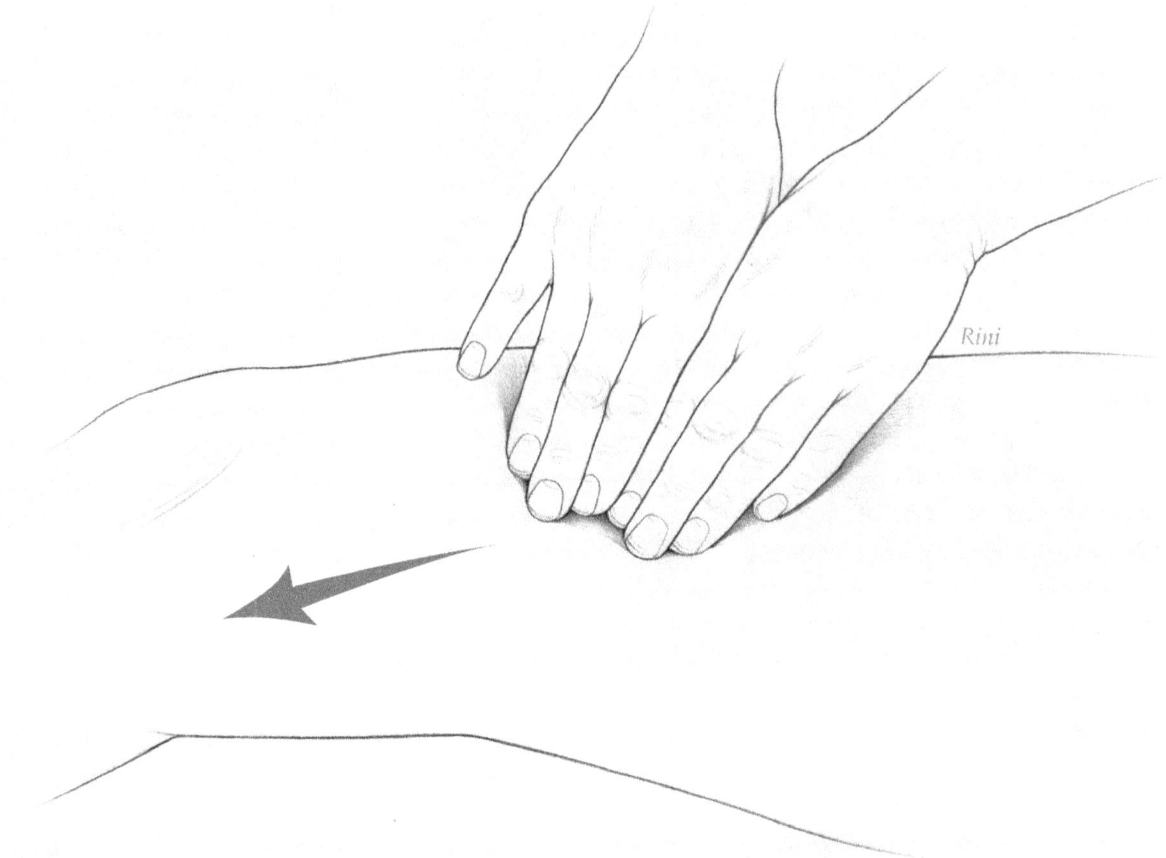

FIGURE 5-5 Stripping (deep effleurage).

Neuromuscular Techniques Using Stretching with Resistance: Muscle Energy Techniques

Voluntary movement, such as resistance against a force applied by the therapist, maintains feedback between bodyworker and client and can increase the sense of control for the client. Incorporating this kind of voluntary movement helps the patient be more consciously aware of the changes occurring in the soft tissue. Resistance against a directed force also models the self-help exercises that can help clients maintain more lasting change. For these reasons, it is common for neuromuscular therapists to complement the release of myofascial TrPs with the use of a number of movement plus resistance maneuvers. These are collectively known as muscle energy techniques (METs).

Specifically, METs are a set of stretching techniques that require clients to voluntarily contract their muscles in a precisely determined direction (Hendrickson, 2003). Clients are cued to use a specific muscle to push against a therapist-applied force. It is believed that the conscious effort on the part of the client helps reprogram nonadaptive autonomic nerve responses exhibited as muscle tension. Active muscle contraction also helps to mobilize the joints and increase ROM. Another clinical use of MET is to reduce the pain and discomfort of TrPs. The next section reviews the background and individual techniques that make up MET.

HISTORY OF MUSCLE ENERGY TECHNIQUES

Muscle energy techniques have now evolved into voluntary contractions of a client's muscle in a precisely controlled direction at varying levels of intensity against a distinctly executed counterforce applied by a therapist (Greenman, 1996). The origins of MET began in the 1940s with Kabat, who developed techniques requiring neurologically impaired patients to voluntarily contract their muscles to strengthen them (Hendrickson, 2003; Kostopoulos and Rizopoulos, 2001). He called these techniques *proprioceptive neuromuscular facilitation (PNF)*. During the 1950s, osteopaths such as Mitchell and Greenman used this kind of coached voluntary movement to mobilize joints and called it MET. More recently, chiropractors such as Janda and Lewit developed a treatment for myofascial TrPs using therapist-guided movement and resistance coordinated with the application of manual pressure. They call their treatment post-isometric relaxation (PIR)

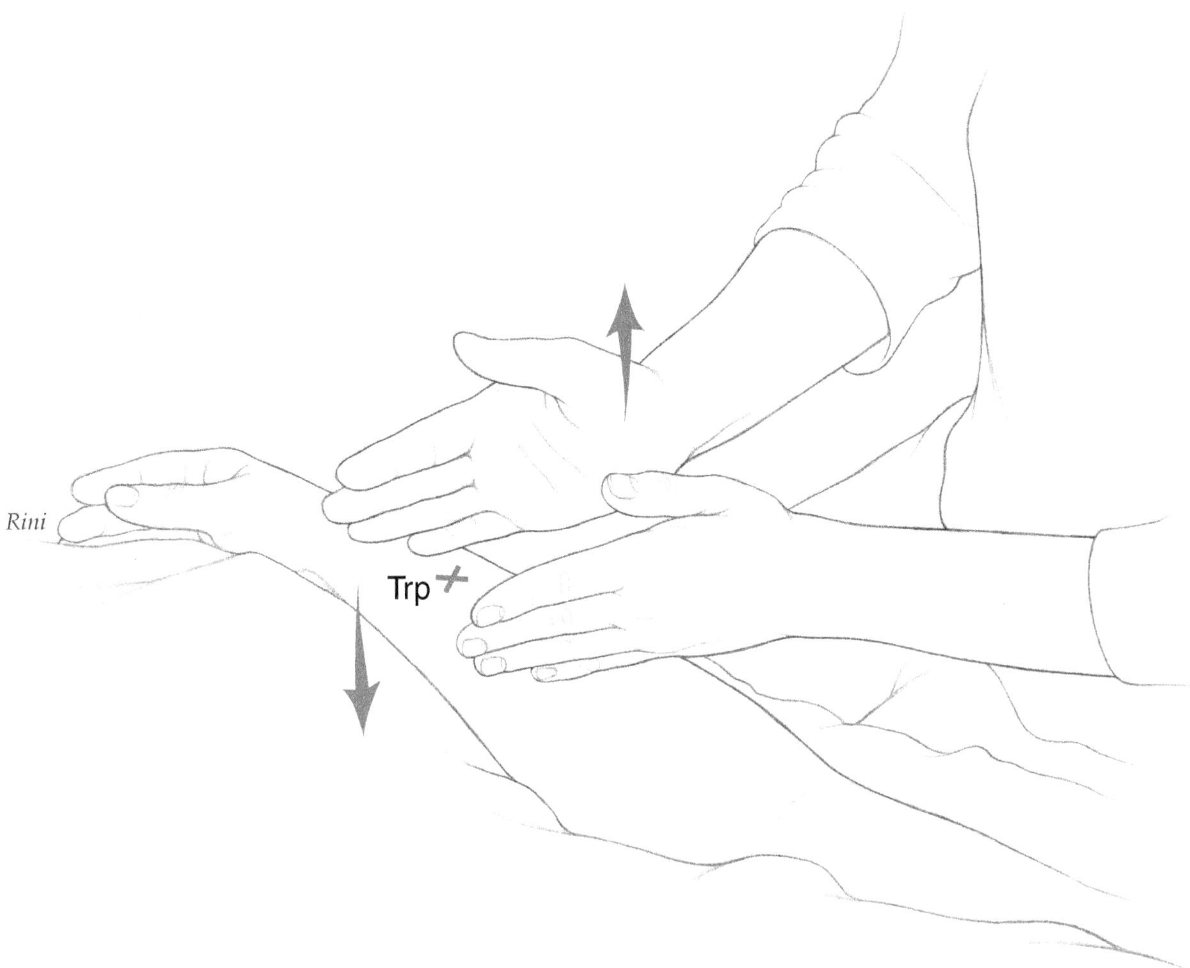

FIGURE 5-6 Percussion and stretch starts with a passive stretch and adds percussion over trigger point. Note that Travell and Simons caution against applying percussion on a stretched muscle to the lower leg!

(Kostopoulos and Rizopoulos, 2001), and it has become one of the most frequently used MET procedures. Osteopaths Chaitow and DeLany (2002a, 2002b) and Greenman (1996) have also made refinements to MET procedures.

BASIC TECHNIQUES

The basic techniques of MET include PIR, contract relax (CR), reciprocal inhibition (RI), and contract relax antagonist contract (CRAC), a combination technique that uses both PIR and RI.

Post-isometric Relaxation

Post-isometric relaxation (PIR) is a name for and literal description of how a target muscle can be relaxed. After a muscle contracts isometrically, it fatigues and loses some of its tone. In essence, the entire muscle, along with its areas of spasm such as TrPs, is "tricked" into relaxing. To perform PIR, lengthen the muscle containing the TrP until you perceive resistance (Figure 5-8). Hold that position, coaching the client to voluntarily resist the lengthening, for 8 to 10 seconds. As the client relaxes, take the muscle into a greater stretch and then repeat the entire process. Repeat a third time and end on stretch/relax. PIR is used to relieve TrPs and lengthen shortened muscles and fascia.

Contract Relax

The process of contract relax (CR) is identical to PIR, except that you do not take the muscle into greater lengthening past the first resistance barrier. The process is simply repeated at the original resistance barrier. CR is used to assess weakness or pain, to relax hypertonic muscles, and to increase sensory awareness in the targeted muscle.

Reciprocal Inhibition

Reciprocal inhibition (RI; antagonist contract) is used when contraction of a muscle is painful even with minimal effort

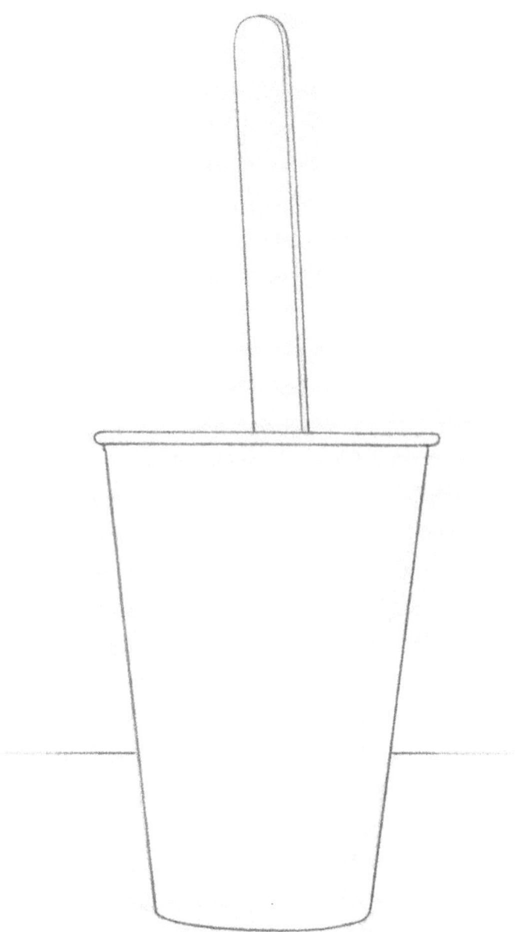

FIGURE 5-7 **Ice friction massage.** Ice popsicles (frozen in a paper cup) are a good way to apply ice friction.

from the client. RI refers to the client's contracting the reciprocal or antagonist muscle to the one you want to relax. This sends a neurologic message to the target muscle to inhibit its contraction because the muscle and its antagonist or opposite muscle cannot both contract at the same time. To perform RI, lengthen (passively stretch) the target muscle until the first resistance barrier (Figure 5-9) and then coach the client to voluntarily resist *shortening* for 8 to 10 seconds. As the client relaxes, lengthen the muscle a little more and then again coach the client to resist your shortening of the target muscle. Repeat the whole process one more time, but always end on the passive stretch/relax.

So, for example, to lengthen the biceps, extend the client's elbow to the point just before pain is felt. Coach the client by saying, "Do not let me move you" and then press on the back of the forearm to bend the elbow. The client's efforts to resist this pressure contract the triceps, which inhibits the biceps from contracting. Then coach the client to relax and wait for her to exhale, signaling relaxation. Repeat this cycle three times (or more, up to five cycles).

Contract Relax Antagonist Contract

Contract relax antagonist contract (CRAC) combines PIR and RI techniques. It sounds complicated, but the therapist simply performs one technique and then the other. So, for example, to lengthen the biceps, begin by taking the client's forearm into extension. Then as you hold onto the front of the forearm and push to further extend the elbow, coach the client to "resist against me." Then switch your hand position to brace the back of the forearm and push to flex the elbow while coaching the client to "resist against me." Repeat this sequence three to five times.

As with RI and PIR individually, it is best to end with a passive stretch of the targeted muscle (in this case, the biceps) because it leaves the client with the feeling of lengthening and relaxing rather than contraction. CRAC is used in chronic conditions only, in which it is used to stretch adhesions, lengthen the CT, and reduce hypertonicity in muscles.

Table 5-3 summarizes the basic MET techniques just discussed.

Advanced MET techniques include eccentric contraction, concentric MET, and MET used to increase the ROM in joints. For more information, see Hendrickson's text on *Massage for Orthopedic Conditions* (2003). Analysis and description of advanced MET techniques is beyond the scope of this text.

RECOMMENDATIONS FOR COACHING

1. *Ask the client to practice resisting against your force. Let her practice making smaller and less intense pushes.* At first, clients tend to make movements that are too fast and too forceful. They need to be coached to resist just enough to engage the muscle and reset the proprioceptors to allow a greater ROM. Large or gross motor contraction can cause pain in itself.
2. *Use imagery or sensory cues* to help the client visualize what she is supposed to be doing. A good cue is to guide the client to "push into my hands" or "resist against me."
3. Guide the client into *breathing comfortably at her own pace, and coordinate your stretch with her exhalation.* Guided easy breathing is particularly beneficial when addressing TrPs that surround muscles that move in inspiration or expiration (e.g., scalenes, QL, serratus anterior, internal and external intercostals).
4. *Combine elements of recommendations 2 and 3* by asking the client to "breathe right into the area underneath my hands."
5. *Help the client visualize the area you are working on.* Show her a picture of the region from an anatomy

TABLE 5-2 Manual Neuromuscular Techniques

Technique	Description	Application
Deep pressure (ischemic compression)	Apply sustained digital pressure on a TrP for 8 to 10 seconds (may be repeated several times with total time not to exceed 1 minute).	Pressure can gradually increase as pain sensitivity decreases. Pressure is released when the TrP tension subsides or when TrP is no longer tender.
Vibration	Begin with compression and add trembling. Use the same time guidelines as with deep pressure.	Pressure is released when the TrP tension subsides or when TrP is no longer tender. Use when deep pressure is not well tolerated or is ineffective.
Deep effleurage (stripping)	Apply effleurage deeply enough to move the underlying tissues without moving the skin along the length of the myofascial taut band, through the TrP region.	Used to relieve the signs and symptoms of myofascial pain.
Percussion and stretch	Start by lengthening the muscle to the first signs of resistance. Then perform percussion on the TrP 10 times (rate less than 1 per second and greater than 1 per 5 seconds).	Particularly helpful for QL (self-applied), brachioradialis, finger extensors, and peroneus muscles. *Not* for anterior or posterior leg compartment muscles.
Ice friction (intermittent cold)	Use water frozen in a paper cup with a stick inserted like a popsicle. Tear back the cup and cover with plastic wrap.	Use unidirectional parallel strokes. Keep the skin dry. Slow application. Use for TrPs that may be located in or around acute areas of inflammation.
Relaxation during exhalation	Coach the client to breathe slowly and deeply, concentrating on relaxing at the site of the TrP during exhalation.	Lengthen the muscle beforehand. Can be used in conjunction with ischemic compression, or with PIR or RI (types of MET) techniques or can stand alone. Use to improve the effect of other neuromuscular techniques or to help the client relax.

MET = muscle energy technique; PIR = post-isometric relaxation; QL = quadratus lumborum; RI = reciprocal inhibition; TrP = trigger point.

chart or text. This encourages conscious and voluntary healing. Clients will better understand where and why you are working and actually see the unobstructed fiber direction of the muscles.

Positioning, Draping, and Support

The stretching of MET involves working with a client from many angles, including in the supine, prone, and side-lying positions. You may also ask the client to shift positions more often than in a relaxation massage, so make sure that you can coach the client in safe and modest turning procedures.

Trigger point release is best done with skin-to-skin contact, so keeping the rest of the body draped and modest is essential. During deep work such as TrP and other neuromuscular techniques, clients must always be draped and comfortably warm to create a feeling of safety so that the work does not feel invasive. Follow basic Swedish massage draping guidelines (see Fritz, 2000). In addition, it is better to use the diaper or Buddha drape for the legs (as opposed to tucking under the opposite leg or not tucking) for extra-secure coverage (Figure 5-10). When draping a client in the side-lying position, remember that the technique is similar to prone or supine draping except that your body must be aligned differently to meet the side orientation. Draping a side-lying client's legs may seem to be a little trickier, but it will work if you slide a thin edge of the drape under the knee, pull it through, and then shimmy it up. Rolling the drape under itself will hold it in place better than folding it over. One therapist in the Portland area recommends clothespins to hold the drape in place.

Support is important with neuromuscular massage. To counter the deep pressure into the table, reinforce with a pillow or bolster directly underneath any areas of focus (Figure 5-11). In general, pillows work better than bolsters because they can more easily conform to the client's shape. A contour body cushion is an excellent appliance for the side-lying position. When the client is on the side, keep the top leg supported by a flat bolster or several pillows and the bottom leg stretched out behind rather than letting the top leg compress the bottom leg (even if separated by a pillow). This avoids needless compression of the arteries and veins of the medial legs.

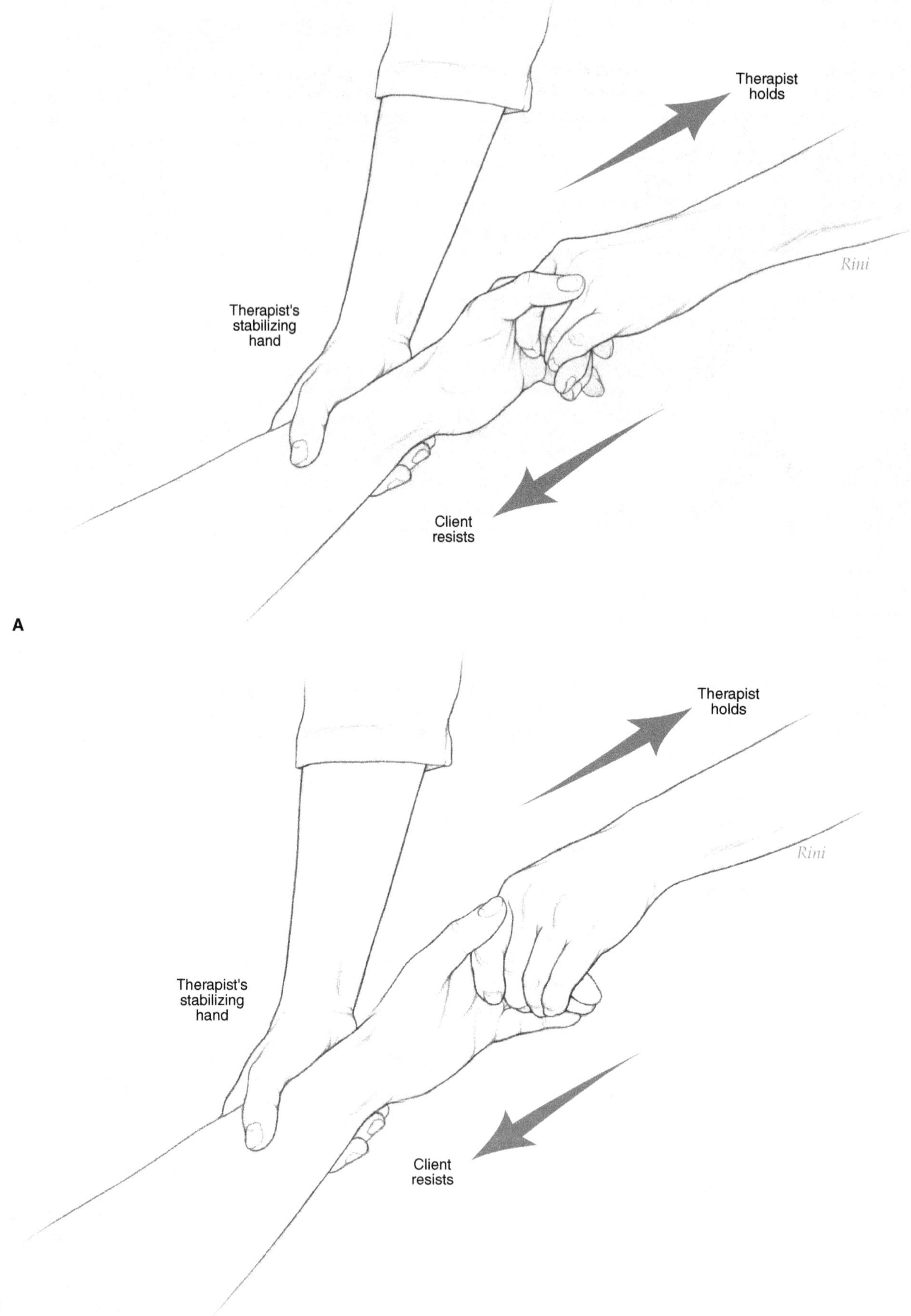

FIGURE 5-8 **Post-isometric relaxation for the finger flexors.** Place one hand on the client's fingers and stretch to extend them. Say "resist against me" (8 to 10 seconds) and then extend more as the client exhales. Repeat two or three times. (**A**) Start position (client). (**B**) End position (client).

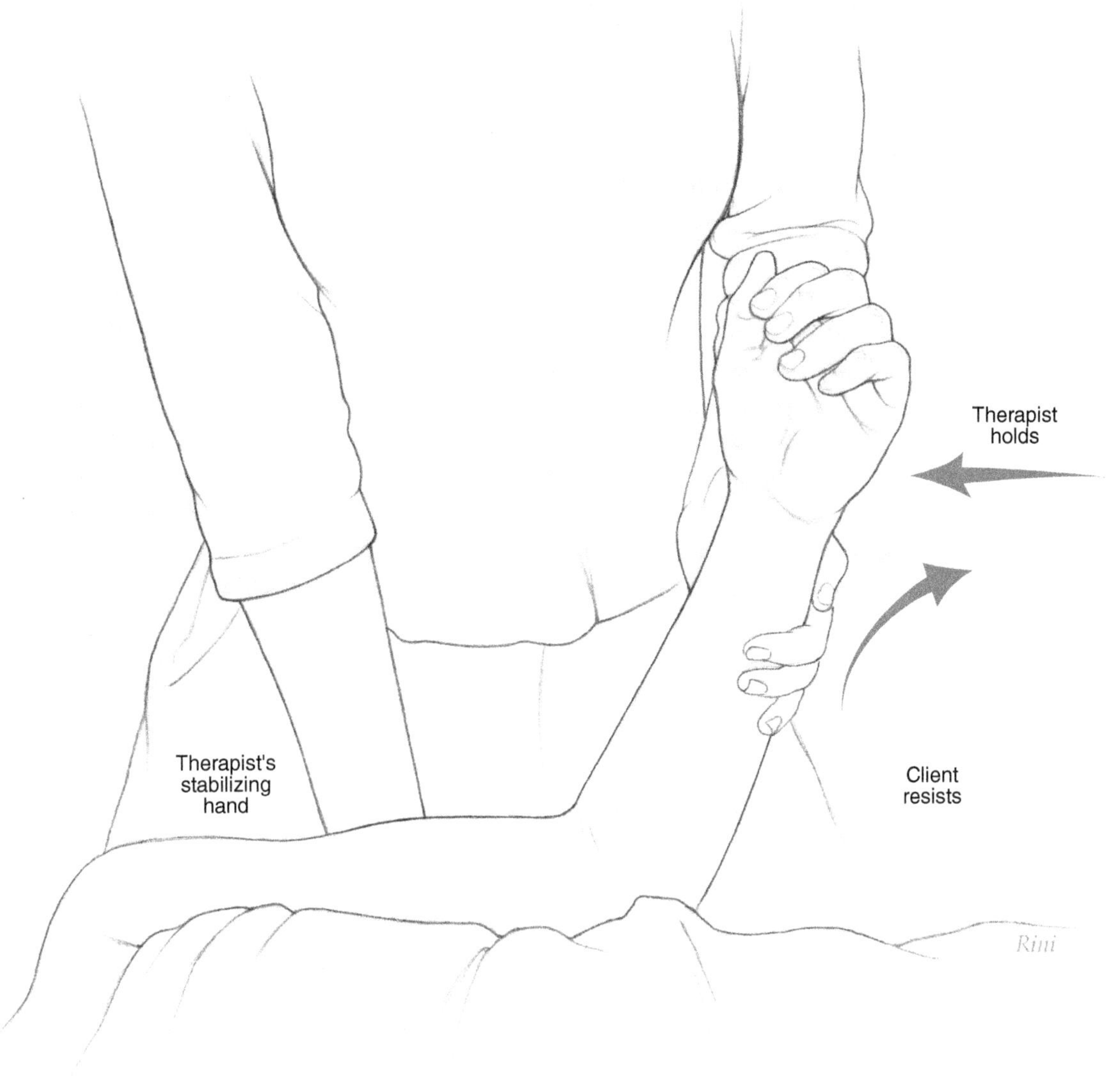

FIGURE 5-9 **Reciprocal inhibition for the biceps.** While pushing the client's forearm to promote elbow flexion, say: "Resist against me." Sustain for 8 to 10 seconds and then release as the client exhales. Repeat two or three times. (**A**) Start position (client).

Treatment Planning and Decision Making

When designing a session or series of neuromuscular sessions for a client, always begin with the needs of the client, as determined by a thorough history and intake procedure. One example of a sample interview form is included as Appendix A. Use the client's responses to individual intake questions as a jumping-off point to generate detailed and specific information about possible contraindications, indications, and requests for relief from discomfort, pain, or stress. Based on this information, you can identify a plan of action (e.g., spending most of the treatment session on the lower legs to address recurrent TrP complaints in the calves), which is then modified as you work with and palpate the tissues directly.

It is not a good idea to perform deep work on more than three areas of the body in any one session. The client's pressure receptors can become overloaded with information about where to focus, and the overload will be counterproductive to creating lasting and effective change. In my practice, I usually identify a few areas to focus on based on the intake procedure and then modify my plan according to the TrPs or spasms that I palpate during the course of the massage. Clients report that such directed work feels more complete than a superficial session that touches all parts of the body but does not pay real attention to any distinct region.

Neuromuscular and TrP work are injury dependent; thus, it would be inappropriate (and impossible) to pre-

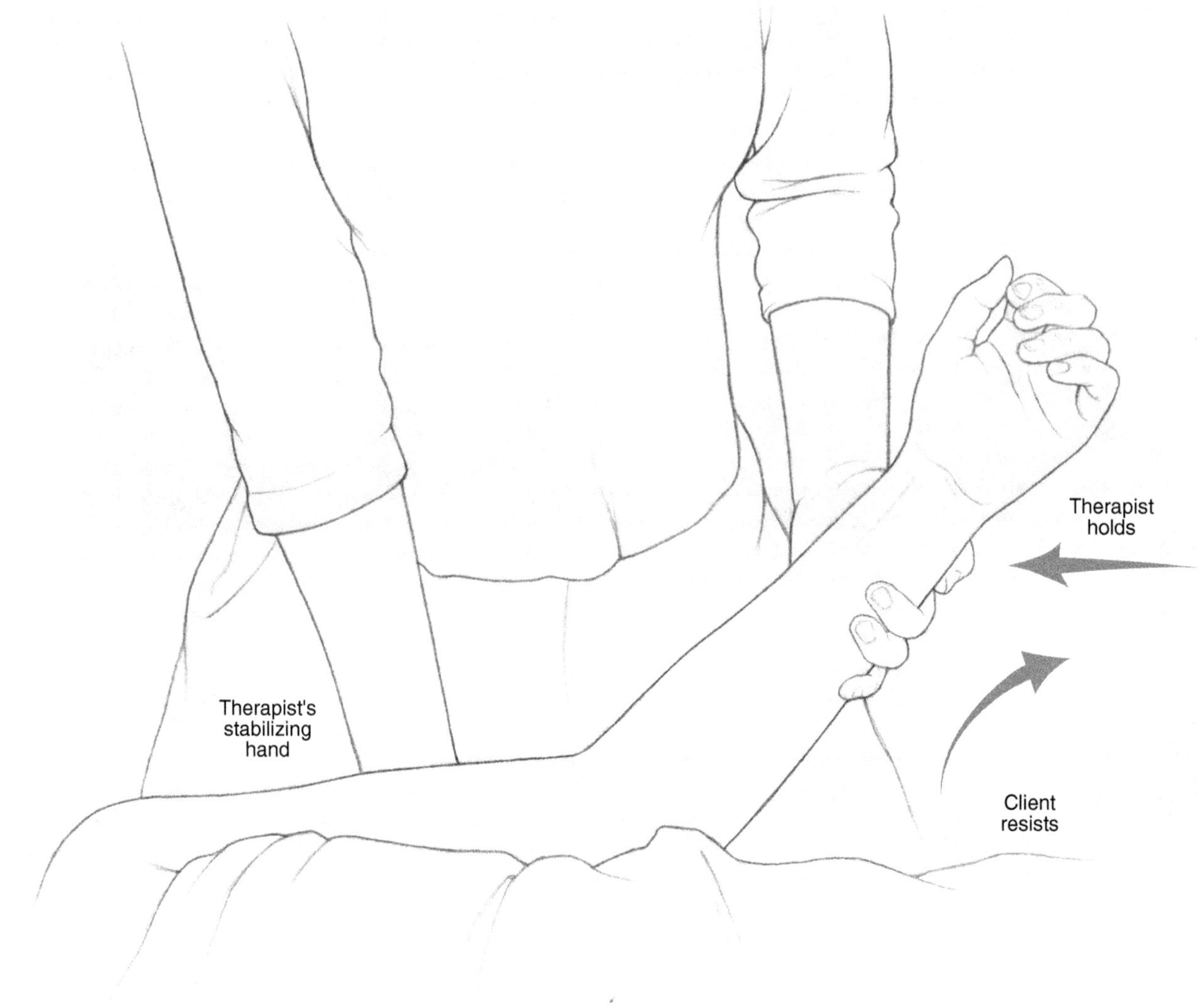

FIGURE 5-9 Reciprocal inhibition for the biceps (continued). (**B**) End position (client).

scribe an effective specific full-body protocol. A good strategy is to cycle through the many tried-and-true techniques until you find the best match for you and your client while considering her specific complaints and condition on the day of the appointed session. For example, some clients do very well with deep pressure with the elbow; others find this procedure too aggressive. Some clients respond well to stripping or deep effleurage on the medial hamstrings one day but not another.

The guidelines that follow, however, are provided for work with neuromuscular clients who present with acute, subacute, or chronic inflammation and mild, moderate, or severe injury.

An acute area of inflammation is typically hot, red, swollen, and painful. This is because blood has moved into the area to help aid in healing the trauma. If there is a specific site within the area that produces referrals upon palpation, this is a classic myofascial TrP. When applying the neuromuscular approach to treat acute inflammation, stick with less aggressive techniques, lighter pressure, and indirect work (e.g., proximal or contralateral to the site). For example, percussion with stretch would be applied very lightly to the inflamed site, if at all. Other tactics would include a shorter application time and discontinuing any technique that causes pain. Most METs, because they stretch the area, are too harsh. Passive exercise is permissible if tolerable, and RI may be used because neither involves active contraction of the agonist. Cold is preferable to heat as an analgesic because in addition to a pain-killing effect, a cold application can reduce heat and swelling.

Subacute injuries are a little less red, hot, swollen, and painful. Thus, treatment strategies are a little more direct and a little deeper, but the therapist should continue to use pain as a boundary that is not crossed.

TABLE 5-3 Basic Muscle Energy Techniques

Technique	Description	Application/Purpose
Post-isometric relaxation (PIR)	Lengthen the muscle until the first resistance barrier. Then coach the client to voluntarily resist *lengthening* for 8 to 10 seconds. As the client relaxes, passively lengthen again. Repeat the process three to five times, ending on a stretch/relax.	Lengthens shortened muscles and fascia and relieves TrPs.
Contract relax (CR)	Similar to PIR, except that the muscle is *not* lengthened past the first resistance barrier. The process is repeated three to five times at the original resistance barrier.	Used to achieve relaxation in hypertonic muscles, to bring sensory awareness to a muscle, and to assess weakness or pain.
Reciprocal inhibition (RI)	Lengthen the target muscle to the first resistance barrier. Then change hand position to push against the antagonist action and coach the client to resist *shortening* for 8 to 10 seconds. As the client relaxes, passively lengthen again. Repeat the process three to five times, ending on a stretch/relax.	Used in acute conditions. If contraction of a muscle is painful, RI can still be used because the opposite muscle is the one that is contracting.
Contract relax antagonist contract (CRAC)	Combines PIR and RI techniques. Do one and then the other. End on the stretch/relax.	Used in chronic conditions only. Used to stretch adhesions, lengthen the connective tissue, and reduce hypertonicity in muscles.

Chronic injuries are older traumas that have not resolved. The tissues generally feel cold in relationship to the surrounding areas, may be whiter or bluer because of ischemia, may be harder because of scar tissue, and are generally not painful. More aggressive techniques are appropriate here, such as deep effleurage (or longitudinal friction, also discussed in Chapter 6). MET techniques are practical strategies for chronic injuries because they use both stretching and resistance. Heat is sometimes used in chronic injuries to soften up the tissue, but it may give the therapist a false sense of flexibility in the tissues. Also be aware of the possibility of encountering a chronic region with an embedded hot spot that was reinjured and is now acutely inflamed.

Severe injuries can be treated as if they were areas of acute inflammation, moderate injuries follow the prescriptions for subacute inflammations, and mild injuries observe the guidelines for chronic inflammations. (These were detailed above.)

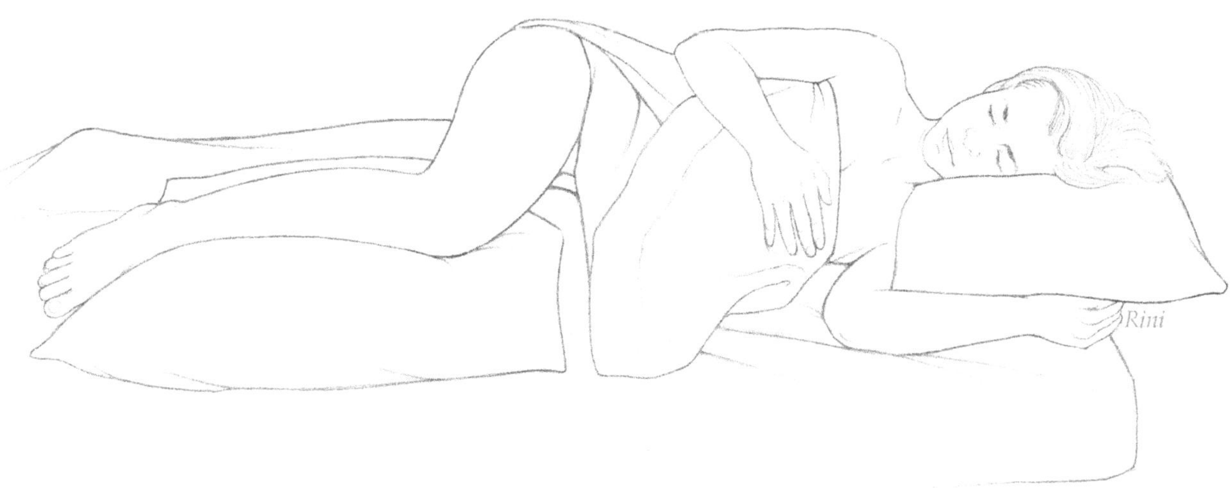

FIGURE 5-10 Diaper drape for the side-lying position.

One Therapist's Experience: The Experience of Performing Neuromuscular Massage

The following is a personal account of my experience using the neuromuscular approach. I hope my words give students a better appreciation of what it feels like to practice the deep pressure TrP release and other manual neuromuscular techniques and MET.

"What I most enjoy about the neuromuscular approach is the intellectual focus of the work. Finding and releasing TrPs is a lot like working as a detective. I begin by analyzing my client's muscular complaints and then hone in on certain clues (e.g., persistent pain deep in the shoulder; functional impairment in the ability to put dishes away on the top shelf). I pursue the evidence by palpating the soft tissues in this region. What I feel in my hands then guides me to collect more clues, this time of a sensory nature (e.g., the tissue here feels like a taut band, and there is a sensitive area in the center of it where the client says "ouch" when I touch it). As I sink into a tender area and ask if the pain or discomfort refers someplace else, I find that I can simply and systematically release the TrPs by following the pain referrals that are reported by my patient. It is almost like playing a game of connect the dots. Listening to the pain elicited from the TrPs and following these referrals until no more tender spots are found seems to provide a good deal of relief for the client and satisfaction for me as a bodyworker. To deepen the experience and improve effectiveness, I watch and facilitate matching the client's breathing (exhalation) to a visualization of the TrP release ("Imagine the tissue softening under my hands as you breathe out"). I see the power of the TrP release, indeed, when the client focuses her breath into tight spots, fills them up, and is able to let go. Sometimes I feel a quivering in the TrP as it is getting ready to soften. When I check on the client's pain level to confirm the shift, pain is invariably reduced.

I also enjoy the "magic" of the MET techniques. The increased ROM in the client's arm after a resisted contraction followed by a stretch is remarkable. And the process is surprisingly gentle. I can still remember one of my AIDS patients from years ago who called me an angel, primarily because of the relief that PIR and RI brought him in his neck and shoulder muscles. Again, breathing is key. Cueing the client to breathe in helped him exaggerate the feeling of resistance and understand what he was trying to let go. Cueing him to breathe out to facilitate a stretch allowed him to relax further into even greater flexibility and ease."

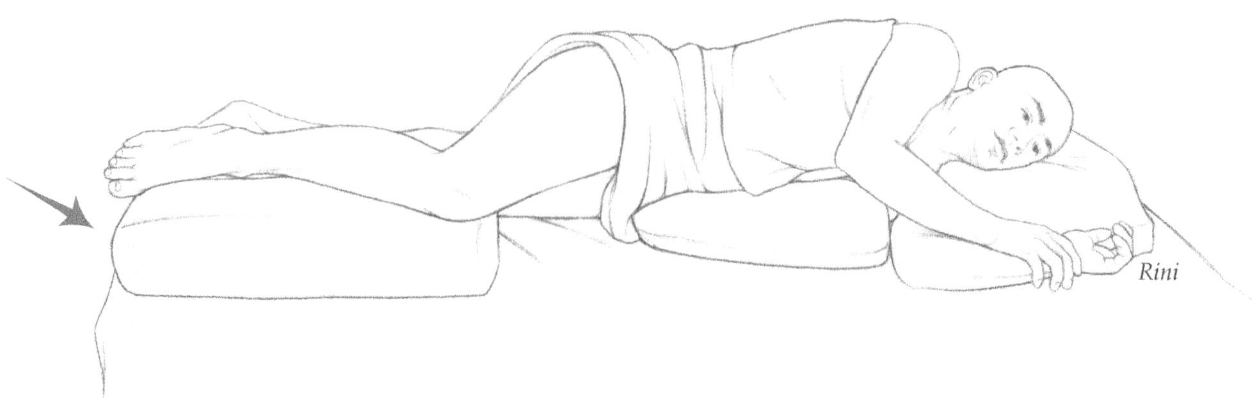

FIGURE 5-11 Supporting the client. Use pillow under the top leg for support when the client is in the sidelying position.

SUMMARY

Myofascial TrPs are hyperirritable areas that are locally tender and may refer pain, tenderness, other autonomic phenomena, or proprioceptive changes when pressed. TrPs produce weakness and prevent complete lengthening in the muscle and may elicit a local twitch response upon compression. They may be active, latent, or satellites. TrPs are not the same as tender points or acupuncture points and are treated according to different theoretical models.

Manual neuromuscular techniques stress the release of TrPs, spasms, and pain, and increasing ROM. They include a wide variety of techniques, including deep pressure, deep effleurage (stripping), intermittent cold (ice massage), relaxation during exhalation, percussion and stretch, and vibration.

Muscle energy techniques activate the proprioceptors to initiate relaxation, lengthening, or facilitation of muscle tone in specific muscles. MET adds the power of the client's voluntary muscle contractions and stretching against resistance to the neuromuscular approach. Basic MET techniques include PIR, CR, RI, and CRAC.

You can customize neuromuscular techniques to any part of the body and can adapt your session to incorporate TrP release as needed, in conjunction with other massage approaches and styles, for an eclectic massage. Because of the nature of the work, specific sample protocols can not be provided without customizing the neuromuscular approach to the specific area of injury. More detailed texts on TrP and neuromuscular applications (e.g., Hendrickson, 2003; Scheumann, 2002; Travell and Simons, 1999a, 1999b) devote entire chapters to describing such protocols. Here, general protocol guidelines for applying neuromuscular techniques to clients with acute, subacute, and chronic inflammation or severe, moderate, and mild injuries are provided.

Review Questions

1. A(n) __________ is an area of hyperirritability that can refer pain and other autonomic phenomena to other locations in the body.
   a. tender point
   b. acupuncture point
   c. satellite point
   d. TrP
2. __________ and Simons were the first to identify specific TrPs, referred pain patterns, and contributing factors.
   a. Barnes
   b. Prudden
   c. Simons
   d. Travell
3. Manual neuromuscular techniques do not include __________.
   a. ischemic compression
   b. percussion with stretch
   c. deep pressure
   d. light effleurage
4. True or false: Myofascial TrPs equate accurately with acupressure points in the human body.
5. True or false: Myofascial trigger points equate accurately with tender points in the human body.
6. __________ TrPs are a source of pain without any outside stimulus, such as pressure from the massage therapist.
7. Latent TrPs may become __________ TrPs when the site is reinjured.
8. Referred autonomic phenomena may consist of pain but may also include sensations such as twitching, __________, __________, and goosebumps, often reported by clients.
9. Techniques that involve a movement combined with an active resistance on the part of the patient are collectively termed __________.
10. Name and describe four METs.

REFERENCES

Alexander D. Soft tissue resistance barriers. Massage Therapy 2003; 42:96–112.

Chaitow L, DeLany JW. Clinical Application of Neuromuscular Techniques. Vol. 1: The Upper Body. Edinburgh, UK: Elsevier Science, 2002a.

Chaitow L, DeLany JW. Clinical Application of Neuromuscular Techniques. Vol. 2: The Lower Body. Edinburgh, UK: Elsevier Science, 2002b.

Danneskiold-Samsoe B, Christiansen E, Andersen RB. Myofascial pain and the role of myoglobin. Scand J Rheumatol 1986;15:174–178.

Danneskiold-Samsoe B, Christiansen E, Andersen RB. Regional muscle tension and pain ("fibrositis"). Scand J Rheumatol 1983;15:17–20.

Ezzo J, ed. Neuromuscular Therapy Update, 1987–1994. Baltimore: St. Johns Neuromuscular Therapy Services, 1994.

Fritz S. Mosby's Fundamentals of Therapeutic Massage. 2nd Ed. St. Louis: Mosby, 2000.

Greenman PE. Principles of Manual Medicine. Baltimore: Williams and Wilkins, 1996.

Hart J. Deep Tissue Massage. Unpublished manuscript, 1999.

Hendrickson T. Massage for Orthopedic Conditions. Baltimore: Lippincott Williams & Wilkins, 2003.

Kellgren HJ. Observations on referred pain arising from muscle. Clin Sci 1938;3:175–190.

Kostopoulos D, Rizopoulos K. The Manual of Trigger Point and Myofascial Therapy. Thorofare, NJ: SLACK Inc., 2001.

Manheim CJ. The Myofascial Release Manual. 3rd Ed. Thorofare, NJ: SLACK Inc., 2001.

Rubik B. Manual healing methods. In: Alternative Medicine—Expanding Medical Horizons. Washington, DC: US Government Printing Office, 1992.

Scheumann DW. The Balanced Body. 2nd Ed. Baltimore: Lippincott Williams & Wilkins, 2002.

Travell JG, Simons DG. Myofascial Pain and Dysfunction: The Trigger Point Manual. Vol. 1: The Upper Extremities. Baltimore: Lippincott Williams & Wilkins, 1999a.

Travell JG, Simons DG. Myofascial Pain and Dysfunction: The Trigger Point Manual. Vol. 2: The Lower Extremities. Baltimore: Lippincott Williams & Wilkins, 1999b.

SUGGESTED READINGS

Dixon MW. Body Mechanics and Self-Care Manual. Upper Saddle River, NJ: Prentice Hall Health, 2001.

Hendrickson T. Massage for Orthopedic Conditions. Baltimore: Lippincott Williams & Wilkins, 2003.

Moore KL, Dalley AF. Clinically Oriented Anatomy. 4th Ed. Baltimore: Lippincott Williams & Wilkins, 1999.

Riggs A. Deep Tissue Massage. Berkeley, CA: North Atlantic Books, 2002.

Schuemann DW. The Balanced Body. 2nd Ed. Baltimore: Lippincott Williams & Wilkins, 2002.

Chapter 6

Direct Connective Tissue Approach

OBJECTIVES

- **Explain the major points of the direct connective tissue approach.**
- **Describe applications of the direct connective tissue approach to superficial fascia.**
- **Describe the application of the direct connective tissue approach to deep fascia.**
- **Discuss positioning, draping, and support.**
- **Discuss treatment planning and decision making.**

CHAPTER OUTLINE

Components of the Direct Connective Tissue Approach
The Direct Connective Tissue Approach to Superficial Fascia
- Anatomy of Superficial Fascia
- Superficial Direct Connective Tissue Techniques
- Soft Tissue Mobilization Techniques
- Optimal Use of Superficial Direct Connective Tissue Techniques

The Direct Connective Tissue Approach to Deep Fascia
- Anatomy of Deep Fascia
- Components of the Basic Deep Direct Connective Tissue Stroke
- Optimal Use of Deep Direct Connective Tissue Techniques

Positioning, Draping, and Support
Treatment Planning and Decision Making
Summary

KEY TERMS

Superficial direct CT massage: The direct CT approach applied to superficial fascia (i.e., loose connective tissue underneath the skin).

Deep direct connective tissue massage: The direct connective tissue approach applied to deep fascia (dense or collagenous connective tissue surrounding muscles, tendons, or ligaments).

Muscle sculpting (longitudinal friction, deep effleurage): Technique that uses deep effleurage or longitudinal friction to lengthen the myofascial in the direction parallel to muscle fibers and/or the epimysium surrounding the whole muscle.

Rolfing: Bodywork style that aims to realign the structural components of the body for enhanced function. Usually requires 10 or more sessions to realign the whole body.

Structural integration (postural integration): Bodywork style that is similar to Rolfing, but instructors are not certified by the Rolf Institute.

Skin rolling: Technique applied to superficial fascia. A type of pétrissage in which the tissue just beneath the skin is grasped between thumb and forefingers and held until a movement of fascia (release) is felt by the therapist.

Compression: Technique applied to superficial fascia; pumping the muscle (and surrounding fascial layer) against the bone.

Stretching: Technique applied to superficial fascia; involves mechanically lengthening the muscle and fascia in a line between your hands.

Scraping: Technique applied to superficial fascia; involves scraping bony or ligamentous areas with your thumb, knuckles, or fingers and imagining that you are smoothing the surface, as if you were shaving off ice.

Soft tissue mobilization: More aggressive direct CT approach techniques; includes cross-fiber friction and the J stroke.

Cross-fiber friction (transverse friction, Cyriax friction): Soft tissue mobilization technique used to prevent or soften adhesions in the contractile tissue between the ligaments and the underlying bone and to smooth roughened surfaces between tendons and their sheaths. To apply, move the client's skin over the underlying tissue in a direction perpendicular to the muscle fibers.

J stroke: A more forceful soft tissue mobilization technique performed to release skin restrictions or adhesions that do not respond to skin rolling. This stroke is used in localized areas only.

Micromovements: Very small regular movements made by the client, usually in response to coaching by the massage therapist. Used to enhance lengthening and release of the client's soft tissue.

Direct myofascial methods include both the neuromuscular approach, discussed in Chapter 5, and the direct connective tissue (CT) approach, which is the subject of this chapter. In the direct CT approach, the therapist applies pressure to the CT to meet resistances in the client's body directly, *as the name implies. The direct CT approach is especially useful for addressing chronically inflamed tissues and chronic pain.*

This chapter describes the application of the direct CT approach to both superficial and deep fascia. The structure of the fascia is reviewed insofar as it affects the application of strokes used in the direct CT approach. The chapter also describes the correct use of deep body mechanics, as well as positioning, draping, and support to enhance the process of soft tissue release. Decision making about where and when to practice direct CT massage is also discussed, and algorithms are provided for adapting the approach to special conditions.

This chapter concludes with two formalized plans for applying the direct CT approach—a standardized 10-session protocol and a two-session protocol—and a chart summarizing technique applications for specific CT and muscle regions.

Components of the Direct Connective Tissue Approach

The direct CT approach involves releasing the muscle tissue by applying sustained pressure to the CT while the client performs micromovements of the joints.

For superficial direct CT massage techniques, encouraging the client to breathe easily without stopping. The breath will create enough movement to propel you through the superficial fascia. The tiny muscular movements that accompany inhalation and exhalation are adequate for this purpose. The way to perform sustained pressure will be described separately for each superficial technique.

For deep direct connective tissue massage techniques, the sustained pressure and micromovements are somewhat more complicated and are explained in more detail in the section on the basic deep direct CT stroke.

The Direct Connective Tissue Approach to Superficial Fascia

This section discusses the application of the direct CT approach specifically to superficial fascia. The therapist chooses this approach for warming tissues or to soften solidified superficial fascia as a prelude to accessing deep fascial adhesions. Also, many times, the primary restrictions in the CT are found in the superficial fascia.

Elements of the direct CT approach can be observed in muscle sculpting, deep effleurage, Rolfing, deep longitudinal friction, postural or structural integration, and John Latz's style of CT massage.

ANATOMY OF SUPERFICIAL FASCIA

When you view an anatomical chart of the musculoskeletal system (see Chapter 3), the fascia is clearly visible. As a rule, muscles are marked in red, leaving the fascia to stand out as the areas marked in white, usually found next

Consider This: Piezoelectric and Thixotropic Effects of Direct CT Massage

As discussed in Chapter 3, the spread of piezoelectricity can be palpable. At times, bodyworkers sense the end result of the piezoelectric response: softening, yielding, and lengthening of the client's soft tissue. Sometimes the client will report a sensation of tingling or electricity that is not numbness and does not feel like a nerve phenomenon. The piezoelectric response may also be recognized as a softening, awareness of relaxation, or electrical sensation inside the therapist's own body. These internal apperceptions often coincide with client reports of physiological changes (e.g., sensations of electrical discharge, ease, relaxing, moving a physical blockage) or psychological shifts (e.g., laughing, crying, sense of letting go, memories).

The shearing of CT created by the downward pressure combined with a forward stretch may be one cause of the piezoelectric effect, discussed in Chapter 3. *De qi* is a well-documented phenomenon in acupuncture in which the therapist perceives the client's body tissues coming up to grasp the acupuncture needle when it is inserted and twisted. This same sort of grasping can occur when using the deep direct CT stroke. Langevin et al. (2001) have theorized that the two-dimensional pull on the CT (i.e., pressure from the insertion of the needle plus twisting it) is responsible for this grasping effect. In the direct CT stroke, the grasping effect results from the combination of pressure vectors, rather than a needle insertion and twist. An alternate type of information transfer (i.e., traveling through the CT) in the human body may begin to account for the alternating grasp and release phenomenon. The writings of Juhan (1998), Oschman (2000), and Langevin et al. (2001) suggest that the CT network is responsible for the grasp and release phenomena of acupuncture and some types of bodywork. Meridians are postulated to be channels of least resistance for processing and refining the body's energy flow (chi or qi). Thus, the shearing effect may partly explain the profound effectiveness and some unusual effects (e.g., twitching, slow arcing of the body, feeling of electricity reported by the client) in the direct CT approach.

Because the piezoelectric charge attracts water molecules, the fascia subsequently becomes longer, more responsive, and generally more supple under the fingers. *Thixotropy* is the term used to describe how material can sometimes be thicker and harder and sometimes more pliable and soft.

to and around the bones. Superficial fascia is readily seen in the lower back, around the joints, in the skull, in the iliotibial band that runs down the lateral aspect of the thigh, and along the anterior midline of the trunk.

As discussed in Chapter 3, superficial fascia lies just beneath the dermis. It can run in any direction. Schultz and Feitis (1996) have identified several distinct areas of superficial fascia where uneven forces of tension create visible folds or horizontal lines of stress in the body. They refer to these as body *retinaculae,* or straps (bands) of CT. The external regions overlying the pelvic floor, respiratory diaphragm, collar bone, and chin are examples of retinaculae (Schultz and Feitis, 1996; Upledger and Vredevoogd, 1983). Schultz and Feitis (1996) also consider the inguinal bands separating the hips from the upper thighs, the umbilical band around the waist, and the band that surrounds the eyes like a mask to be retinaculae.

Because retinaculae seem to act as focal points of physical stress, bodyworkers may find working at and around these areas a particularly fruitful way to begin myofascial massage for clients with myofascial pain or discomfort (Figure 6-1).

SUPERFICIAL DIRECT CONNECTIVE TISSUE TECHNIQUES

The direction of the superficial CT fibers is not determined by the direction of muscle because the CT fibers do not surround muscle tissue at this level. Thus, superficial direct CT strokes can be performed in any direction.

A number of techniques are used to soften, warm, and bring blood into superficial CTs. Some of these have familiar names and may be similar to procedures you have already learned in Swedish or deep tissue classes. It is important to note, however, that superficial direct CT strokes have a more specific intent (softening and freeing the superficial fascia) and may be performed differently (specifically, so that they never cause pain) than versions that you may have already been exposed to. Skin rolling,

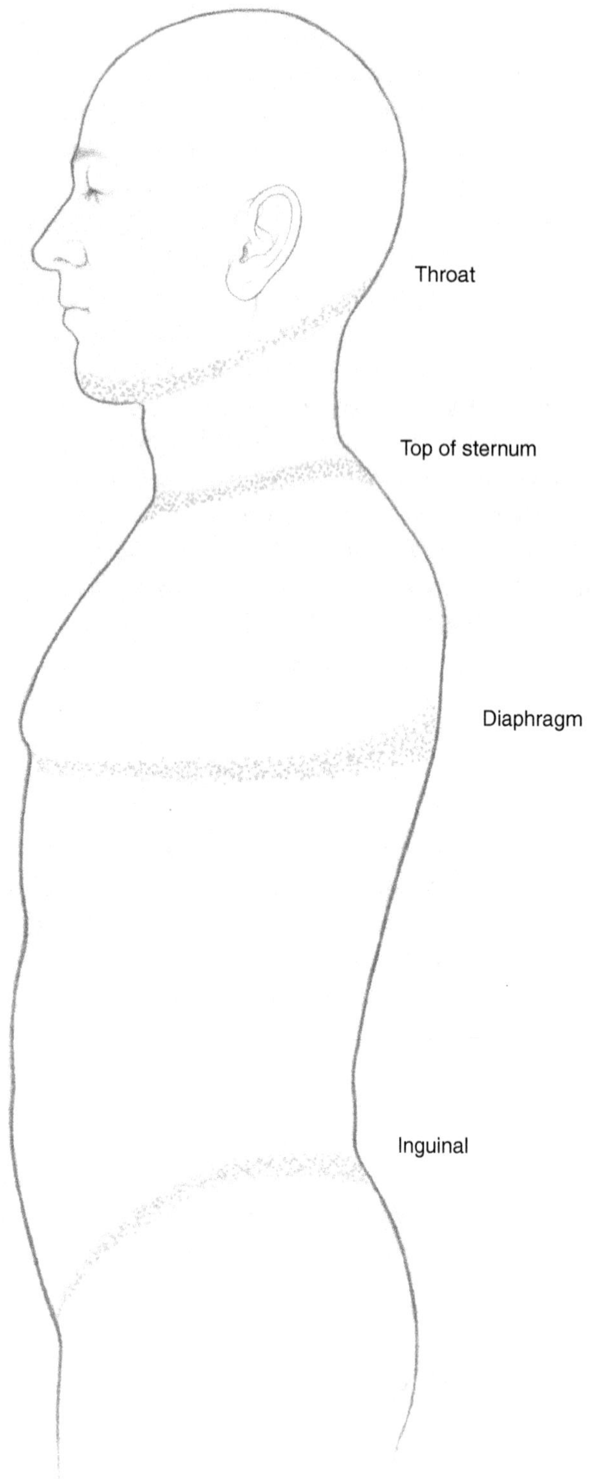

FIGURE 6-1 **Retinaculae.** In this side view, you can see retinaculae, or body straps, at the inguinal, diaphragm, top of the sternum, and throat areas.

compression, stretching, and scraping are the superficial strokes described in this chapter. Table 6-1 summarizes these techniques.

Skin Rolling

Skin rolling is a type of pétrissage in which the tissue just beneath the skin is grasped between thumb and forefingers (Figure 6-2). To prevent wear and tear on your thumbs, keep your thumbs in line with the wrist when performing skin rolling. It is important to let the release of the client's tissue (perceived as movement under your hands) guide the speed of the stroke. Too often, skin rolling is taught as a "scrape and burn" technique that does not wait for or follow the release (or lack thereof) in the client's CT. Whereas the skin of biologically young clients moves quickly and easily, many clients have some binding down of the fascia. Although people with biologically older CT really need skin rolling for the blood it brings into bound down tissues, quick, easy skin rolling for them is not possible. Properly applied skin rolling for such clients may actually feel more like skin folding, bending, or even just holding as you wait for the tissue release.

Compression

Compression is a technique in which the therapist pumps the muscle (and surrounding fascial layer) against the bone (Figure 6-3). It is not mashing, compacting, squeezing, or punching. Properly applied, it is more easily tolerated than skin rolling.

Use compression as a means to listen to and follow the tissue, rather than just pushing and sequentially letting go of the push. Listen to the natural rhythm of your client's body and release when her body is ready, not before or after. "Following the natural rhythm" does not mean imposing your rhythm on the client but rather listening to and following her lead.

Compression has two special advantages that make it especially useful at the start of a myofascial massage. It can be used for warming the tissues all over the body, as a substitute for effleurage, and it can be performed through a sheet, so that the client can remain covered.

Stretching

Stretching is another stroke that may be used for those who are having difficulty tolerating skin rolling. It means mechanically stretching the muscle and fascia in a line between your hands (or your hand and a second barrier) as the hands pull in opposite directions. Place your two hands

TABLE 6-1 Superficial Direct Connective Tissue Techniques

Technique	Description	Application
Basic Strokes		
Compression	Press the muscle against the bone.	Can be used for warming the tissues, rather than effleurage; all over the body; can be performed through the sheet.
Skin rolling	A type of pétrissage, capturing the superficial fascial layer between your thumb and fingers. Wait to feel the tissues release before gathering up more tissue.	All over the body, often used on the back; can move in any direction because the superficial fascial fibers run in all directions.
Stretching	Place both hands on the client's body and lean forward to separate the superficial fascia between the hands.	Used in areas where the fascia is particularly tight or when skin rolling cannot be performed because of pain, such as the lumbar region, near the sternum (as raking), or on IT band.
Scraping	Use knuckles, thumb pads, or other tools (body parts) to smooth the tissue, rubbing off the mineral deposits or "crunchies."	Used on bony areas, or a particular variation can be used on the IT band.
Soft Tissue Mobilization Techniques		
Cross-fiber friction	Apply force down into the muscle and move the fingers slowly in a direction perpendicular to the muscle fibers (like strumming a guitar).	Aligns fascia or scar tissue along parallel lines. This provides more strength and flexibility for the soft tissue.
J stroke	Evaluate skin mobility by pulling in all directions using the fingerpads. When a restriction or resistance is found, use counterpressure. The hook of the J can go in either direction.	Used to increase skin mobility and can be used throughout the body.

IT = iliotibial.

along the sheath where you intend to stretch and then lean forward over the two hands, letting the shifting weight of your own body draw your hands (and the superficial fascia underneath them) apart (Figure 6-4). This procedure affords the best opportunity to facilitate a "natural stretch." Stretching lengthens the fascia underneath your two hands by manually spreading the two ends, like pulling Silly Putty or taffy.

Listening is also important in stretching because it guides you in finding the line of resistance, meeting that line of resistance with the pressure of your hand (or other tool), and then waiting for the line of resistance to move. When you incorporate listening, you will not stretch or push past the limits of the tissue.

Use stretching in areas where fascia is particularly tight or when skin rolling cannot be performed because of pain, including regions such as the lumbar fascia of the back, around the scapulae (shoulder blades), and in between the pectoral (chest) muscles overlying the sternum (breastbone). When stretching is applied over the breastbone, the fingers are spread to accommodate the ribs, and the stroke is called *raking*.

Scraping

Scraping is an unusual stroke that requires you to scrape bony or ligamentous areas with your thumb, knuckles, or fingers, imagining that you are smoothing the surface, as if you were shaving off ice (Figure 6-5). It involves sinking down through CT layers to smooth the underlying tissue free of lumps and bumps. Although it seems to run counter to guidelines that students are taught in Swedish massage, scraping can be used directly over the ankle bones, knee bones, or any bony areas. It can also be used on ligamentous areas such as the iliotibial band. The trick here is to actively solicit client feedback. Ask your client to let you know if scraping feels good in the area that you selected or if the stroke feels irritating. Say, "Do you find this work annoying, or does it feel good?" The response will be a clear indication to either continue or stop immediately. Clients will either like the technique and answer that they think it is freeing something or they will find it irritating. Needless to say, do not continue scraping or any other stroke that is irritating the client, aggravating a problem, or simply is not especially helpful.

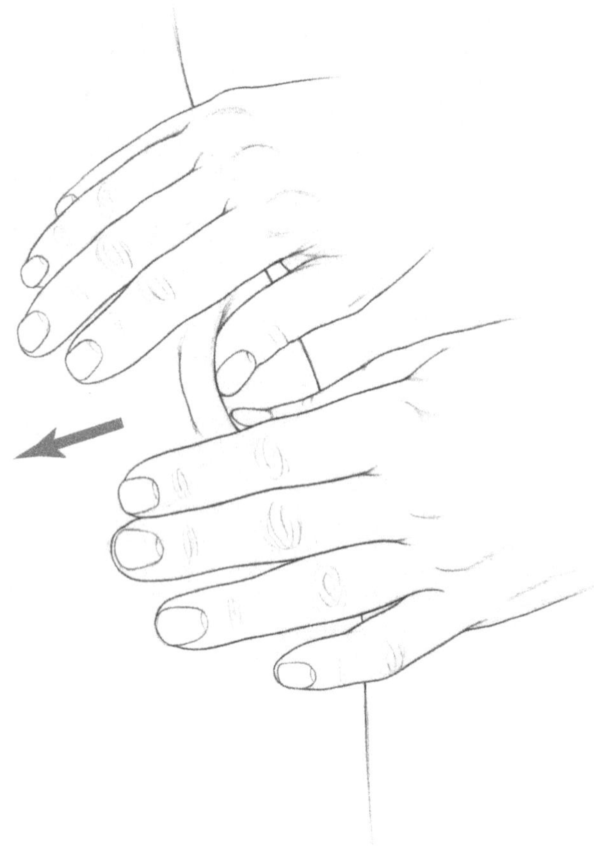

FIGURE 6-2 Skin rolling. Keep the thumbs relaxed and in neutral position when practicing skin rolling.

SOFT TISSUE MOBILIZATION TECHNIQUES

Several authorities (Barnes, 1995; Manheim, 2001) promote additional superficial CT techniques that are collectively termed soft tissue mobilization. Most soft tissue mobilization techniques are variations on skin rolling (e.g., applied to scars) or stretching (applied to any area of the body). Two techniques (J stroke and cross-fiber friction) are described here. Refer to Table 6-1 to review these soft tissue mobilization techniques.

Cross-fiber Friction (Transverse Friction, Cyriax Friction)

Cross-fiber friction (transverse friction, Cyriax friction) is used to prevent or soften adhesions in the myofascial unit, between the ligaments and the underlying bone, and to smooth roughened surfaces between tendons and their sheaths. Note that Travell and Simons (1999a, 1999b) specifically *exclude* cross-fiber friction as a treatment for trigger points (as discussed in Chapter 5).

To perform cross-fiber friction, move the client's skin over the underlying tissue in a direction perpendicular to the muscle fibers (Figure 6-6). Prepare for cross-fiber friction by trimming the fingernails short and rounded on the edges, so that you do not scratch the client. Also, you will find it easier to perform cross-fiber friction when your hands and the client's skin are free of lotion or oil. Effective cross-fiber strokes sweep across the muscle fibers and must be long enough to cross the entire myofascial unit. Locate the specific area that you wish to soften by palpating for taut bands, pain response, or crepitation ("crunchiness") or by noting an area of restricted motion. The client's skin and the therapist's finger(s) should move as one unit.

For chronic injuries, a recommended duration is 2 minutes of easy cross-fiber friction followed by 6 to 8 minutes of deeper pressure and having the client follow the procedure with 20 to 30 repetitions of a small movement of the targeted muscle. Finish with a 5-minute or less application of cold (ice pack wrapped in a towel) over the area to counteract any swelling that might arise from the therapeutically induced local inflammation. For acute injuries, carry out the light application *only*, for 4 to 5 minutes, and conclude with a cold application. *Pain is a sign for caution.* If you notice your client wincing or tensing up at your touch, you must reduce your pressure. If the client continues to tense, discontinue the cross-fiber friction.

J Stroke

The J stroke is a more forceful technique performed to release superficial CT restrictions or adhesions that do not respond to skin rolling. It can be used to increase skin mobility anywhere in the body; however, it should be applied in specific areas and should not be used as an overall skin release. Performing the J stroke over a trigger point may cause a reactive muscle spasm, negating the release (Manheim, 2001).

To prepare, position the client to allow maximum slack in the target area and make sure your hands and the client's skin are free of lubricants. To perform the stroke, use the finger pads to pull in all directions to evaluate skin mobility. When you feel restriction or resistance, pull away from the restriction, ending with a motion like the hook of the letter J (Figure 6-7). The hook is drawn with a quick, abrupt motion crossing the restriction. It can go to either side. Use the palm of your hand to recheck skin mobility in all directions. If the restriction is not completely released, repeat the J stroke at right angles to the first application. Test again and if needed, repeat the sequence in a starburst pattern until the restriction softens.

The client may report a burning sensation in the area. Hyperemia is likely because the stroke promotes local

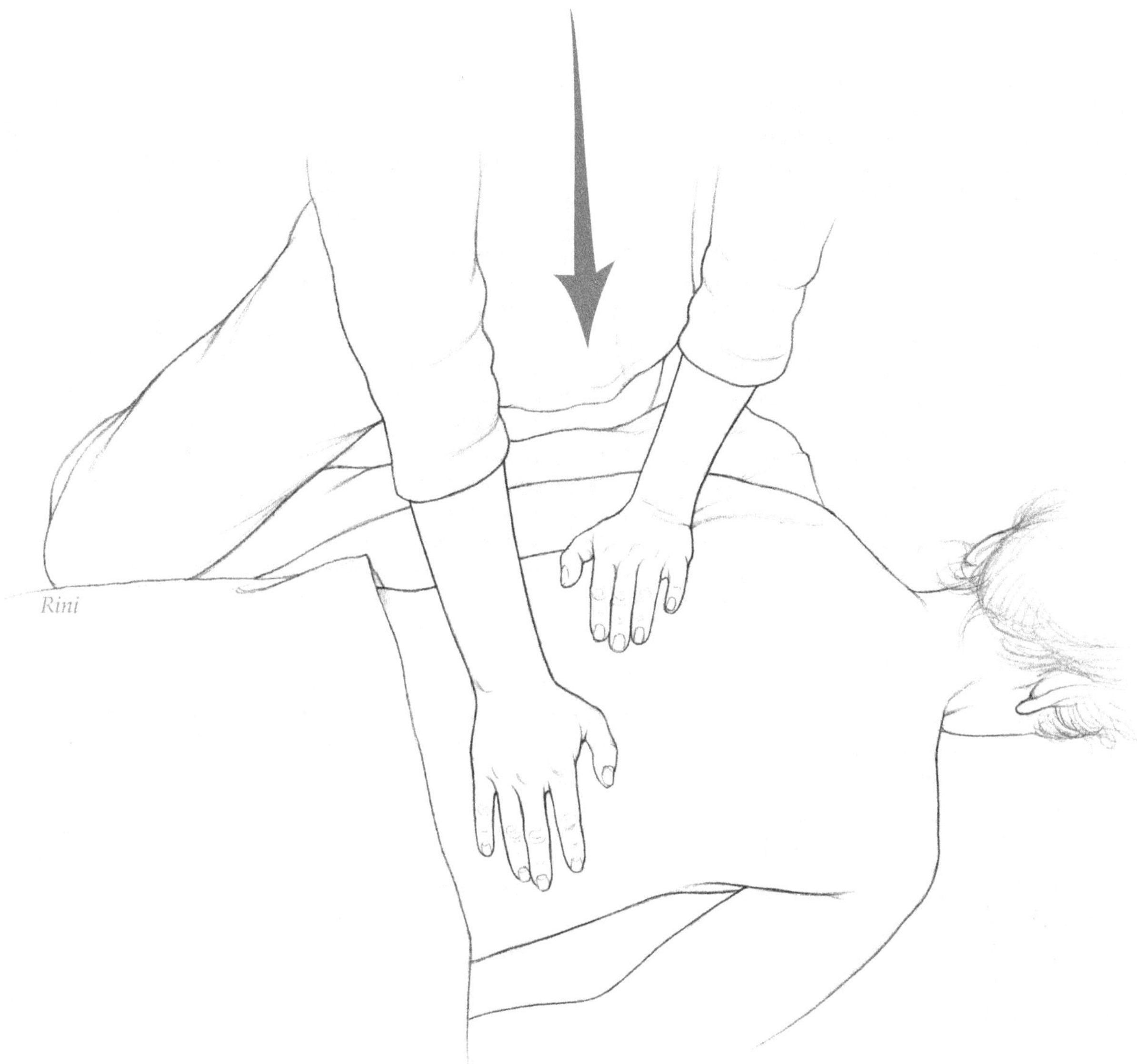

FIGURE 6-3 **Compression.** In compression, the force comes from sinking into the client's tissue with the whole body rather than pressing with the arms and shoulders.

inflammation. The J stroke, however, should not cause injury or pain. Instruct the client to ice the area at home two or three times for the first 24 hours and continuing, if needed, another 24 hours to reduce any accompanying swelling or subsequent pain.

OPTIMAL USE OF SUPERFICIAL DIRECT CONNECTIVE TISSUE TECHNIQUES

The following recommendations summarize the important elements involved in effectively applying all superficial CT strokes.

1. Keep your pelvis, shoulder girdle, wrists, and hands in line. This allows your body to work in unison rather than fighting against yourself.
2. Do *not* poke, push, or shove the tissue. Instead, allow time for the tissue to move before rushing on.
3. Sink into the tissue past the surface of the skin until you feel that you have accessed superficial CT. Note: This may differ widely for different clients. Some clients will not let you into the superficial fascial layer; their skin feels like hard armor. Other clients have biologically young superficial CT, and the skin over it moves freely like a wrinkly Shar-Pei dog.
4. Do *not* spend more than 1 minute being stuck without movement. If you cannot follow a movement, change the placement of your hands (even if only 1/2 inch),

One Therapist's Experience: The Experience of Performing Direct CT Massage

A standard assignment in my direct CT class is to write a case study report that includes client feedback and what it actually feels like to be a therapist administering the direct CT approach. The following is an excerpt from one student report. This account may provide additional insight into what it might be like to incorporate direct CT techniques into other kinds of massage.

"The process of learning to work with the direct CT approach to myofascial massage has been a challenge. It has required me to step outside my comfort zone with massage and asked me to be even more aware of both my client and myself.

. . . In our second session, we focused on B's legs since she had talked about having some problems with shin splints . . . working the rest of her body with the Swedish method . . . when we got to B's legs, I coached her with some micromovements, alternating dorsi and plantar flexion. Sure enough, she wanted to make much bigger movements than we needed to accomplish our task, but it didn't take that long for her or me to get the hang of it. First we used the release beginning just below the knee, moving in a cephalic direction. We began the second focus just above the ankle and moved inferiorly. She appeared to have a little fuller ROM [range of motion]. I gave her one exercise for her back and shoulders and another general body (stretch). We practiced them together so that I could be sure she understood how and why to do them.

. . . At the beginning of our third session, B reported that she hadn't had any problems with shin splints since our last session. I was very excited to hear that. It gave me a sense of validation that maybe I'd helped give her body the direction it needed to readjust itself. During this session, the focus was on her shoulders and chest. She complained of some tightness. This time, we really went in deep. I used the direct CT approach on serratus and pec minor. I also worked bilaterally down her sternum with raking. We used movement of breath in all three spots. During work on the sternum and pec minor, both places were like "wow" moments for us. I felt like the work was smooth and intense all at once. I wanted to just jump out of my skin when I got down into the pec minor and knew which muscle I was touching. B let out a nice sigh of relief and commented that she didn't even know that she had muscles there or that they even needed to be massaged. On ending our session, I cautioned her that we had done some really deep work and that she should be sure to ice the area and drink *lots* of water when she got home.

In looking back over the sessions, I think the most exciting thing was teaching B about her own body while I was learning to work on it at the very same time. The partnership between client and practitioner inherent in this type of work is so exciting. I can't wait to continue exploring it."

and try again. If you cannot find a good orientation to the tissue after several tries, try a less invasive superficial CT technique (e.g., stretching or compression).

5. If the tissue moves freely at first contact, you do not need to apply additional superficial CT techniques. The work you have done to assess the fascia, however, will warm the tissues and feel good to the client.
6. Know the anatomical structures that you are palpating (i.e., muscles, lumbar fascia, bones) and use that knowledge to guide your pressure and choice of superficial CT techniques as you free the fascia. For example, the lumbar fascia is traditionally less moveable than the fascia that lies over the erector spinae muscles, just superior. You might then conclude that the lumbar fascia may be more responsive to stretching than to skin rolling.
7. Keep your feet closer together than you would in Swedish massage so that the stability of your own body does not prevent you from perceiving small movements of the superficial fascia.
8. If you feel movement in the tissue, follow the direction of that change. As the tissue lengthens, it will feel as if the client's body is moving you along.
9. If your body feels out of line, stop and readjust your position. As you take your hands away, ask the client to breathe and move the area in a comfortable way. Use

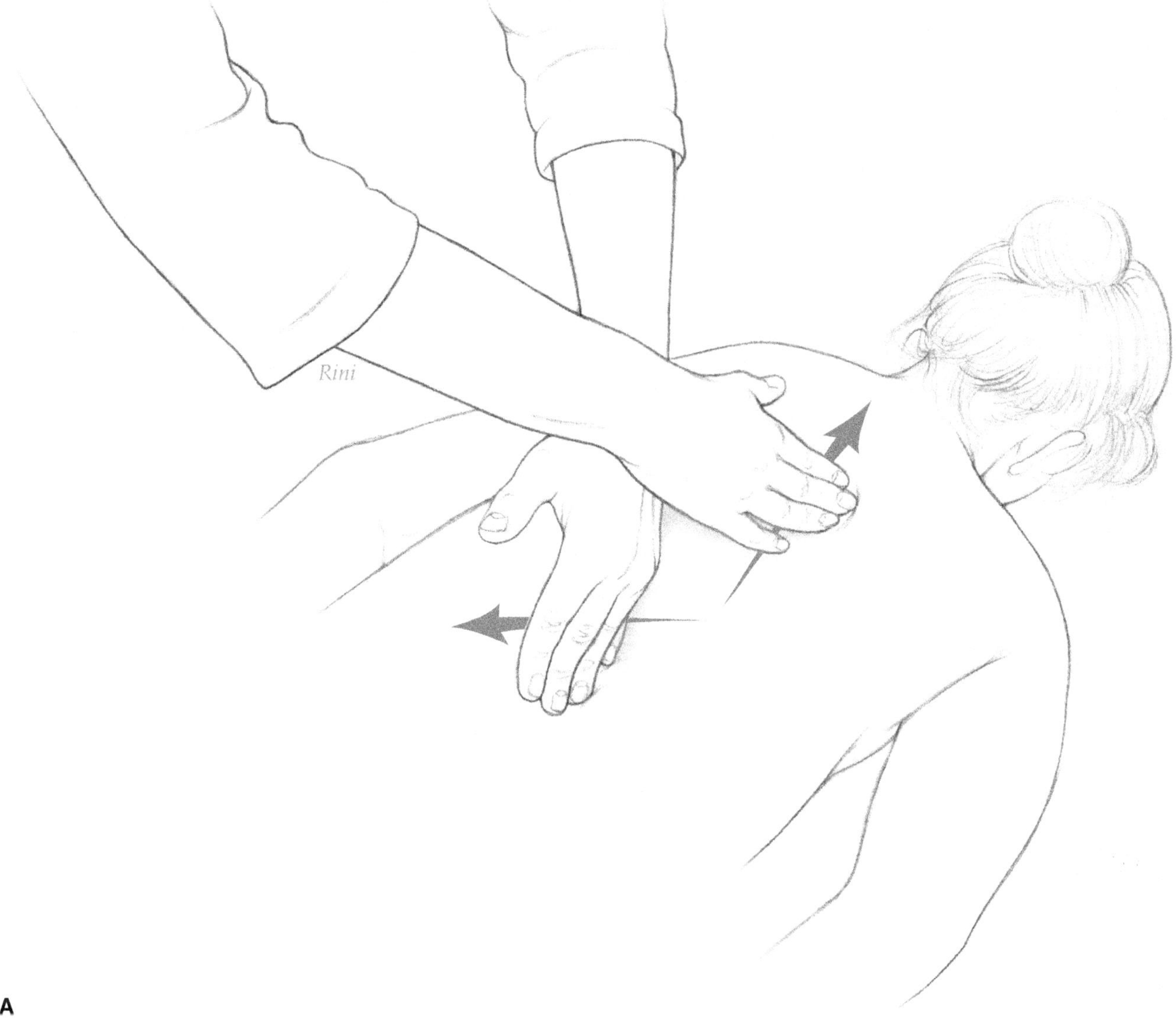

FIGURE 6-4 **Superficial direct CT stretching.** (**A**) Incorrect technique in which the hands are held stiffly, with only the sides touching the client's body.

this time to stretch and breathe for yourself as well. When you reconnect, you will be fully present with your client rather than halfway there.

10. Breath cues (e.g., telling your client to continue to breathe easily) increase your client's awareness and decrease the pain level.
11. Movement cues are not necessary when releasing superficial fascia; the movements of breathing will suffice. If you do wish to add movement cues, use the guidelines provided in the Coached Micromovements section later in the chapter.
12. Have clients ice any areas that were worked heavily (or provide this service as part of the myofascial massage). Rub the ice over the area for 5 minutes (ice friction) or leave a pack on for 10 minutes (or less if it becomes uncomfortable). Suggest that the client apply the ice at least twice on the day of the massage and one to three times the next day to prevent swelling and pain.

The Direct Connective Tissue Approach to Deep Fascia

This section discusses the application of the direct CT approach specifically to deep fascia. The therapist chooses this approach to access deep fascial adhesions and chronically inflamed tissues. Clients who require or request deep direct CT massage often suffer from old injuries or

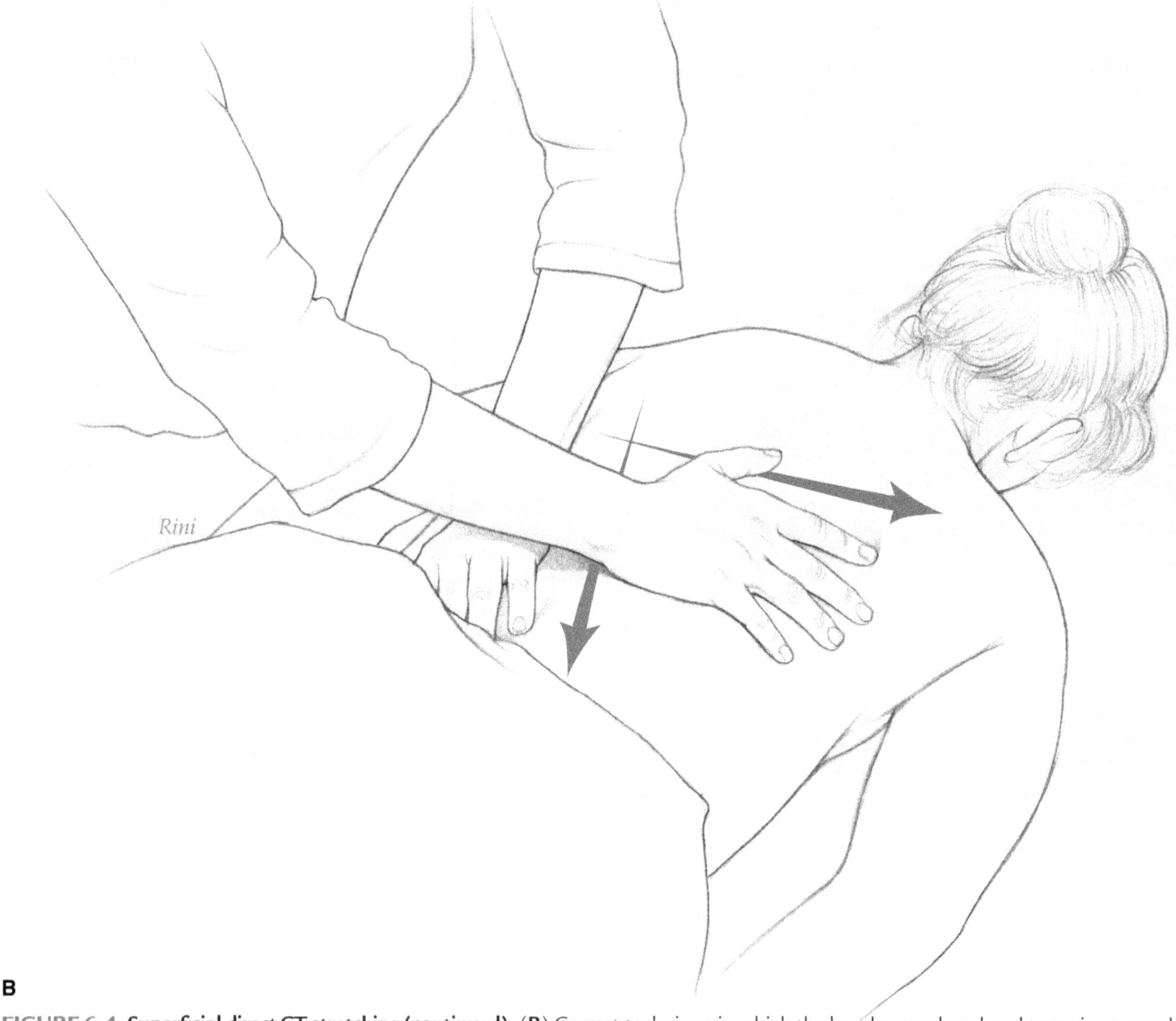

B

FIGURE 6-4 **Superficial direct CT stretching (continued).** (**B**) Correct technique in which the hands are relaxed and torso is centered over the client's body.

chronic postural distortions that have bound down the CT, either locally or distally to the original trauma.

ANATOMY OF DEEP FASCIA

Deep fascial planes have (at least) three distinct depths or levels, distinguishable by the predominant direction of the muscle fibers at that level. These are the superficial plane of the deep fascia, the middle plane of the deep fascia, and the deep plane of the deep fascia. Sometimes the superficial plane of the deep fascia is coexistent with what we know simply as the superficial fascia. For example, the lumbar fascia on the lower back can be considered both superficial fascia and the superficial layer of the deep fascia (Figure 6-8).

In some cases, especially in the regions bordering the bones, the deep plane of the deep fascia comes up to meet and is contiguous with the superficial fascia and the superficial layer of the deep fascia (e.g., the extensor retinaculum around the ankle; Figure 6-9).

As discussed in Chapter 2, deep fascia wraps every single muscle cell (as endomysium), fascicle of muscle cells (as perimysium), and each muscle in its entirety (as epimysium). Sheaths of deep fascia make up the walls, called *septae,* between and within muscles. These septae thus determine a large part of how bodyworkers can effectively align themselves to apply deep direct CT strokes.

It is important to remember that retinaculae, ligaments, tendons, and tendon sheaths, along with the endomysium, perimysium, and epimysium, are all continuous structures of CT. Manual therapists who address the fascial wrappings of soft tissue with deep direct CT strokes establish an orientation to the myofascia that therapeutically aligns their application of pressure to muscles and tendons and by

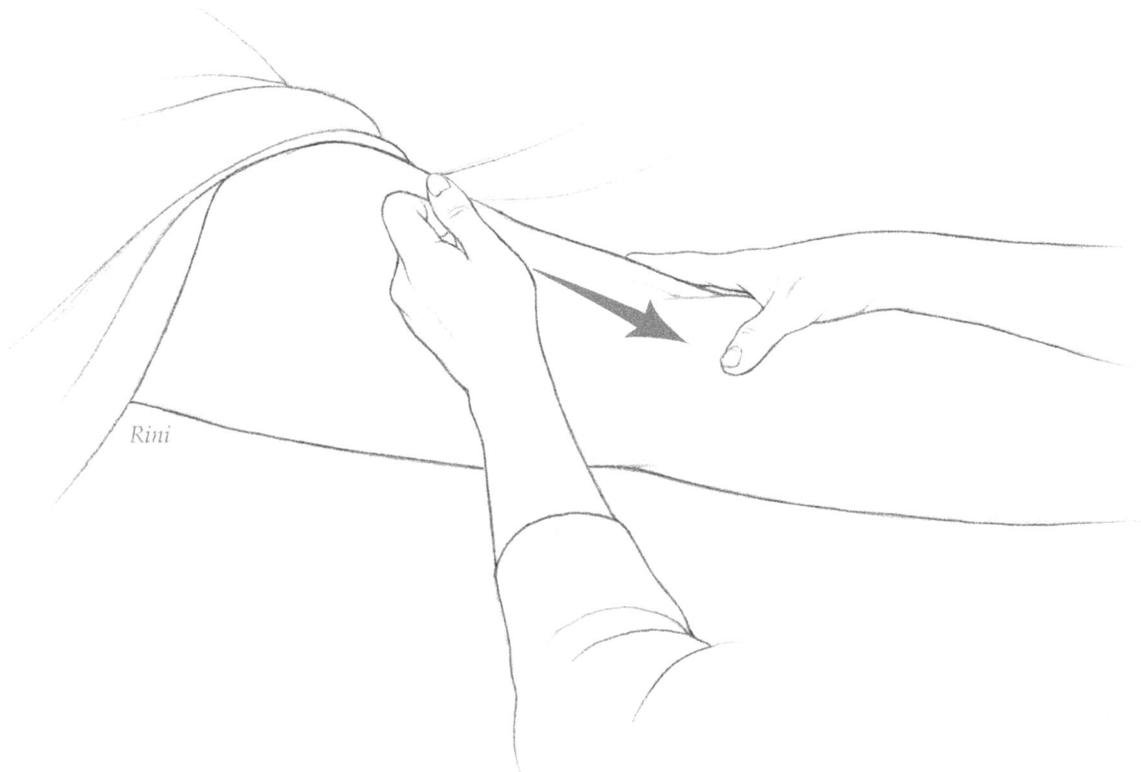

FIGURE 6-5 **Scraping.** Use a steady rhythm when "scraping" the IT band.

extension, onto bones. Bodyworkers who do not realize the importance of the protective sheath and concentrate only on relaxing muscles take longer to effect change; what change they do effect is less likely to last. When a muscle is manually relaxed but guarded by a tight CT binding that will not move, that muscle is prevented from maintaining its fully relaxed length. In this case, muscles become far more prone to return to a shortened, contracted state after the massage.

COMPONENTS OF THE BASIC DEEP DIRECT CONNECTIVE TISSUE STROKE

All deep direct CT techniques are variations on one fundamental stroke, which combines sustained pressure in a precise direction while coaching the client in micromovements of the nearby joints. See Table 6-2 for appropriate applications and a summary description of the deep direct CT stroke.

Sustained Pressure

Sustained pressure follows a line of contact composed of two distinct directions of force and intent. One of these descends vertically down toward the bone, penetrating as deeply as the client's tissues allow. This component of the pressure is applied by waiting for the fascia to soften, not by forcing. The other direction of force and intent is directed along the skin surface, following the line of the fascia (Figure 6-10). Because CT wraps around individual muscle fibers, bundles, and whole muscles, knowing the general anatomical direction of muscle fibers is invaluable in applying direct CT strokes. The anatomical orientation of the muscle fibers provides a basic roadmap for lengthening dense CT.

The actual route of pressure varies with the depth of the fascia being accessed. This is because muscle fibers (and the CT that surrounds them) tend to be aligned in different directions depending on how deep they are in the body. For example, the fiber direction of the trapezius and its fascia lie in a different direction than the rhomboid fibers just beneath it.

Individual kinks that can be palpated in the myofascia also cause the therapist's route to diverge from the standard muscle fiber direction portrayed in anatomy books. It sounds almost too simple, but the route of your resultant pressure is determined to a large extent by the way that the CT will move most easily. Trial and error, along with a great deal of patience, is needed to palpate this ease of movement. After you grasp the process of following ease of movement (i.e., the easiest direction of movement), it is surprisingly easy to just follow the tissue in the way that "it wants to move."

The trick to administering sustained pressure involves leaning a controlled amount of body weight into the client's

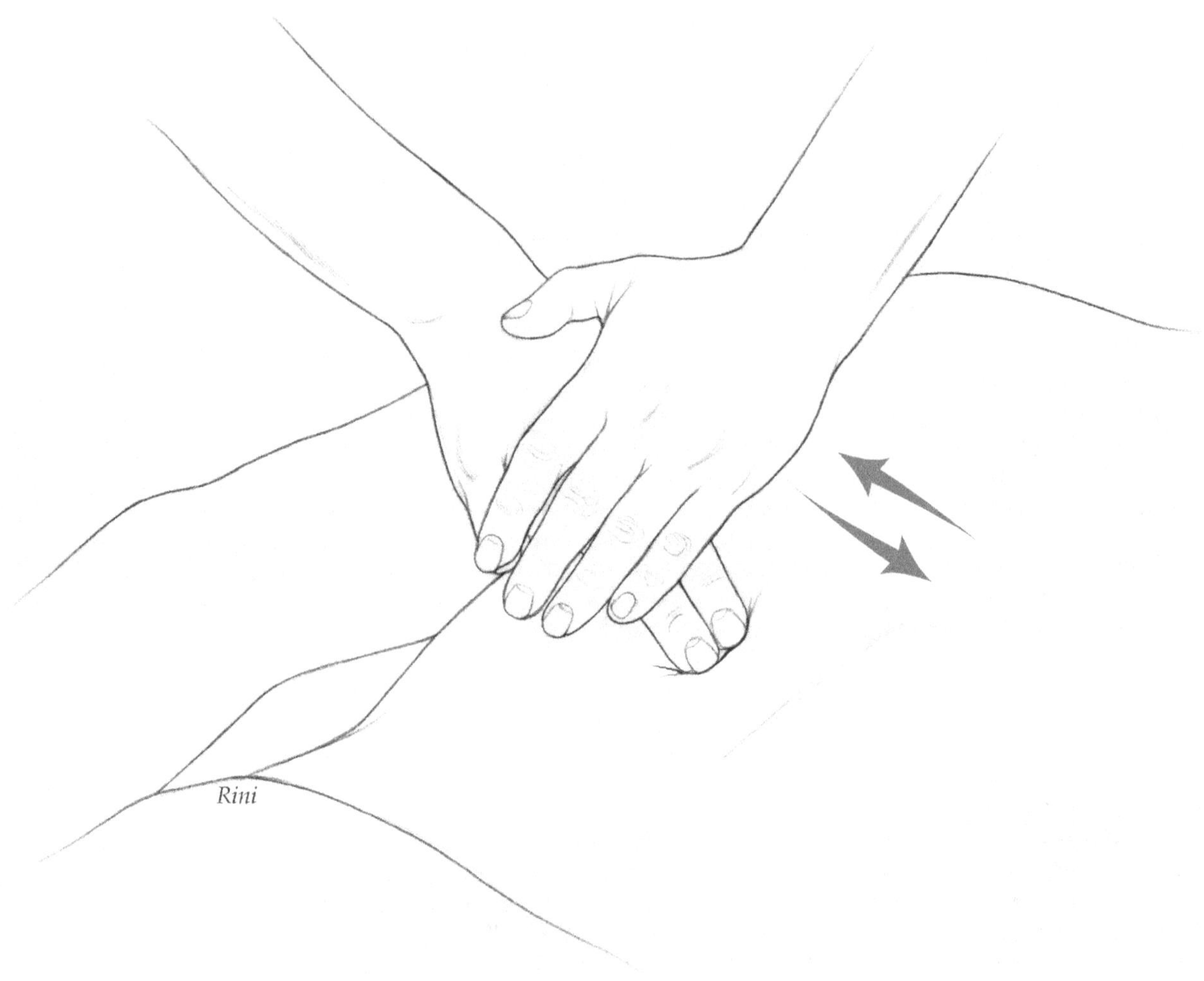

FIGURE 6-6 **Cross-fiber friction.** Apply cross-fiber friction with (**A**) braced fingers.

body. This feels somewhat like "controlled falling." The depth of your stroke is determined by the angle of your lean in conjunction with the tissue resistance that you meet. By leaning only until you feel resistance, you will never push past a safe and appropriate pressure, and your work will not hurt the client. "Controlled falling" does not involve muscular effort. It is painless for the bodyworker because you are leaning into the force of gravity. On the other hand, it ensures that you are leaning deeply enough to effect a real change on the CT.

"Controlled falling" is effective only when your body is in alignment and when you face in the direction of the stroke. Check your alignment all the way from the sole of your foot through your ankle, knee, hip, shoulder, nose, and top of the crown. Your eyes can still look down at the client for nonverbal clues of release (e.g., sigh, deep breath, stomach rumbling, faint smile) or discomfort (scowl, shudder, scrunched-up face), but your head should remain in line with the direction of the lengthening stroke. In a kind of sympathetic mirroring of the intended lengthening of the client's soft tissue, your body also lengthens vertically from the bottom of your feet to the top of your head and extends out through the arms as you move through the deep direct stroke. According to Latz (2003), aligning your body with your force smoothes out and lengthens shortened fascia like wrinkles on a sheet.

The ability to remain at ease in your body and your hands is imperative when you are applying the basic stroke. You cannot feel tiny releases in the CT unless your body stays soft and relaxed enough to fall into the tissue when it lengthens. Then you can easily recognize tissue releases because you feel like you are just falling forward a little more. A state of ease also encompasses remembering to continue breathing and elongating the CT comfortably and easily. When the CT lengthens and you fall forward, it is time to reposition yourself for the next step in release. Repositioning means shaking off tension, remembering to take a breath (and cueing your client to do the same), and perhaps moving forward a tiny step. It may also mean using a different part of your body as the main tool or stepping to the other side of the table to get a better angle.

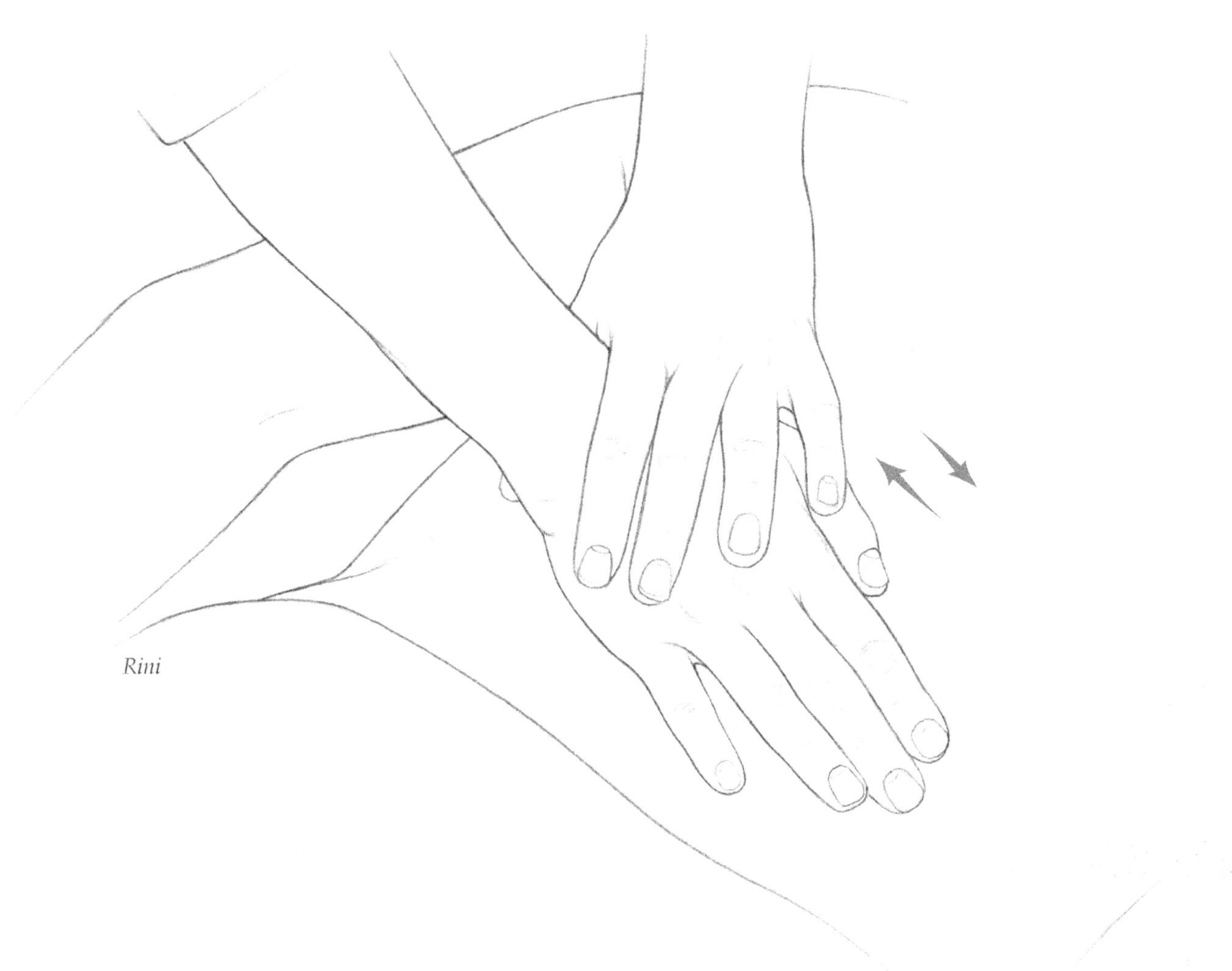

FIGURE 6-6 **Cross-fiber friction (continued).** (B) Apply cross-fiber friction with whole hands or other parts of your body.

The two lines of force are administered simultaneously; thus, there is really only one resultant impetus in the deep direct CT stroke. This composite impetus is an oblique line of entry into the body, which minimizes the perception of invasive contact and maximizes stretching in the CT's collagen fibers. Whereas a downward vector alone would immobilize the tissue, the composite stroke allows for an edge of the fascial net to be held in place while the rest of the net is stretched out from that base.

Coached Micromovements

Micromovements are very small movements of the nearby joints that the client initiates according to therapist instructions. These movements enhance the ability of the client's soft tissue to lengthen and release and make it easier for the CT to absorb the mechanical stretching of the direct pressure. Micromovements need to be precisely coached by the therapist so that the client does not make too big or too fast a movement. Movements that are too forceful or quick are counterproductive because they tend to push the therapist's hands (or other tools) away from the site.

Coaching the client in specific micromovements helps engage the tissue that is beneath the therapist's hands (or elbow, knuckles, or forearm). Also, when the client makes very small movements, it helps the bodyworker to better sense the line of restriction in the CT. (It is easy to feel where the movement stops.) In addition, asking for movement maintains interaction between the bodyworker and client and can thereby increase the sense of control for the client. Asking for movement helps create conscious

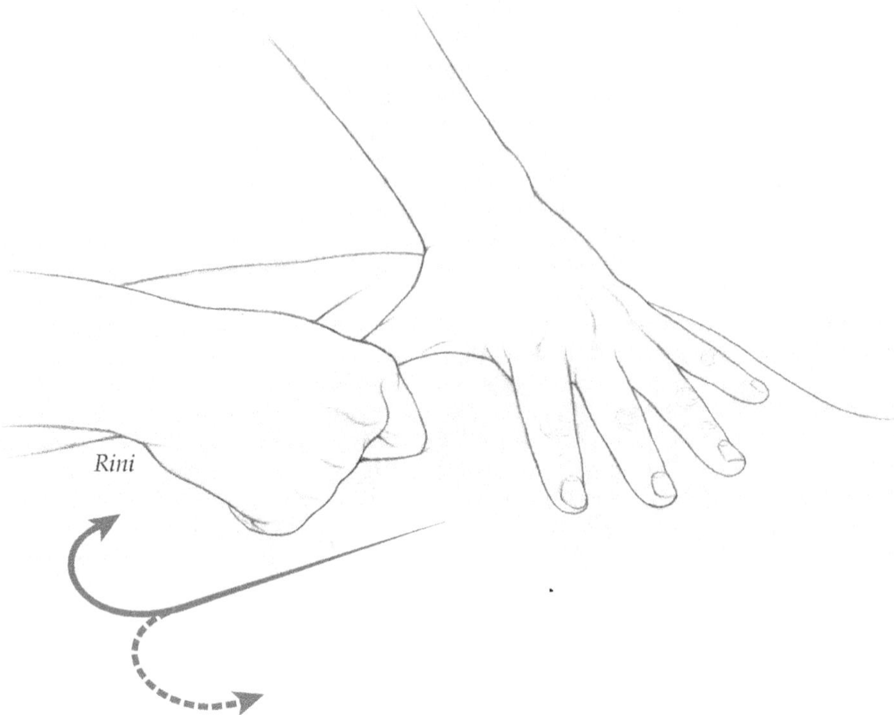

FIGURE 6-7 **J stroke.** Use your dominant hand to draw the J, which can go to either side.

awareness of the changes that are occurring in the client's CT and facilitates the utilization of self-help exercises that help maintain more lasting change. Together, coaching the client in micromovements and active stretches during the breaks from hands-on applications will stir up congealed CT and make it more pliable and soft.

OPTIMAL USE OF DEEP DIRECT CONNECTIVE TISSUE TECHNIQUES

The following recommendations summarize the important elements involved in effectively applying sustained pressure with the deep direct CT stroke.

1. Take time to position your body behind restricted planes of fascial tissue. Keep your pelvis, shoulder girdle, wrists, and hands in the same line. This allows your body efforts to work in unison rather than fighting against yourself.
2. Do *not* poke, push, or shove the tissue. Instead, allow time to sink into the tissue and feel your way into the line that leads out of the restriction.
3. Let your hands sink past the surface of the skin toward the bone until you feel that you have accessed the CT. Note: This may differ widely for different clients. Some clients will only let you in to the superficial fascial layer, just beneath the surface of the skin. Other clients will let you deep into the deep fascia that spirals directly into bone.
4. After you sink to the right depth, apply a second pressure (like longitudinal friction) at a perpendicular angle. The CT wrappings of the muscle will determine the exact direction. Thus, your second pressure will tend to follow the direction of the muscle fibers. See Table 6-3 for precise descriptions of the predominant muscle (and CT) fiber directions. Because CT can get twisted and may not always follow the muscle fiber in every detail, you must palpate for the direction that most easily leads you out of restriction.
5. Do *not* spend more than 1 minute in each placement. If you cannot follow a movement, change the placement of your hands (even if only 1/2 inch), and try again. If you cannot find a good orientation to the tissue after several tries, move to a different area.
6. Deep and superficial fascias merge around the attachments of muscles on the bones. This makes the bony margins an especially good place to begin your work to find your way into restricted fascias.
7. Know the anatomical structures that you are palpating (i.e., muscles, ligaments, tendons, vessels, bones) and use that knowledge to guide pressure and movement.
8. Keep your feet closer together than you would in Swedish massage. It is as if you are practicing "controlled falling" into the tissue.

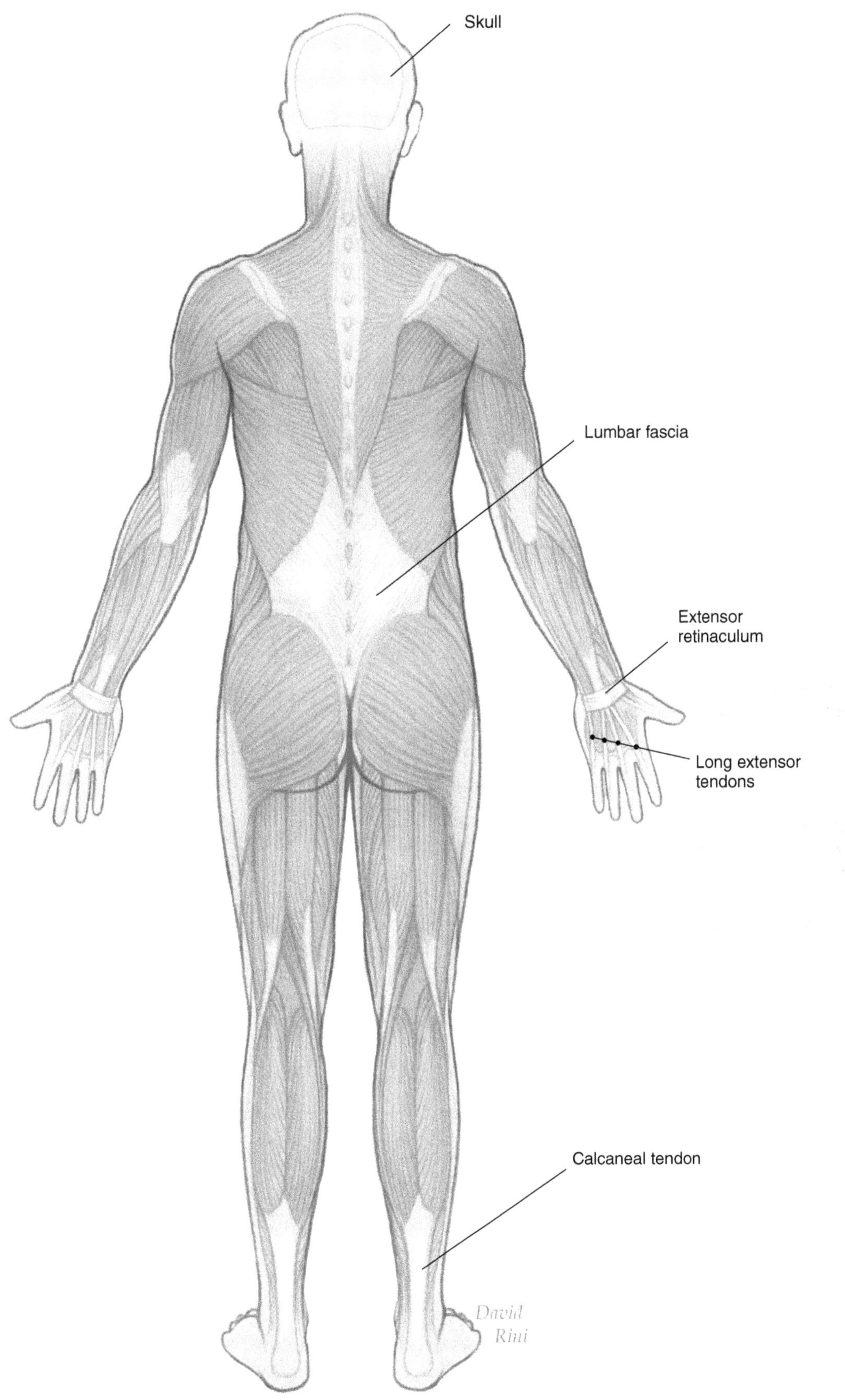

FIGURE 6-8 Lumbar fascia. You can access both the superficial layer of the deep fascia and the superficial fascia at the location of the lumbar fascia.

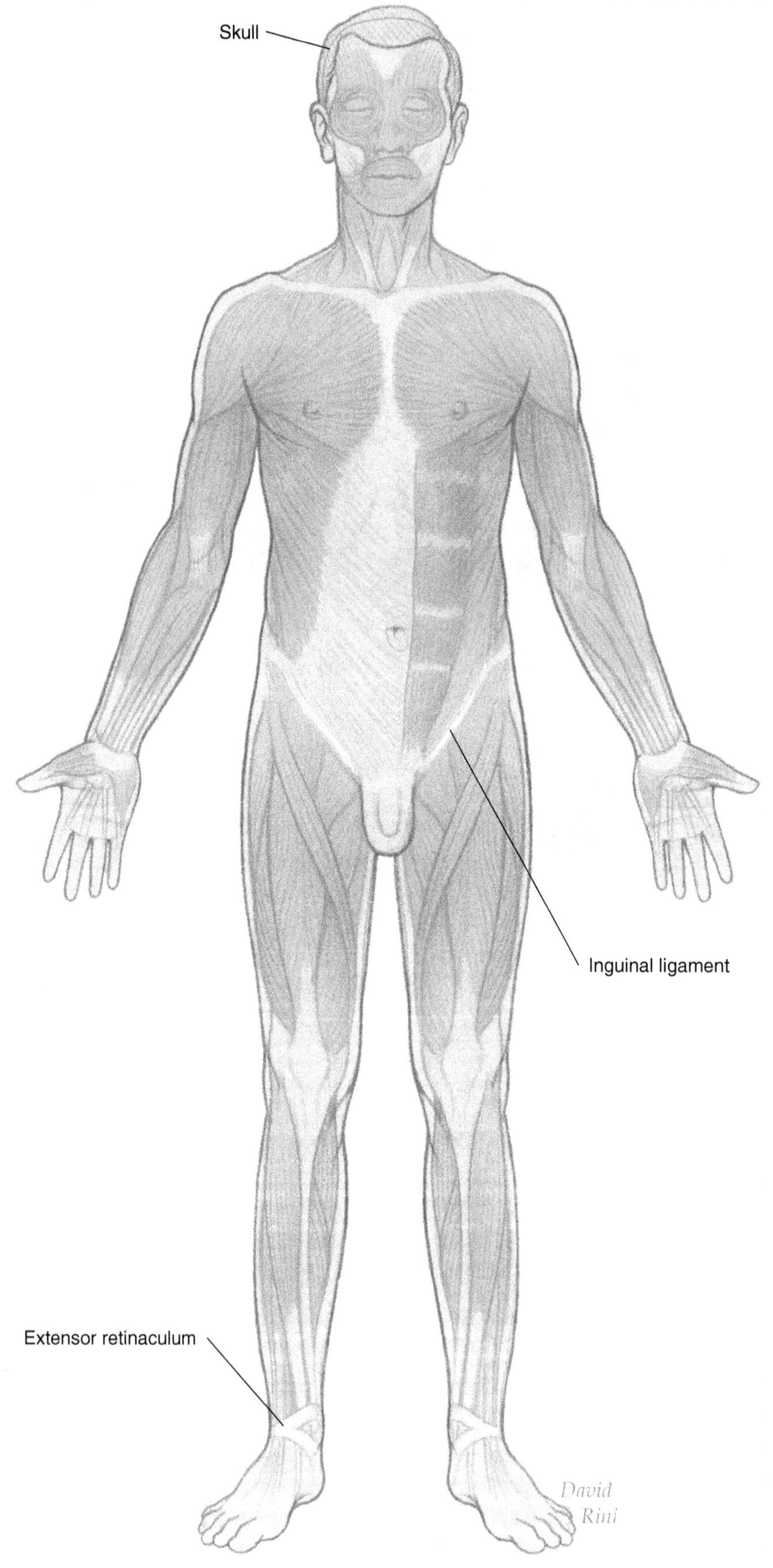

FIGURE 6-9 Extensor retinaculum of the ankle. You can access both the superficial layer of the deep fascia and the superficial fascia at the location of the extensor retinaculum of the ankle.

TABLE 6-2 Deep Direct Connective Tissue Technique

Technique	Description	Application
The basic stroke	A composite of two vectors of force. One vector sinks down to the bone. The second vector is perpendicular to the first and moves along the edge of myofascial fibers. Coached micro-movements make the stroke more effective. Break physical contact to coach breaths and larger voluntary movements.	The most direct way to stretch chronically injured tissue, scar tissue, or old injuries that do not resolve. *Do not use over areas that are red, hot, swollen, or painful!*

9. If you think that you feel a release in the tissue, give yourself permission to believe in and follow that change.
10. You are looking for a softening or lengthening in the area where you are working. As the tissue lengthens, it will feel as if the client's body is moving you along.
11. If your body feels out of line, stop and readjust your position. As you take your hands away, ask the client to breathe and move the area in a comfortable way. Use this time to stretch and breathe for yourself as well. When you reconnect, you will be fully present with your client rather than halfway there.
12. Breath cues (e.g., telling your client to continue to breathe easily) increase your client's awareness and decrease the pain level.
13. Movement cues (described shortly) engage the stuck layer and make it easier to free restrictions without pain.
14. Have the client ice any areas that were worked deeply (or provide this service as part of the myofascial mas-

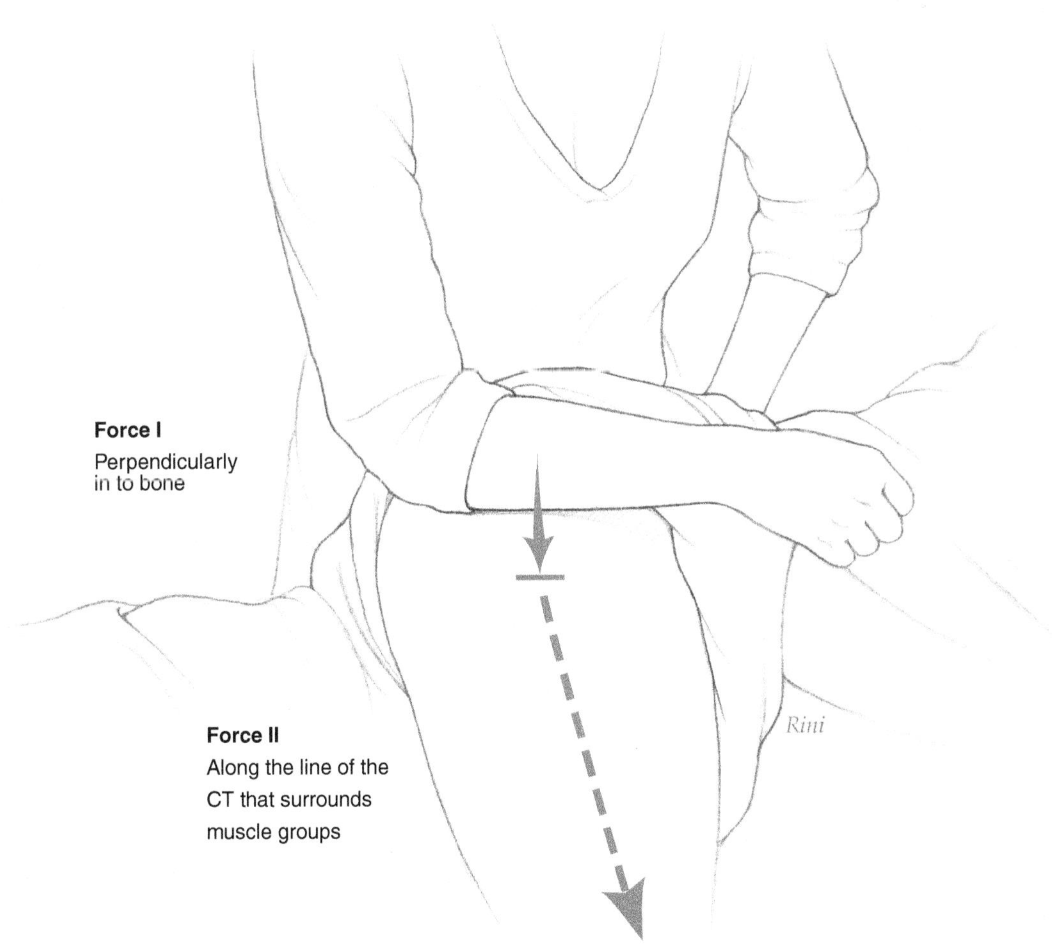

FIGURE 6-10 **Basic deep direct CT stroke.** Shown are the two types of force that combine in the basic deep direct CT stroke.

TABLE 6-3 Deep Direct Connective Tissue Applications (by Region)

Region	Direction of Force	Therapist's Body Tools	Client Position	Movement Cue
Lower Leg (Lateral Side)				
Ankle bones (extensor retinaculum)	Cephalic (toward the head)	Knuckles	Side-lying	Point and flex your ankle.
Interosseus membrane between tibia and fibula	Cephalic	Knuckles, fingers (if not painful to therapist)	Side-lying	Point and flex your ankle. Press into my hand.
Achilles tendon	Cephalic or caudal (toward the feet)	Knuckles, elbow	Prone (can use your own leg as a bolster)	Tuck your tailbone under (move your hips forward and back).
Plantaris	Pressure into the bone; no other vector	Fingers, elbow; tool must be focused	Prone with flexed knee	Point and flex your ankle.
Calf muscles (gastrocnemius and soleus)	Caudal (toward the feet)	Thumb	Prone	Point and flex your ankle.
Thigh				
Quadriceps	Cephalic or caudal	Forearm	Supine	Flex and extend your knee.
Septum between quadriceps and adductors	Caudal	Fingers	Supine	Flex and extend your knee. Push into my hand (placed at lateral or medial thigh).
Piriformis and biceps femoris	Caudal	Elbow or fingers at attachments, forearm at muscle belly	Prone	Flex and extend your knee. Flex and extend your hip.
Medial hamstrings, semitendinosis, semimembranousus	Cephalic	Elbow at attachments, fists at muscle bellies	Prone	Flex and extend your knee. Flex and extend your hip.
Adductor magnus	Cephalic	Elbow at attachments, fingertips at muscle bellies	Side-lying	Push into my hand (placed at lateral or medial thigh).
Hip and Lateral Posterior Thigh				
Iliac crest and greater trochanter	Caudal	Elbow, ulnar side of forearm	Side-lying	Tuck your tailbone under. Press into my hand.
Quadratus lumborum	Pressure into the bone, no other vector	Fingers, knuckles, forearm	Side-lying	Extend your leg from the hip. Reach your arm overhead.
Gluteus medius or tensor fascial latae, down the iliotibial band	Caudal	Forearm, knuckles, full hands	Side-lying	Lengthen your leg from the hip joint. Press into my hand.
Trunk				
Psoas	Pressure into the muscle	Fingers	Supine	Breathe in and out.
Rectus abdominus	Diagonally, cephalic, and medial	Fingers	Supine	Tuck your tailbone under. Breathe in and out.
Lumbar fascia	Diagonally, cephalic, and medial	Elbow	Prone	Tuck your tailbone under.
L5 to S1 joint (sacrum)	Cephalic	Cupped hand	Prone or supine	Breathe in and out.

(*continued*)

TABLE 6-3 Deep Direct Connective Tissue Applications (by Region) (continued)

Region	Direction of Force	Therapist's Body Tools	Client Position	Movement Cue
Sacrotuberous ligament (just medial to ischial tuberosity)	Pressure into the bone, no other vector	Fingers	Prone	Tuck your tailbone under.
Paraspinal fascia	Caudal	Fingers, knuckles	Prone or seated	Tuck your tailbone under. Push your feet into the floor (when seated).
Neck and Shoulder				
Trapezius	Caudal	Forearm	Seated	Turn your head to the side. Press into my hand.
Sternocleidomastoid	Caudal	Backs of fingers	Supine	Turn your head to the side.
Scalenes	Caudal	Fingers, thumb	Supine	Turn your head to the side.
Pectoralis minor	Cephalic	Fingers, knuckles	Supine	Reach your arm overhead.
Serratus anterior	Caudal	Fingers, knuckles	Supine	Reach your arm overhead.
Subscapularis	Medial, reaching anterior to scapula	Fingers, knuckles	Supine	Reach out with your elbow.

sage). Rub the ice over the area for 5 minutes (ice friction) or leave a pack on for 10 minutes (or less if it becomes uncomfortable). Suggest an ice application at least twice on the day of the massage and one to three times the next day to prevent swelling and pain.

The following recommendations for optimal use of movement cues summarize the essential aspects of applying micromovements to the basic deep CT stroke. Many of these suggestions have been adapted from Shea (1995). Shea trained as a Rolfer and currently teaches a popular form of myofascial technique.

1. Ask the client to *practice* the movement before applying pressure. The way that the client chooses to perform the micromovements may provide clues as to where the CT net is immobile or stuck. The micromovements practice may also highlight areas where movement is not continuous or easy.
2. Ask for *smaller* and *slower* movements. At first, clients tend to make movements that are too fast and too large. Clients need to be coached to make just enough movement to engage the layer that is stuck and to move slowly enough to keep it engaged. Large or gross motor movement tends to throw the therapist's pressure out to the superficial fascial layer.
3. Use *imagery* to help clients visualize what they are supposed to be doing. Some suggestions that promote slower and smaller movements include: "Let me see half of that movement," "Show just the first inch of movement," and "Just think about making the movement."
4. Ask for *one movement at a time* until you find the right one. The right movement is the one that engages the tissue, the one where you feel the movement under your hands. Asking for more than one movement at a time confuses clients unless they are already comfortable with the idea of moving during massage. When you and your client feel more confident with having the client move during massage, (i.e., when you both perceive the benefits of moving, including lengthening, freedom, enhanced relaxation, more awareness of the stuck body areas), you can ask the client to add in a second motion.
5. Select micromovements that move the joint closest to where you are applying pressure. For example, if you are massaging the medial hamstrings from the knee up to the thigh, begin by asking the client to "bend and straighten the knee just slightly." As you work toward the thigh, there may be a point where you lose the sensation of being moved along and guided by the client's knee micromovements. If so, switch the focus to the hip attachment of the hamstrings by instructing the client to "bend and straighten at the hip."
6. Another good instruction for movement is to suggest that clients breathe comfortably at their own pace. Easy breathing is particularly beneficial when addressing the fascia that surrounds muscles that move in inspiration or expiration (e.g., scalenes, quadratus lumborum, serratus anterior, internal and external intercostals).

7. Another good cue is to guide the client to push into (or away from) your hands with very tiny movements. You could effectively coach this movement by saying "move into my hands" or "let your bone come toward me."
8. Combine elements of recommendations 6 and 7 by asking the client to "breathe right into the area underneath my hands."
9. Help clients visualize the area you are working on. Show them a picture of the region from an anatomy chart or text. This engages conscious and voluntary aspects of healing into your session. Clients will better understand where you are working and actually see the unobstructed direction of the muscle fibers and fascia that lie in that area.
10. Use a mirror to show clients how their fascia holds and displays tensions. Do this before and after a session to point out improvements that the client could model after the myofascial massage and between sessions.
11. Ask the client to walk and notice how easy (or difficult) it is to move both before and after a session. It is better to emphasize what the client *can* do as opposed to what the client cannot. Your words will be more healing and empowering if they focus on ease of movement rather than stuck points or difficulties. This does not mean ignoring difficulties but rather acknowledging the freedom that was achieved within the boundaries that exist now.

See Table 6-2 for appropriate applications and a summary description of the deep direct CT technique.

Positioning, Draping, and Support

The direct CT approach involves working with a client from many angles, including in the supine, prone, and side-lying positions. You may be asking the client to shift positions even more often than in a neuromuscular massage, so make sure that you can coach the client in safe and modest turning procedures. Furthermore, the direct CT approach works best when there is skin to skin contact, so keeping the rest of the body draped and modest is essential. During deep work, clients must always be draped and comfortably warm, to ensure that the work does not feel invasive. Follow basic Swedish massage draping guidelines (see Fritz, 2000) and be sure to use the diaper or Buddha leg drape for extra-secure coverage. To drape the legs of a side-lying client, slide a thin edge of the drape under the knee, pull it through, and then shimmy it up. Roll the drape under itself to hold it in place or if you like, use a clothespin to hold the drape in place (see Figure 5-10). When applying direct CT techniques to a client in the side-lying position, remember that you must align your body differently to meet the same tissues from the side.

Propping is imperative with the direct CT approach. One component of your force in the deep direct CT technique always sinks down to the table. Thus, it is important to place a pillow or bolster directly underneath any bony areas where you apply this stroke. In general, pillows are preferable to bolsters because they conform more easily to the client's shape. A contour body cushion is an excellent tool for putting the client in a side-lying position. Whenever the client is in a side-lying position, remember to keep her top leg from compressing the bottom leg. Position the client's bottom leg out straight and place the bolster underneath the top leg, which is bent forward. Bolstering the top leg in this manner, rather than placing a pillow between the two legs, avoids compression of the medial leg arteries and veins (see Figure 5-11).

Treatment Planning and Decision Making

When designing a session or series of sessions, always begin with the specific needs of the client, as determined by a history and intake procedure. Client responses to standard questions may trigger more detailed and specific queries about possible contraindications, indications, discomforts, and pain. Based on this information, identify a plan of action (e.g., spending most of the treatment session on massaging the lower legs because of recurrent shin splints), which is then modified through palpating the current condition of the tissues as you work.

The deep direct CT approach is especially effective for reducing chronic inflammation from old injuries that have not healed correctly. Areas of chronic inflammation are easily identified as being colder, harder or stiffer, lighter, whiter or bluer in color (this relative difference in color can be detected even in persons of color). Chronically inflamed tissues are quite likely not painful until touched directly.

The basic deep CT stroke can be adapted to any region or segment of the body that requires attention. The key is to know where muscles are divided by septae and to be aware of the general direction of muscle fibers that lie beneath your hands. Remember that your basic deep CT stroke is determined by the direction of muscle fibers because your goal is to lengthen the CT sheaths that cover them.

Your contact tool is determined by the targeted body part and tissue condition. The forearm provides a very broad contact, whereas the elbow provides a contact that is pointed and focused (Figure 6-11). The radial (fleshy) side of the forearm provides a wide diffuse contact, while the ulnar (bony) side provides a wide but more concentrated contact. Simply

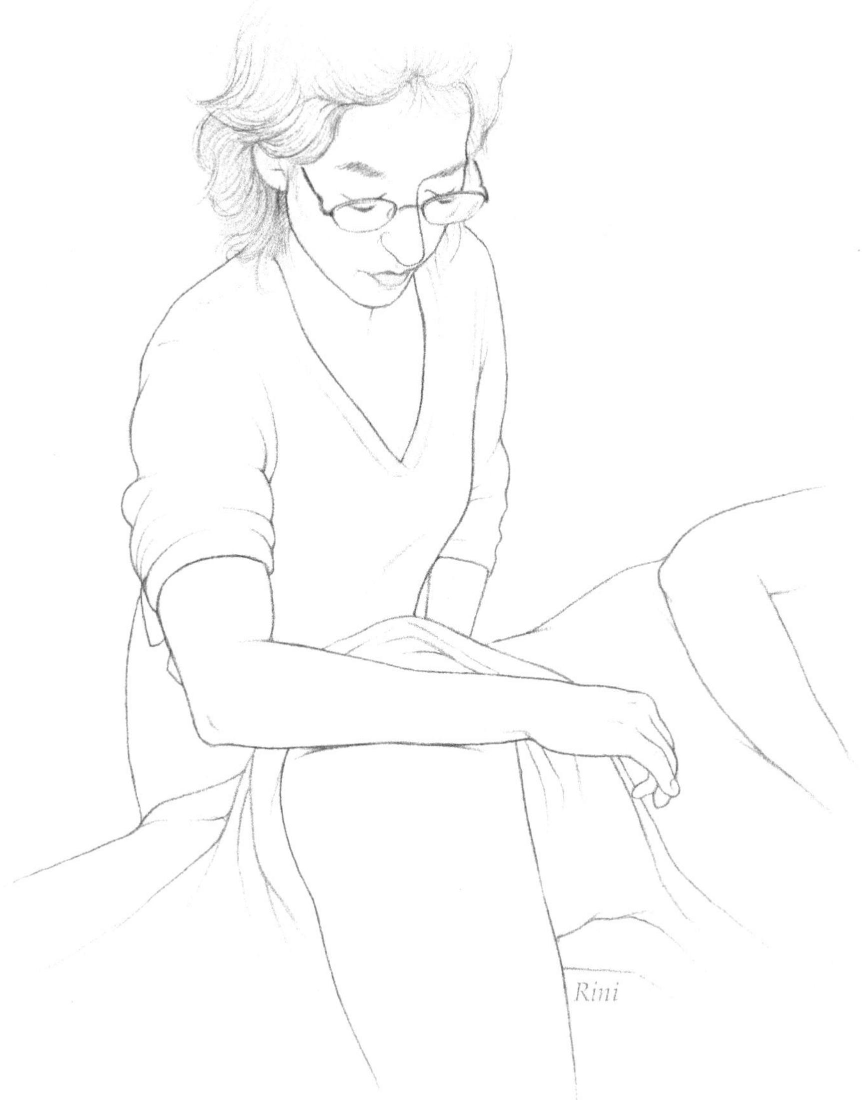

FIGURE 6-11 **Forearm and elbow as contact tools.** (**A**) Using the medial or ulnar sides of the forearm as a tool.

flexing the arm can take you through a continuum that increasingly concentrates your efforts on more specific areas with a more and more penetrating or keen touch.

Table 6-3 provides an overview of how to position yourself and your client and what part of your body to use as the contact tool for any specific body region that needs a deep direct CT approach. It is important to remember that such charts can really only give a starting orientation for the application of the deep direct CT stroke. Body awareness of your own discomfort will help to modify the strokes so that they are most effective for you. "Fiddling" around with your body position is actually at the heart of myofascial massage work. It means lining up your body so that you meet the resistance head on, which helps you listen to the client's body in the most effective way.

It is *not* a good idea to perform deep direct CT techniques on more than three areas of the body (two is better) in any one session. Pressure receptors can become overloaded with information about where to focus for lasting and effective change. In my practice, I usually identify a few chief complaints or target areas during the interview and spend the majority of the session working with these or along a fascial line that moves out from the area of an initial complaint, like unraveling a knot in a sweater. Do not forget to attend to the rest of the body (in addition to the regions of focus) through holding, compression, or some

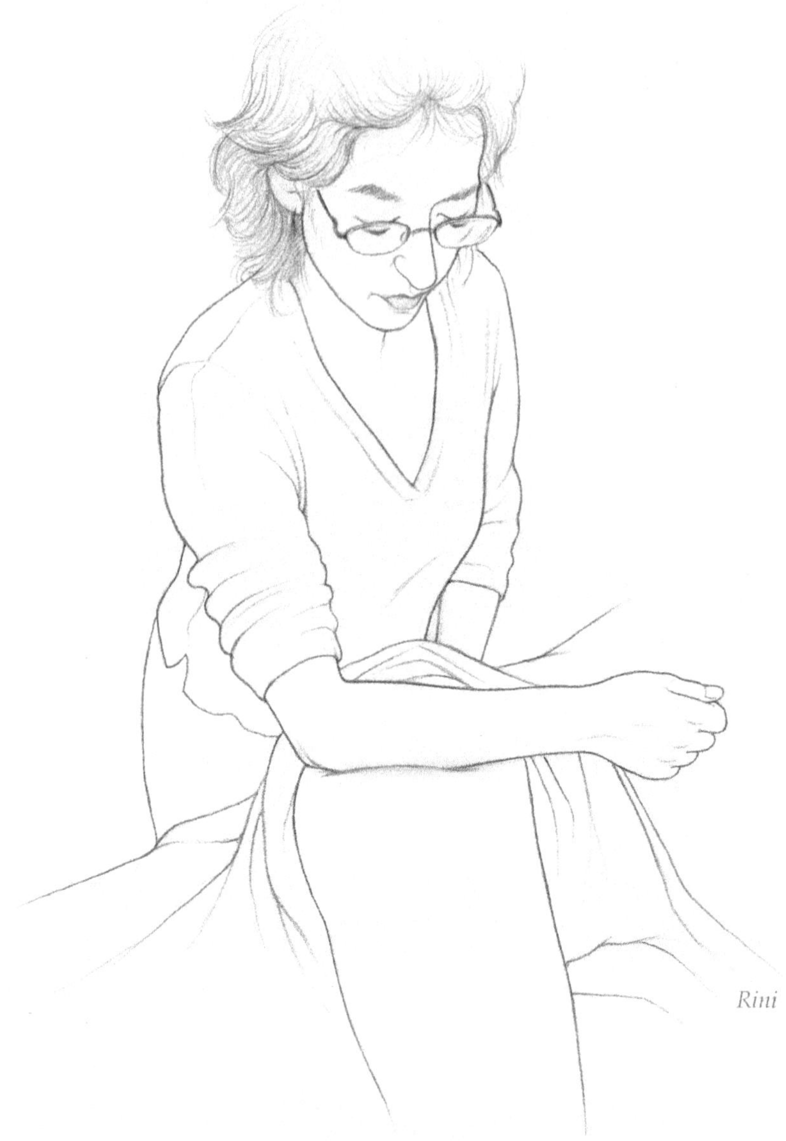

FIGURE 6-11 Forearm and elbow as contact tools (continued). (**B**) Using the lateral or radial sides of the forearm as a tool.

other contact. (The indirect CT approach, described in Chapter 8, combines well with direct CT massage.) The direct CT approach takes patience; you will need to devote more time and attention to identified focus area than if you were using Swedish massage. It takes time to tap into the CT layer and listen to where it is drawing your hands; however, clients report that such directed work feels more complete than a superficial session that touches all parts of the body but does not pay real attention to any distinct region.

You could choose to use a plan for a 10-session Rolfing-like approach to resculpt the body (see p. 108). (Use Table 6-3 to identify how to position yourself and your client for each area of focused deep direct CT work. Table 6-3 also suggests which body part to choose when contacting each specific target area and which direction to face as you apply each deep direct CT stroke.)

Alternately, Shea (1993) has suggested a two-session protocol for bodyworkers who prefer to address the entire body in a proscribed plan (see p. 108).

SUMMARY

The direct CT approach is especially useful for dealing with chronically inflamed and painful areas. This approach is reputed to have more immediate and longer-lasting therapeutic effects than other types of massage for these kinds of issues. Direct CT work involves using sustained pressure

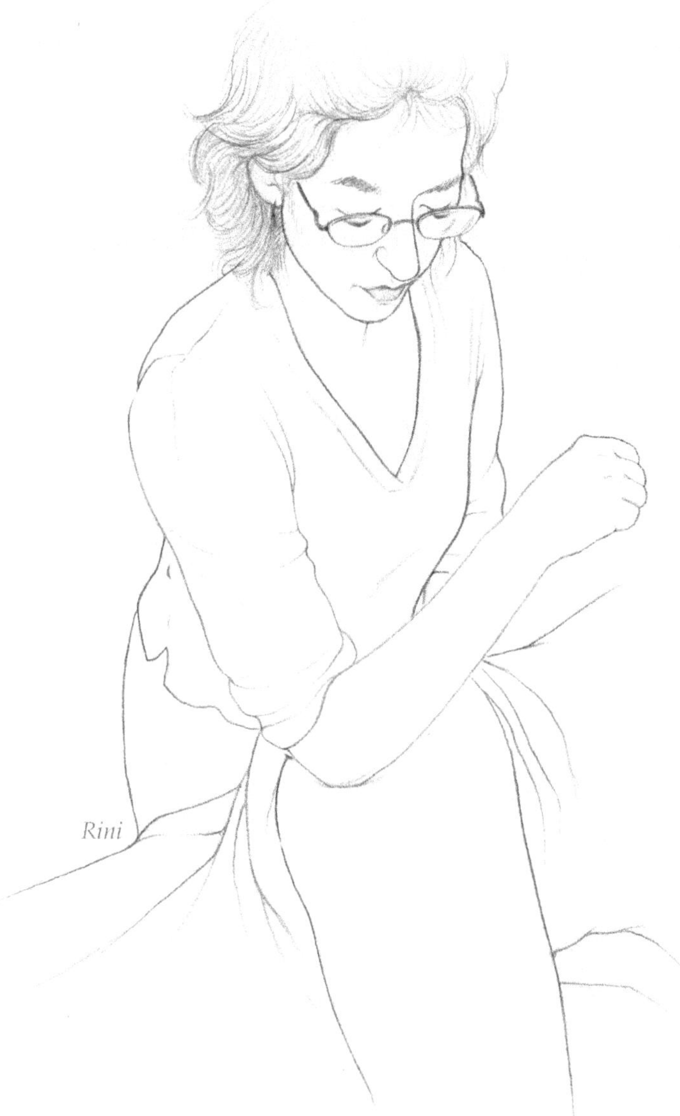

C

FIGURE 6-11 **Forearm and elbow as contact tools (continued).** (C) Bending at the elbow allows the therapist to focus more pressure on a smaller area.

with coached micromovements. Elements of the direct CT approach can be observed in muscle sculpting, deep effleurage, Rolfing, deep longitudinal friction, postural or structural integration, and John Latz's style of CT massage.

Direct CT massage can target the superficial fascia, which is the loose CT just under the skin. Superficial fascia can be readily identified on muscle charts as the whitest areas near the bones (e.g., lumbar fascia at the low back, extensor retinaculum around the ankles). Superficial direct CT strokes include skin rolling, compression, myofascial stretching, and scraping ligaments such as the iliotibial band or the CT that lies over bone.

Direct CT massage can also target the deep fascia. There are at least three identifiable planes of deep fascia. The superficial plane of deep fascia is found around superficial muscles such as the trapezius and in large CT-only areas such as the lumbar fascia. The middle plane surrounds deeper muscles such as the rhomboids and quadriceps. The deep plane surrounds even deeper muscles, such as the adductors and psoas. In certain places in the body (e.g., at the extensor retinaculum around the ankle), all three deep planes and the superficial fascia are accessible. The depth of the fascial plane and the lie of the muscle fibers at that level determine the optimal direction of a deep direct stroke.

The basic deep direct CT stroke is described as the convergence of two vectors. The composite impetus results in an oblique line of contact that converts the downward vec-

TEN-SESSION PROTOCOL

1. **Session 1:** Superficial direct CT focused on the back and areas of major complaint
2. **Session 2:** Deep direct CT focused on the feet and the lateral side of lower leg
3. **Session 3:** Deep direct CT focused on the back and the medial side of lower leg
4. **Session 4:** Posterior and medial thigh up to the gluteal muscles
5. **Session 5:** Lateral sides of the trunk, hips, and thigh
6. **Session 6:** Anterior trunk and back
7. **Session 7:** CT surrounding deep muscles of the truck and hips (psoas, piriformis, and other external rotators; quadratus lumborum)
8. **Session 8:** Upper extremities, chest, and shoulders
9. **Session 9:** Neck
10. **Session 10:** Seated work integrating entire spine (neck and back)

Note: Although structural integration and Rolfers often include intraoral bodywork in their formalized 10-session treatments, work inside the mouth is not described in this chapter. It is an advanced application of myofascial massage and thus, is outside of the scope of this overview text. See Shea (1993) for a written description of intraoral deep direct CT techniques.

TWO-SESSION PROTOCOL

1. **Session 1 (superficial focus):** The client is in the side-lying position, and bodywork is concentrated on the lateral malleolus, interosseus membrane, greater trochanter and iliotibial band, back, and neck.
2. **Session 2 (deeper focus):** The client is in the prone position, and bodywork is concentrated on the Achilles tendon, hamstrings, ischial tuberosities, back, and neck.

tor into a more forward stretching movement, maximizes the stretch on the collagen fibers that make up dense CT, and minimizes any invasive or compressive contact.

Take time to align yourself, incorporate breaks to encourage breathing and active stretch, and cue the client to perform micromovements to optimize the effectiveness of the deep direct CT stroke.

You can customize the basic deep direct CT stroke to any part of the body and can adapt any massage to incorporate some direct CT techniques, as needed. You can also address the entire body with the direct CT approach in 10 sessions. Alternately, you could address superficial and deep planes of fascia with a two-session plan.

Review Questions

1. The direct CT approach to myofascial massage is exemplified by ____________, ____________, and ____________.
   a. Rolfing, deep longitudinal friction, and postural integration
   b. rocking, rolling, and gliding
   c. trigger point release, muscle energy techniques, and percussion with stretch
   d. effleurage, pétrissage, and tapotement
2. Which is *not* a direct technique for releasing superficial fascia?
   a. stretching
   b. compression
   c. raking
   d. basic deep direct CT stroke
3. The direct CT approach is typically used for ____________ inflammation.
   a. acute
   b. subacute
   c. chronic
   d. all kinds of
4. The direct CT approach involves sustained ____________ with movement.
5. Name three possible strategies to use during a session with a client who is experiencing an overload of physiological change from direct CT bodywork, as evidenced by tremoring or giggling during the session.
6. Name a physiological change (other than tremoring or giggling during the session) that you might observe if your client has not had enough time to integrate a change in his or her stress level.
7. True or false: To maintain efficient body mechanics in the direct CT approach to myofascial massage, a good rule is to keep your feet facing out and wider than you would in performing Swedish strokes.
8. True or false: Maintaining contact in the direct CT approach means that you should always keep one hand on your client's body during sessions.

REFERENCES

Barnes JF. Myofascial Release Handbook. Paoli, PA: MFR Seminars, 1995.

Fritz S. Mosby's Fundamentals of Therapeutic Massage. 2nd Ed. St. Louis: Mosby, 2000.

Juhan D. Job's Body: A Handbook for Bodywork. Barrytown, NY: Barrytown, Ltd., 1998.

Langevin HM, Churchill DL, Cipolla MJ. Mechanical Signaling through Connective Tissue: A Mechanism for the Therapeutic Effect of Acupuncture. Burlington, VT: Department of Neurology, University of Vermont, 2001.

Latz J. Key elements of connective tissue massage. Massage Therapy 2003;4:44–53.

Manheim CJ. The Myofascial Release Manual. 3rd Ed. Thorofare, NJ: SLACK Inc., 2001.

Oschman JL. Energy Medicine: The Scientific Basis. Edinburgh, UK: Churchill Livingstone, 2000.

Schultz RL, Feitis R. The Endless Web: Fascial Anatomy and Physical Reality. Berkeley, CA: North Atlantic Books, 1996.

Shea M. Myofascial Release: A Manual for the Spine and Extremities with Intra-oral Supplement. Juno Beach, FL: Shea Educational Group Inc., 1993.

Travell JG, Simons DG. Myofascial Pain and Dysfunction: The Trigger Point Manual. Vol. 1: The Upper Extremities. Baltimore: Lippincott Williams & Wilkins, 1999a.

Travell JG, Simons DG. Myofascial Pain and Dysfunction: The Trigger Point Manual. Vol. 2: The Lower Extremities. Baltimore: Lippincott Williams & Wilkins, 1999b.

Upledger JE, Vredevoogd JD. Craniosacral Therapy. Seattle, WA: Eastland Press, 1983.

SUGGESTED READINGS

Myers TW. Anatomy Trains: Myofascial Meridians for Manual and Movement Therapists. London: Churchill Livingstone, 2001.

Riggs A. Deep Tissue Massage. Berkeley, CA: North Atlantic Books, 2002.

Rolf IP. Rolfing: Establishing the Natural Alignment and Structural Integration of the Human Body for Vitality and Well-Being. Rochester, VT: Healing Arts Press, 1989.

Schultz RL, Feitis R. The Endless Web: Fascial Anatomy and Physical Reality. Berkeley, CA: North Atlantic Books, 1996.

Chapter 7

Hatha Yoga to Supplement Direct Methods

OBJECTIVES

- Discuss how hatha yoga is an important supplement to direct myofascial massage methods.
- Describe the background and history of hatha yoga.
- Discuss research, styles, and goals pertaining to hatha yoga.
- Demonstrate understanding of some basic hatha yoga techniques.
- Discuss how direct myofascial massage can be reinforced with recommendations that encourage the safe practice of hatha yoga.

CHAPTER OUTLINE

KEY TERMS

Yoga: Sanskrit word from the root *yug* (to join, yoke, or concentrate together). A method or discipline that seeks to join the body, mind, and self (soul) or the union between the individual self and the transcendental self.

Ayurveda: Sanskrit term meaning knowledge of the way to live or knowledge of longevity. A comprehensive system of healthcare that emphasizes the interrelatedness of body, mind, and spirit, and seeks to restore an individual's innate harmony. Therapies include foods, herbs, and lifestyle changes, as well as asanas (postures), pranayama (breathing practices), and mantras (sacred sounds) specific to a patient's unique constitution.

Hatha yoga: Branch of yoga that emphasizes the practice of physical postures called asanas (asans) and breathing exercises called pranayama.

Asanas (asans): Physical postures used in hatha yoga; can include standing poses; forward, backward, and lateral bends; spinal twists; and seated, reclining, and inverted poses.

Pranayama: Breathing exercises that enhance the flow, effectiveness, and balance of asanas. Sometimes considered a meditation practice.

Prana: Life energy that travels freely throughout the body.

Chapters 5 and 6 introduced two distinct hands-on approaches to treatment with myofascial massage. Although the approaches are somewhat different, neuromuscular and direct connective tissue (CT) techniques both meet resistance in the tissues with a direct counterforce. As we discussed, it is an art for the myofascial therapist to find the right amount of resistance to meet the soft tissues where they are. In turn, the massage client kinesthetically learns to respond to the pressure by letting go rather than fighting back and further tightening the muscles. Client awareness can be further enhanced through a program of self-care that reinforces meeting resistance in the soft tissues and waiting there to allow the body to let go. Such kinesthetic learning is exactly what is conveyed by the practice of hatha yoga.

The art of letting go of a resistance is not adequately reinforced by handing the client a list of stretches to perform between massage sessions. Awareness of the breath and focusing the mind on target areas of resistance are crucial to helping the client physically and psychologically understand how to let go. Thus, this chapter presents the discipline of hatha yoga, including its clinical uses, goals, and techniques, as a complement to the direct method of myofascial massage.

Hatha yoga can help clients to feel and meet resistance in the soft tissues without pushing past the pain barrier. For example, think of an easy "neck sidebend" in which you lean the head to one side until you feel some holding back. The challenge is not to push past the holding to force the myofascia to lengthen. Instead, the task is to be patient and wait to experience what kind of holding there is without trying to fight or change it. Just stay with the feeling of being with the resistance. When you wait and breathe and meet the resistance without shirking from it or fighting it, after a while, the body softens and you can lean the head to the side a little farther. In hatha yoga, small movements, initiated by the breathing actions, work together with the constant pull of gravity to soften restrictions, without the need for additional or excessive force. This process mimics almost exactly the combination of client micromovements and controlled pressure applied by the direct CT therapist working to soften myofascial restrictions.

It is important to keep in mind that diagnosis and prescription are outside the scope of practice for massage therapists. Thus, any hatha yoga routine should be prescribed by a licensed and qualified professional (i.e., a yoga therapist, physical therapist, physical trainer, or exercise physiologist). However, understanding the goals and benefits of hatha yoga stretches, and how to recommend and inspire their appropriate use, will greatly improve the clinical practice of direct myofascial massage methods.

Background and History

In *The Yoga Sutras*, a 2,000-year-old treatise on yogic philosophy, the Indian sage Patanjali defines yoga as "that which restrains the thought process and makes the mind serene." Yoga has been practiced in India for thousands of years and is traditionally used by spiritual seekers as a system of self-development for purification of the body and mind (Feuerstein, 2001). Practitioners describe yoga as a preventive as well as curative system of healing for the body, mind, and spirit.

Yoga is closely related to ayurveda, the traditional healthcare system of India. Ayurveda is the healing side of yoga, and yoga is the spiritual tradition from which ayurveda emerged. Through ayurveda, one supports yoga by maintaining the body and mind in a state of balance and well being. Ayurvedic therapies include foods, herbs, lifestyle changes, and asanas (postures), pranayama (breathing practices), and mantras (sacred sounds) specific to each patient's unique constitution.

Ayurvedic texts describe eight components or arms of yoga that encompass a philosophy of life:

1. *Yama* (self-restraint)
2. *Niyama* (routines)
3. *Asanas* (postures and physical exercises)
4. *Pranayama* (the use of breathing to achieve focus)
5. *Pratyhara* (withdrawal of mind from sense organs)
6. *Dharana* (concentration)
7. *Dhyana* (meditation)
8. *Samadhi* (emancipation)

This chapter examines the asanas and pranayama insofar as they relate to the practice of myofascial massage. It is not intended to teach the entire eightfold path. Please consult a yoga text for a complete discussion of the yoga system.

Hatha yoga emphasizes the practice of physical postures called asanas (asans) and breathing exercises called pranayama. Asanas can include standing poses; forward, backward, and lateral bends; spinal twists; and seated, reclining, and inverted poses. Pranayama breathing exercises enhance the flow, effectiveness, and balance of asanas. Together, asanas and pranayama can provide a system of movement and self-care that complements the use of the direct method of myofascial massage.

Clinical Uses and Mechanism of Action

Regular practitioners of hatha yoga claim that a balanced program of postures will improve the physiologic function of nerves, muscles, glands, and visceral organs (Farrell et al, 1999). Traditionally, hatha yoga is believed to work with the breath to facilitate the intake, assimilation, and movement of prana, or life energy, that travels freely throughout the body. Breath is thought to be the link between the body and the mind and thus, the key to achieving both physical and psychological wellness (Sovik, 2000). Practitioners believe it cleanses the body of toxins, clears the mind, energizes the body, releases muscle tensions, and increases muscle flexibility and strength (Feuerstein, 2001). Yoga purportedly increases strength by toning the muscles and by correcting the tightness and weakness that might otherwise result in conditions such as torn ligaments and pulled hamstrings (Globus, 2000).

The exact mechanism action of yoga is not known. It is thought that the autonomic nervous system becomes more balanced with yoga, resulting in lessened energy demands on the body. Preliminary research suggests that the efficiency of the cardiovascular and respiratory systems is also significantly enhanced (Mishra et al, 2001).

RESEARCH ON YOGA

Since scientific research on yoga began in the 1920s, nearly 2,000 studies on yoga (including postures, breathing exercises, and meditation) have been published, primarily in India (Achterberg et al, 1994). Many of these studies support the effectiveness of yoga in reducing symptoms of a variety of diseases and promoting other beneficial physiological changes. Most studies of yoga, however, are small, poorly designed, and inadequately controlled, and many include co-interventions, leading to questions about the accuracy of the conclusions (Luskin et al, 2000).

Studies have found that yoga has a wide range of beneficial physiological and psychological effects on numerous body systems. After yoga training, the cardiovascular system appears to function more efficiently, showing increased endurance and aerobic power, improved blood flow, lowered systolic and diastolic blood pressure, and decreased heart rate (Pandya et al, 1999). In a landmark study, cardiologist Dean Ornish and his colleagues (1983) showed that yoga training plus dietary changes reduced cholesterol levels by an average of 14 points in 3 weeks and increased the work efficiency of the heart. Another study found reductions in blood pressure, heart and respiratory rate, and body weight among healthy physical education teachers who had already exercised an average of 9 years before receiving 3 months of yoga training (Telles et al, 1993).

Yoga has been found to lead to positive changes in respiration, including increased chest expansion, vital capacity, and tidal volume (Kant et al, 2000; Sovik, 2000; Udupa and Singh, 1972). No clear evidence yet exists that yoga improves the symptoms of asthma, although several published studies have investigated this subject (e.g., Ernst, 2000; Holloway and Ram, 2001).

Additional documented physiological changes that occur after practicing yoga include better ability to cope with stress (Baldwin, 1999; Schell et al, 1994); decreasing levels of serum cortisol and increasing levels of alpha wave activity in the brain (Kamei et al, 2000); changes in brain activities, including improvements in cortical activities and inhibition of limbic activities (Pandya et al, 1999); enhanced metabolic function (e.g., increased oxidation of fats and improved anabolic functions; Pandya et al, 1999); increased levels of mental and physical energy (Wood, 1993); increased spinal and hamstring flexibility (Baldwin, 1999); and significantly decreased hyperglycemia in non–insulin-dependent diabetics (Jain et al, 1993). Some of these physiological changes, such as lowered sympathetic tone, are assumed to occur via improved regulation by the autonomic nervous system (Pandya et al, 1999).

The practice of hatha yoga alone or with other ayurvedic therapies has been noted in ayurvedic texts to be beneficial in treating certain diseases and conditions such as hypertension, bronchial asthma, anxiety, depression, neurosis, gastrointestinal disorders, headache, and insomnia. The Indian literature reports that hatha yoga is beneficial for both acute and chronic pain management (Farrell et al, 1999). It attributes pain reduction to the increased flexibility and strength, decreased stiffness, increased body awareness, and decreased stress that comes from performing postures (Udupa and Singh, 1972).

Garfinkel and colleagues have evaluated yoga for osteoarthritis of the hand (1994) and for carpal tunnel syndrome (1998). In the 1998 study, in 8 weeks, the yoga groups had significant improvement in grip strength and pain as compared with the groups receiving wrist splinting or no treatment. The pilot study found significantly greater reductions in pain and increased finger range of motion in the yoga group.

In addition, the National Institutes of Health has funded the following studies related to yoga, which have not yet published results:

1. Efficacy of Yoga for Self-Management of Dyspnea in COPD (Virginia Carrieri-Kohlman, University of California, San Francisco).

2. Yoga as a Treatment for Insomnia (Sat Khalsa, Brigham and Women's Hospital, Boston, MA).
3. Effects of Yoga on Quality of Life during Breast Cancer (Alyson Moadel, Yeshiva University, New York, NY).
4. Evaluating Yoga for Chronic Low Back Pain (Karen Sherman, Center for Health Studies, Seattle, WA).
5. Yoga and Peak Flow Rates in Pregnant Asthmatics (Judith Balk, Magee Women's Health Corp., Pittsburgh, PA).
6. Effect of Yoga on Asthma (Prem Kumar, Tulane University, New Orleans, LA).
7. Ayurvedic Meditation and Yoga for Adolescents with Ulcerative Colitis (Lonnie Zeltzer, UCLA, Los Angeles, CA).

STYLES OF HATHA YOGA

Popular styles of hatha yoga practiced in the United States include:

- *Ashtanga,* or power yoga, with an emphasis on building strength, stamina, and flexibility
- *Bikram* or hot yoga, which includes 26 postures done in a 100°F or warmer setting
- *Iyengar* yoga (founded by yogi BKS Iyengar) a technically precise system that emphasizes the use of props such as blocks, bolsters, and straps to help people maintain proper alignment in poses
- *Jivamukti* (a variation of ashtanga) which emphasizes spiritual training, including chanting, meditation, and readings
- *Kripalu,* sometimes called the "yoga of consciousness"
- *Kundalini* yoga, which coordinates classic stretching postures and breathing exercises with chanting and meditation to stimulate the release of kundalini energy
- *Sivananda* yoga, named after the yogi who brought it to the West, is taught worldwide and advocates the rigorous application of postures, breathing exercises, relaxation, vegetarian diet, and study of scriptures
- *Viniyoga* (Feuerstein, 2001), which focuses on the health of the spine and on the function of each posture, rather than how accurately the practitioner executes each posture and uses a special breathing technique in conjunction with the postures to help the practitioner focus on the spine and feel internally how the body is responding to the movement into and out of a posture

GOALS OF YOGA TRAINING

Swami Rama (1979) identifies the fundamental teaching of yoga as "that man's true nature is divine, and with this realization comes liberation from all human imperfections."

The goal of "self-realization" obviously encompasses much more than the goal of releasing myofascia through applying direct pressure and micromovements. The goals of yoga and the direct method of myofascial massage, however, are compatible. The experience of meeting a physical resistance and letting go mirrors the experience of finding spiritual, emotional, intellectual, or other barriers that can be met and transformed.

Furthermore, the direct pressure used during tablework can be likened to the hatha yoga practice of adopting and holding a pose in the face of the body's resistance. Likewise, the direct CT technique of "coached" or conscious micromovements is akin to the hatha yoga practice of moving the body in synch with conscious breath.

The next section explores the specific techniques of hatha yoga.

Hatha Yoga Techniques

What follows is an elementary explanation of some basic techniques of hatha yoga, which are themselves only a small part of a highly evolved and complex discipline. It is strongly suggested that students interested in practicing yoga on a regular basis seek a qualified teacher and read additional texts. It is also strongly suggested that yoga practitioners demonstrate and practice with clients when recommending yoga poses and stretches as self-care. Some valuable books on hatha yoga practice can be found in the suggested readings at the end of this chapter.

BREATHING

Mastery of breathing (pranayama) is an important aspect of yogic training. In fact, learning to control breathing patterns can have direct, immediate value for increasing relaxation. For simplicity, breathing suggestions are incorporated into pose descriptions in this chapter. Pranayama is not presented here as a separate technique.

MEDITATIVE POSTURES

Meditative postures stabilize the body by aligning the torso, neck, and trunk. They provide an erect, very stable posture that allows for maximum relaxation with awareness: "body relaxed, mind alert." Meditative postures are believed to facilitate a clear pathway for breathing and the transmission of electrical impulses throughout the nervous system and the flow of energy (possibly by way of meridians or channels running through the CT).

The *comfortable pose* (*Sukhasana*) is the basic meditative posture. Sit with the legs extended forward. Comfortably

One Person's Experience: The Experience of Performing Hatha Yoga

Fifteen years ago, I taught hatha yoga to students at a large university in our nation's capital. A standard assignment in my class was to write a report about what it actually feels like to practice hatha yoga on a regular basis. The following is an excerpt from one student report. This account may provide additional insight into what it might be like for clients who supplement their direct myofascial massage sessions by practicing hatha yoga.

"Yoga has helped me come in contact with my own body, understand how it works, and love it more. Spending 10 to 20 minutes a day stretching out my body and relaxing my mind allows me the time to enjoy myself and appreciate my life. It helps me think more clearly about my schoolwork and my interpersonal relationships. Asanas have allowed me to understand how each muscle, joint, and ligament works and how to cope if they tense up. Oftentimes during the day when I don't have time to be alone, I go into the bathroom of the Marvin Center, stretch out, and take 10 deep breaths. If it is nice out, I take a break from my studies and treat myself to a 5-minute walk. I really feel the air entering my body when I breathe in and all of the bad energy leaving when I breathe out.

Yoga has helped me concentrate more efficiently on my work. I am less impatient and tense the night before an exam than I used to be. Before taking yoga, I was like many of my friends and classmates, forever busy, running around doing work, and worrying about papers and exams. I was keeping ungodly hours studying, but I was not able to concentrate fully on my work. Yoga has allowed me the opportunity to step out of my frantic collegiate life and simply enjoy myself. I now need that special time by myself to work productively in the outside world. Yoga to me is like another world that no one can touch."

cross the legs under the thighs, as demonstrated in Figure 7-1.

The *corpse pose* (*Savasana*) is another important resting pose. Many of my students and clients claim this as a favorite pose. To practice Savasan, lie down on a mat with your arms at your sides or slightly out from your body, with your palms facing up (Figure 7-2). With your eyes closed, scan your body for tension. Relax your face, your shoulders, your stomach, and any other areas of the body that hold tension.

ASANAS

The *salutation to the sun* (*Surya Namaskar*) is a series of asanas that are said to stretch and limber muscles throughout the body, but particularly the spine and legs. Each posture is counterbalanced in the next asana. It can be practiced alone or with other asanas. After two repetitions of the series, breathe easily and rest for at least 1 minute in Savasana.

1. *Mountain pose* (Figure 7-3A): Stand with feet shoulder-width apart and raise your arms in a circular arc over the head. Slowly let your arms come down and into a point in front of your chest. Hold your palms together

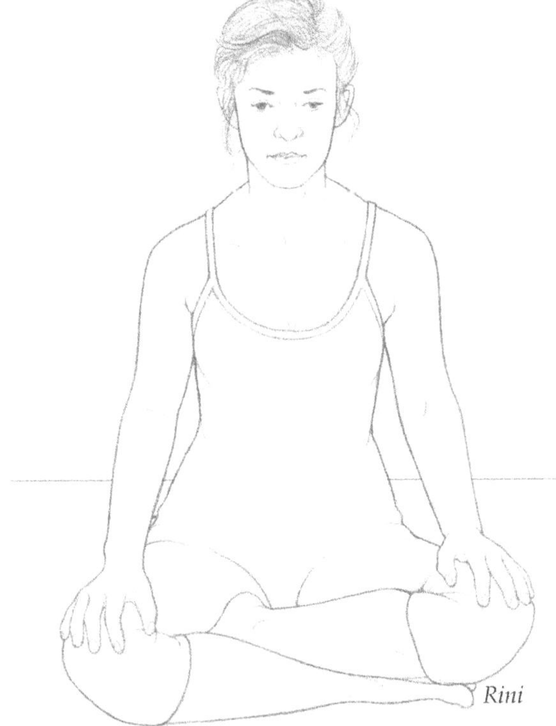

FIGURE 7-1 **Comfortable pose (*Sukhasana*).** Sitting with the legs crossed is the basic meditative posture.

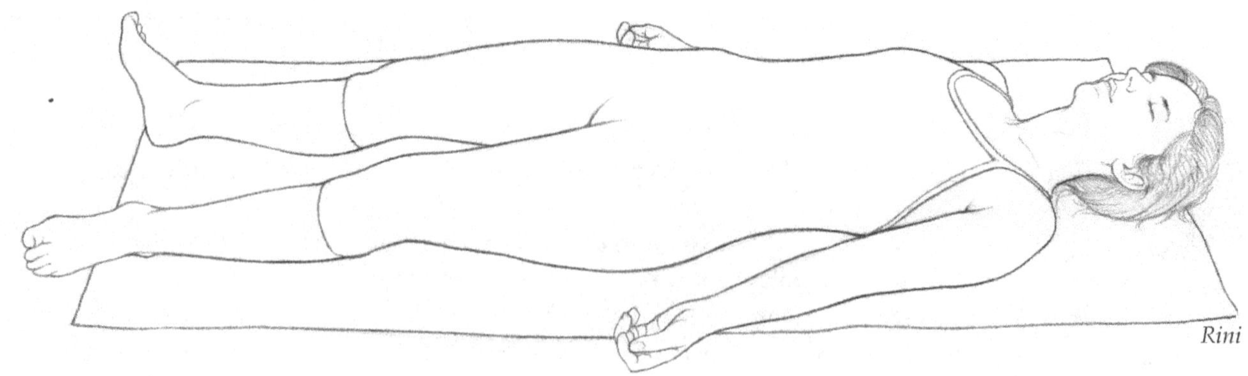

FIGURE 7-2 **Corpse pose (*Savasana*).** To practice this pose, lie down (like a corpse) with your palms facing up and relax any tensions that you notice.

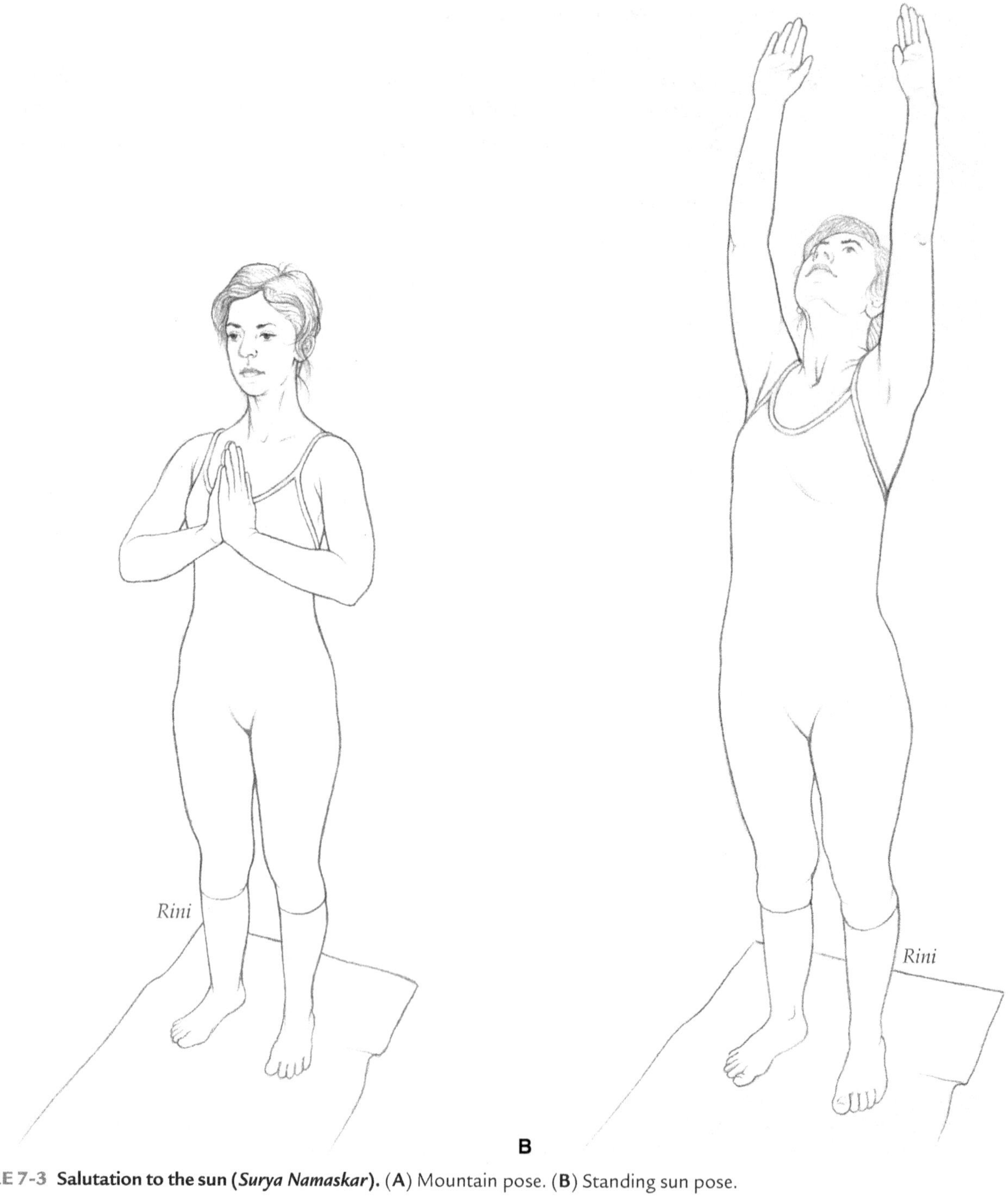

FIGURE 7-3 **Salutation to the sun (*Surya Namaskar*).** (**A**) Mountain pose. (**B**) Standing sun pose.

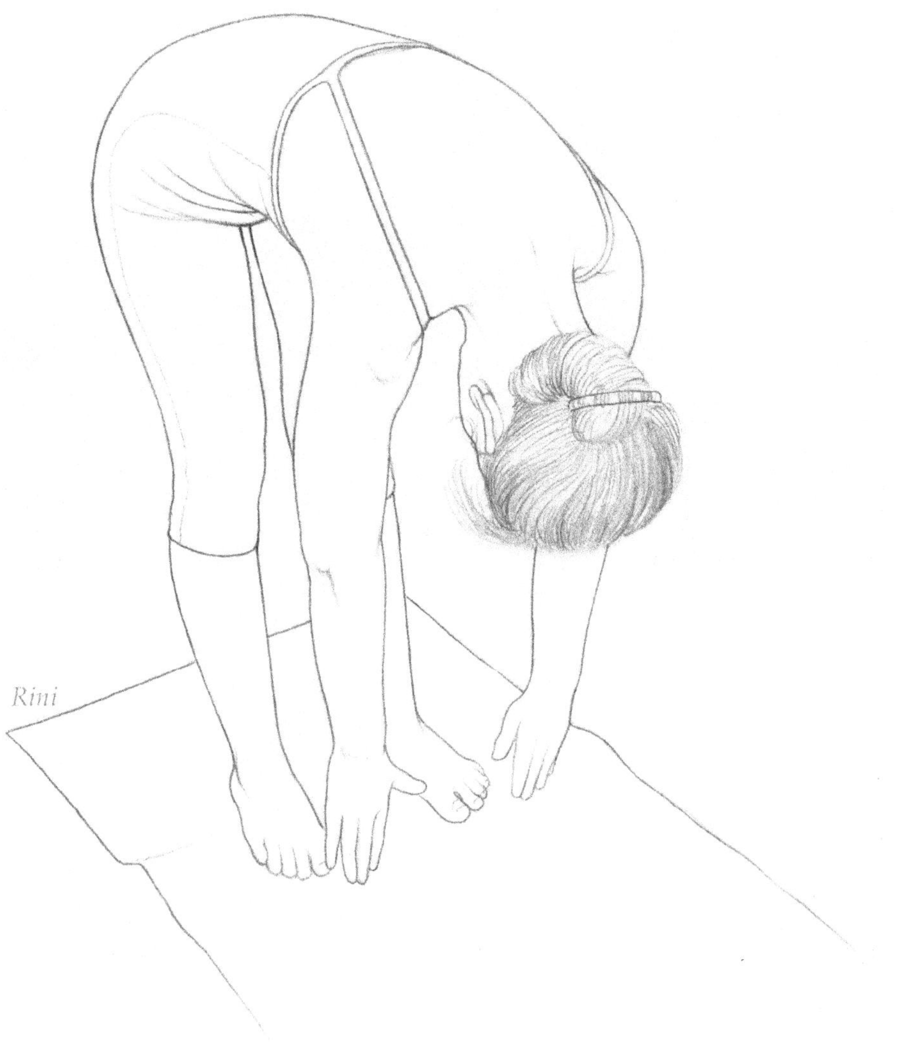

C

FIGURE 7-3 **Salutation to the sun (*Surya Namaskar*) (continued).** (C) Standing sun pose.

and exhale. Think of lengthening throughout the entire spine. Breathe in as you rotate your shoulders backward and breathe out as you let your shoulders down. Then breathe easily, allowing your body to relax any tension out of your body. Maintain the pose as you feel the air entering your nose on the in breath and your feet solidly on the ground ("strong as a mountain") during the outbreath.

2. *Standing sun pose* (Figure 7-3B and C): Raise your arms directly overhead and then back. Push from the waist and keep your legs straight and slightly arch the back. Keeping the line of your back straight, reach out forward and then down toward your toes. Keep your knees slightly bent. Reach only as far as comfortably possible.
3. *Forward lunge* (Figure 7-3D): Place your palms on the floor and then bring your right foot between your hands. Extend your left leg behind you and lower your knee to the floor. Inhale as you extend your leg and feel the stretch in the left groin area.
4. *Downward dog* (Figure 7-3E): Bring your right foot back to meet your left foot and exhale. Raise your hips and buttocks high, keeping your head and eyes directed toward your toes. Keep your arms fully extended.
5. Lower your knees, chest, forehead, and belly to the floor, in that order (Figure 7-3F). Slowly exhale throughout.
6. *Cobra pose* (*Bhujanangasan;* Figure 7-3G): Lie on your stomach with your toes together, forehead on the floor, and palms down next to your armpits. Your elbows will be up in the air. Begin to breathe in and raise just your head. Continue to lift your chest and then your stomach, curling your spine rather than pushing with your arms. Use mostly your back muscles to lift rather than your arms, although your arms are available for balance and support. Hold the pose for a moment, breathing gently (like a cobra). Start to breathe out and

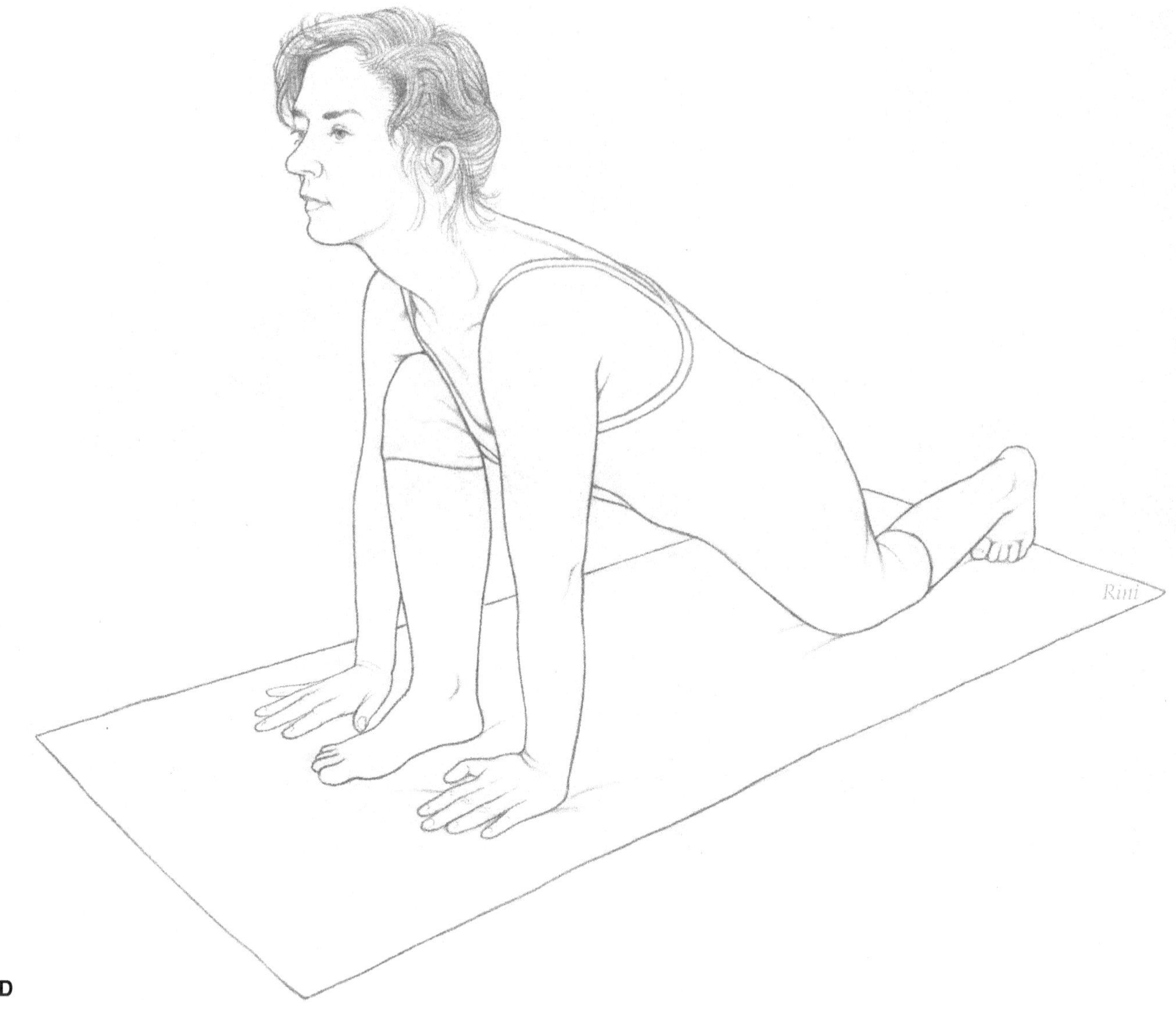

FIGURE 7-3 Salutation to the sun (*Surya Namaskar*) (continued). (**D**) Forward lunge.

uncurl slowly. Your stomach touches the ground first, then your chest, and finally your head.

7. Repeat the downward dog pose.
8. Repeat the forward lunge, but this time step forward with the opposite foot.
9. Repeat the standing sun pose.
10. Return to the mountain pose.

Although the *salutation to the sun* can be practiced in its own right, to flex and limber the entire body, some clients may want to focus on specific areas that presented resistance in a neuromuscular or direct CT session. Use the following asanas (and adaptations) as self-care suggestions for specific body regions.

Sidebends (variation on *Trikosana;* for latissimus dorsi, internal and external obliques, and iliotibial band): Begin in the *mountain pose* and then widen your stance farther apart. Raise your right arm and hand straight above your head. Rotate your head to look up at the right arm. Sidebend at the waist and extend your left arm and hand down to your left ankle (Figure 7-4). As you reach down, rotate your left foot out to protect your knee. Breathe in as you slowly reach up to the right. Hold this feeling of tension for 8 to 10 seconds. Breathe out and feel a good even stretch without overstretching. Repeat two or three times on each side.

Adapted sidebend (for latissimus dorsi): From a standing position, reach up behind your head and take hold of your right elbow with your left hand. Keep your knees slightly bent and gently pull your right elbow overhead as you laterally flex your trunk to the left (Figure 7-5). As with all of the stretches, breathe in while moving into position and breathe out as you hold the position and feel the muscles letting go. Repeat on the other side.

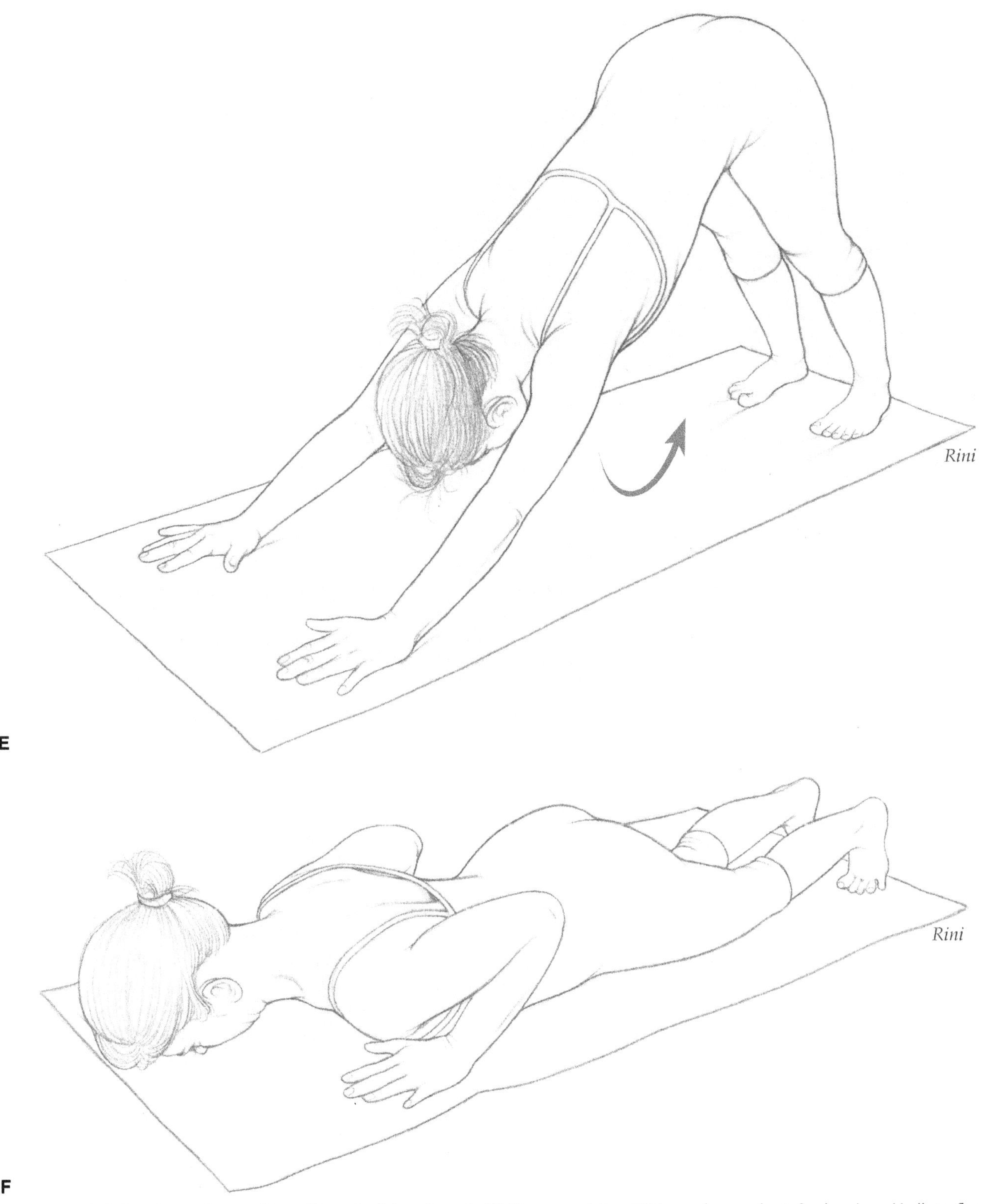

FIGURE 7-3 **Salutation to the sun (*Surya Namaskar*) (continued).** (**E**) Downward dog. (**F**) Lower knees, chest, forehead, and belly to floor.

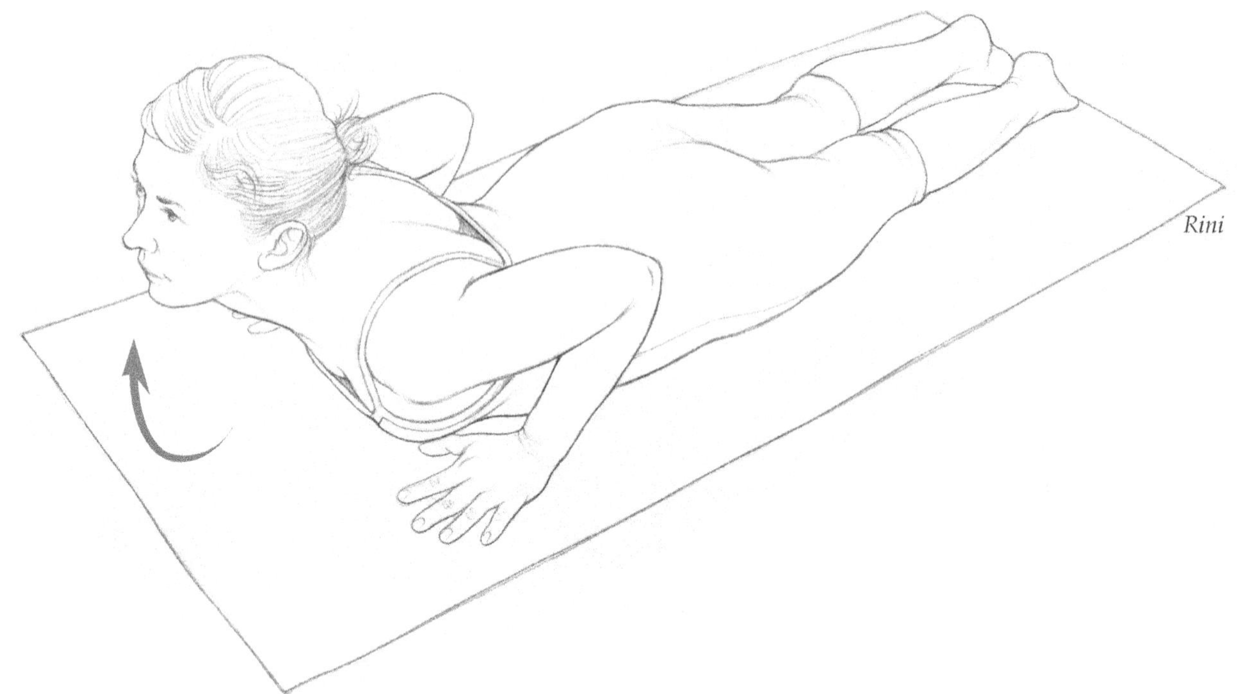

FIGURE 7-3 **Salutation to the sun (*Surya Namaskar*) (continued).** (G) Cobra pose (Bhujanangasan).

Adapted head of the cow (*Gomukhasana;* for deltoids and triceps): Stand with feet shoulder length apart and spine straight. Hold your right elbow with your left hand behind your head and give yourself a pat on the back (Figure 7-6). Do this slowly. As with all of the stretches, breathe in as you move into the pose, and breathe out as you hold the position and feel the muscles letting go. Repeat, reversing the positions of your arms. Notice if one side feels tighter than the other.

Adapted hands over head (*Araha Chakrasana;* for pectoralis muscles). To stretch your chest and shoulders, clasp your hands behind your back (Figure 7-7). Straighten your elbows and pull your shoulders down from your ears. Open your chest and lift, pretending to squeeze an imaginary grapefruit between your shoulder blades. This will bring your arms up behind you. Turn your elbows medially while straightening your arms. Do not tilt your torso forward. (Optional: Lean forward while slowly raising hands over head.) Hold for 8 to 10 seconds. This is great for rounded shoulders and gives an immediate feeling of energy. Exhale as you raise your clasped hands over head and inhale as you release and return to simple standing.

Thigh stretch (*Bandha Konasana*): Sit on a mat or cushion and begin with your knees bent and the soles of your feet touching. Breathe in as you allow your hips to rotate out (your knees will move away from each other to the sides) and completely relax as you exhale (Figure 7-8). This comfortable position stretches the groin muscles. Let the pull of gravity do the stretching. Maintain the position for 8 to 10 seconds. Repeat two or three times.

Adapted thigh stretch: Sit on a mat or cushion with your legs extended out to the sides. Inhale as you allow your hips to rotate out (your legs will extend out to the sides) and lean forward slightly (Figure 7-9). This adapted pose focuses on lengthening the long adductor muscles. Exhale as you hold the stretch for 8 to 10 seconds. Repeat two or three times. You may feel the tendons stretching at their attachments at the pubic bone or at the knee joint. If you wish, you could massage these attachments while holding the pose and breathing easily to get even more release.

You can do a variation of this stretch with a partner by facing one another and holding hands. As one partner leans back (leading with the back of the spine), the other is pulled forward into the stretch. Come out of the position into a straight-up resting pose after 8 to 10 seconds. Repeat with the opposite partner leaning back.

Intense floor stretch (*Uttibitisan*): Lie down on a mat or futon with your legs extended and your arms extended overhead. Inhale as you point your fingers and toes and exhale while you reach as far as is comfortable in opposite directions with your arms and legs (Figure 7-10). To also stretch the abdominal obliques, let your arms and legs extend out from the center of your body in an X shape. Alternate your reach so that you are reaching first the left arm and left leg, then the right arm and right leg, then the diagonal through the left arm and right leg

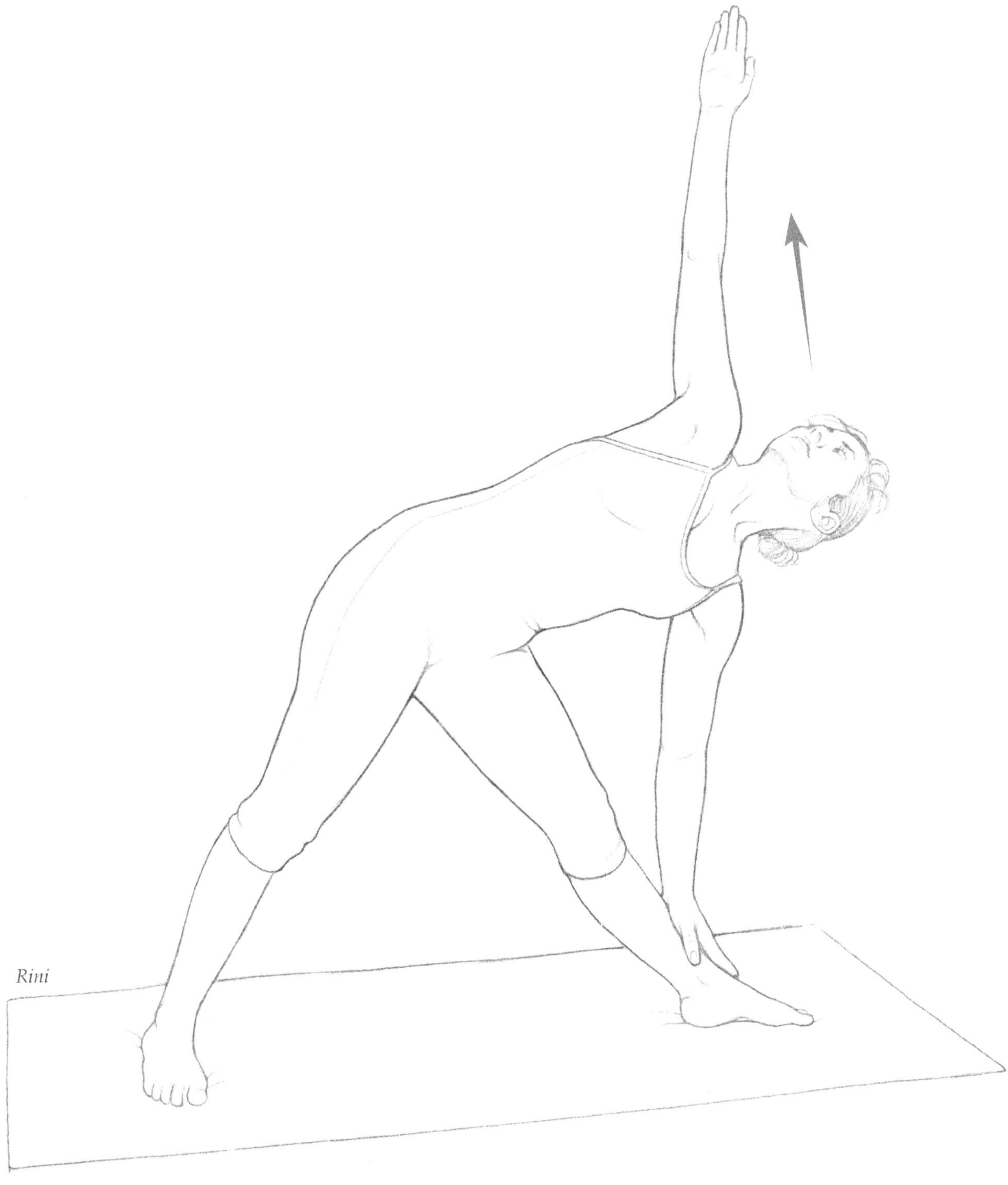

FIGURE 7-4 **Sidebend (variation of *Trikosana*).** Sidebends strengthen the stabilizing muscles of the feet, legs, hips, and spine, and can help even out differences in the paraspinal or hamstring muscles by gradually lengthening the shorter side.

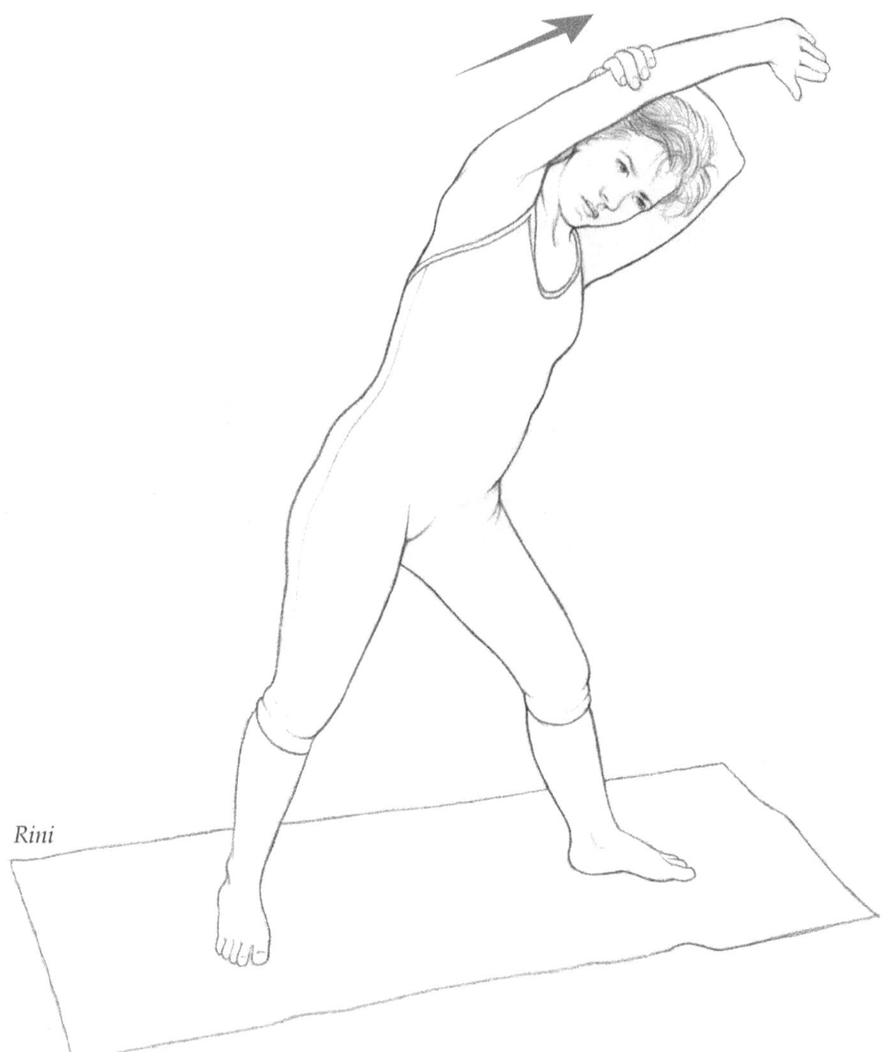

FIGURE 7-5 **Adapted sidebend.** From a standing position, reach behind your head and pull your right elbow overhead with your left hand as you bend your trunk to the left.

and the diagonal through the right arm and left leg. Now stretch in all four directions at once. Breathe in as you reach and breathe out as you hold the position for 8 to 10 seconds. Repeat each variation two or three times.

Knee squeeze (*Pavanamuktasana;* relieves low back pain and strengthens abdominal muscles): Lie on your back on a mat or futon and keep your back flat with your arms at your sides. (You could place a rolled-up towel underneath the lumbar curve for support.) Breathe in as you raise your right knee to your chest. With your lungs full, wrap your arms around your knee (Figure 7-11). Hold your breath in and squeeze your knee to your chest. Exhale and slowly relax, straightening your left leg. Repeat two or three times on each side.

Adapted sun pose (reclining, not sitting; *Pasdhimottanasan;* for hamstrings): Lie down on a mat or futon with one leg extended and the other knee bent with the sole of that foot flat on the floor. Lift the extended leg up to a vertical position. Place your hands behind the thigh or the lower leg (Figure 7-12). Hold a towel in both hands and hook it across the foot if you cannot reach behind your leg. (Note: Avoid putting pressure just behind the knee.) Make sure that your lower back muscles remain flat on the floor. Breathe in as you extend your leg and breathe out as you feel the stretch in the back of your thigh. Pay attention to whether the tension is focused on the tendon attachments at the hip or at the knee. If you wish, massage these attachments during the stretch to achieve more release. Remember to keep your straight leg straight. Sacrifice elevation for straightness. Now flex your knee and ankle and let your leg relax toward your chest. After resting for a moment, straighten your leg again, allowing it to stretch farther this time. Release and flex again and then stretch even farther.

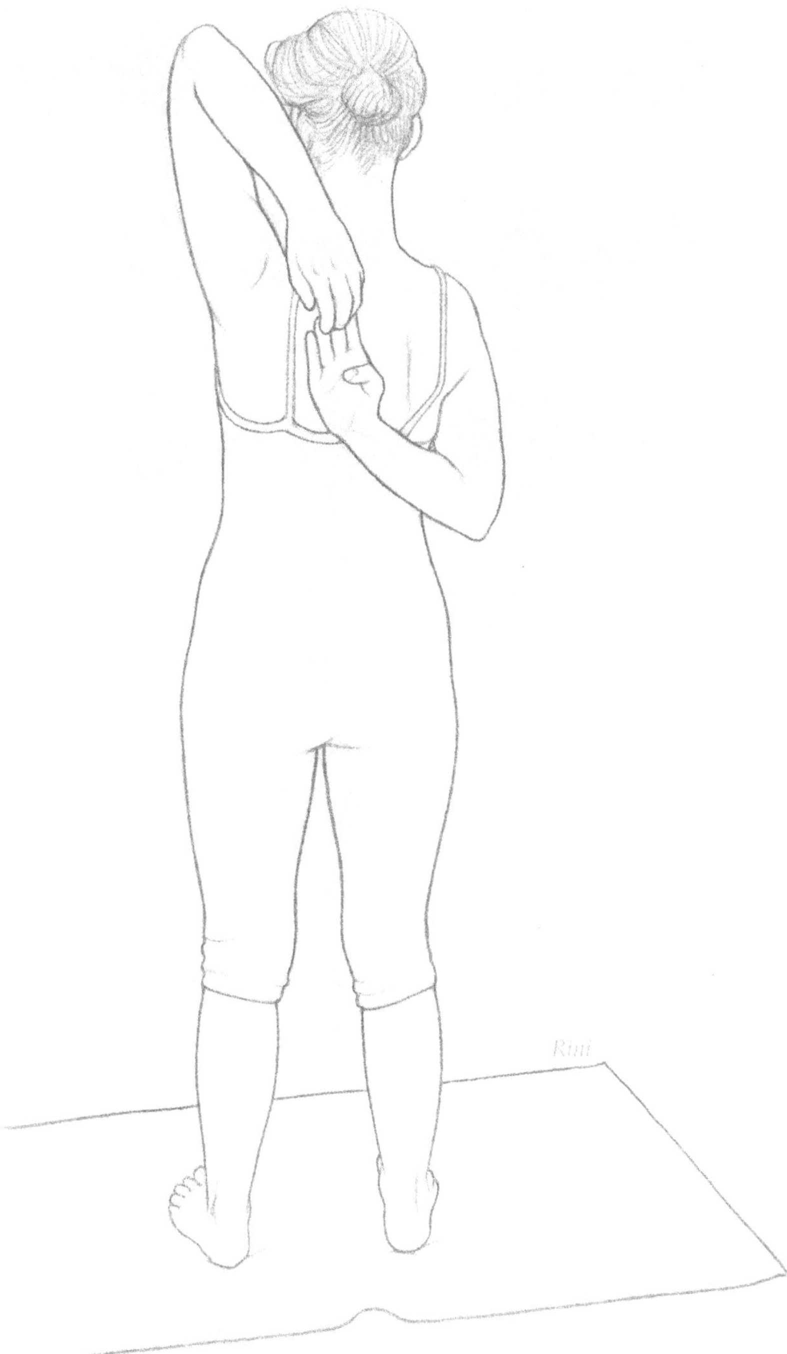

FIGURE 7-6 Adapted head of the cow (*Gomukhasana*). Hold your right elbow with your left hand behind your head and give yourself a pat on the back.

Adapted spinal twist (*Ardha Matsyendrasan;* for entire back): Start seated on a mat or cushion with both legs bent at the knee in front. Weave your right leg under your left, so your right knee rests on the floor and your right foot is next to your left hip. Place your left foot on the outside of your right knee (Figure 7-13). You will always be twisting away from the raised leg. Reach over the lifted (left) leg with your left arm and hold on to the outside of your right thigh with your left hand. Straighten your spine, look forward, and breathe in. Breathe out and twist to the right, keeping your head erect and eyes focused on a spot at eye level as far to the right as you can comfortably see. Hold the position for 8 to 10 seconds, breathing gently. Then release and switch sides.

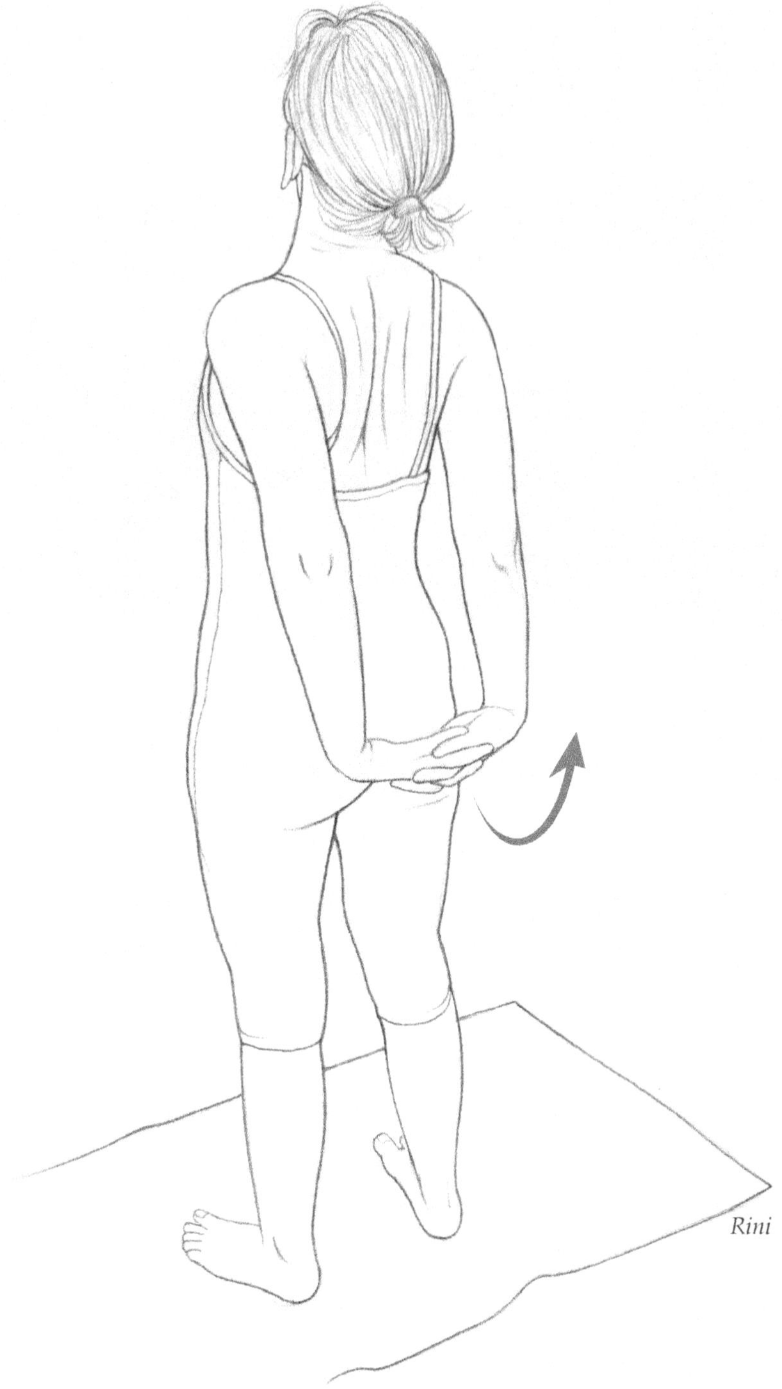

FIGURE 7-7 **Adapted hands over head (*Araha Chakrasana*).** Clasp your hands behind your back and squeeze your shoulder together to lift your arms behind you.

RECOMMENDATIONS FOR OPTIMAL USE

You may wish to put together in one document these suggestions as a self-care handout for clients. Distribute a copy when recommending and demonstrating specific hatha yoga asanas.

1. Do not push past a level of mild resistance. Stretching should feel good, like a cat stretching after a nap. Many of us incorrectly learned to associate pain with

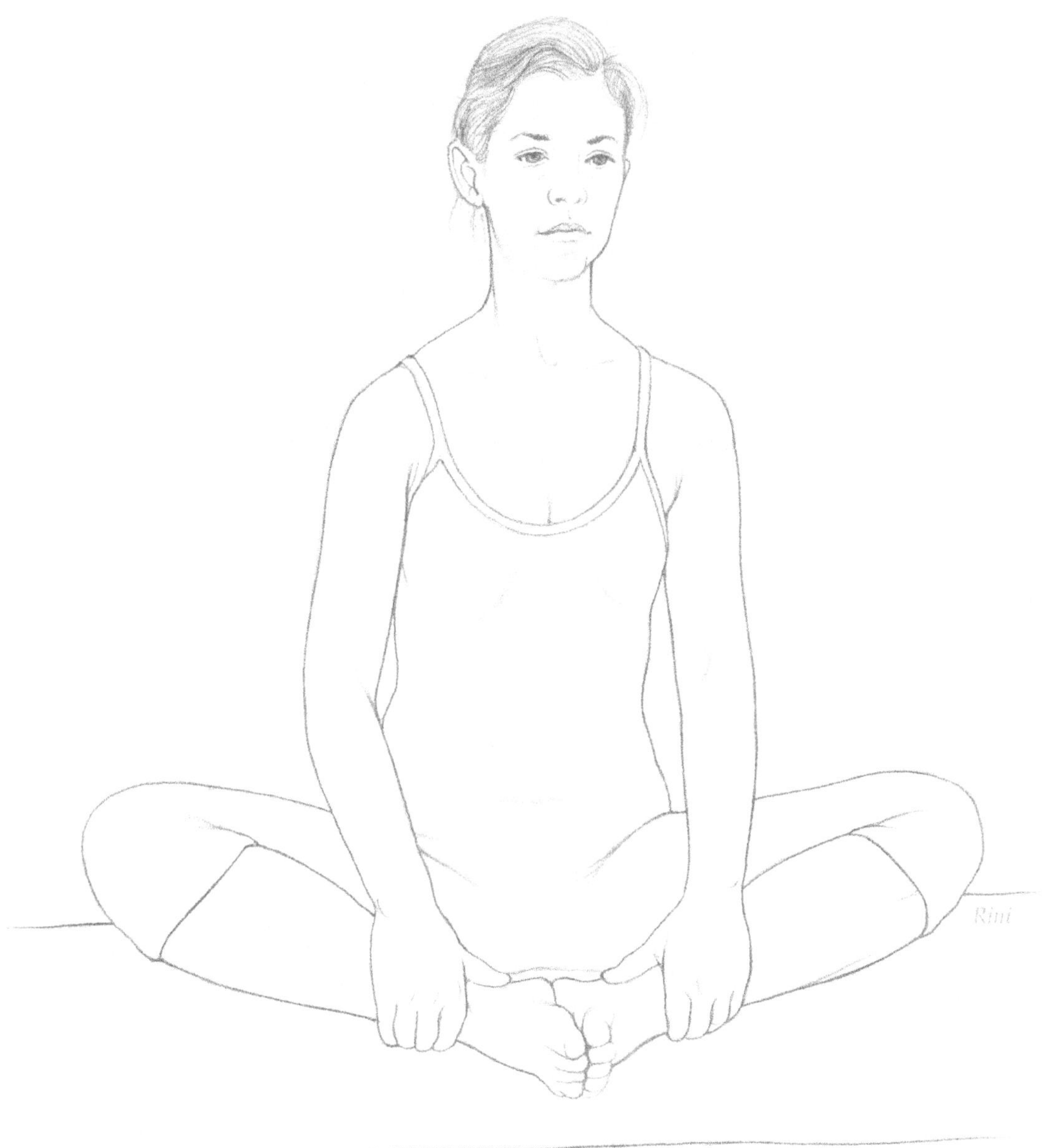

FIGURE 7-8 **Thigh stretch (*Bandha Konasana*).** Sit with your knees bent, hips rotated out, and the soles of your feet touching. This allows gravity to stretch the short adductor muscles of the hip.

physical improvement and were taught that the more it hurts, the better. That "no pain, no gain" adage is a myth. Pain is an indication that something is wrong.

2. Listen to your body's signals. A sharp, acute pain is a warning to immediately stop what you are doing. Any pain that does not go away after 4 or 5 days is a cue to seek medical attention.
3. If you think that you feel a resistance in the tissue, first sense and feel the breath move into the places of tension (e.g., neck, lower back, or behind the knees). Then consciously let go of the tensions by breathing out and imagining the tight area loosening and letting go.
4. If your body feels out of line, readjust your position. Breathe and move the area in a comfortable way. When you return to the asana, you will be fully present rather than halfway there.
5. After every few poses or after three repetitions of salutation to the sun, rest comfortably on your mat or futon in corpse pose (Savasana).
6. Conscious breath (pranayama) will increase your awareness, engage the stuck layers of myofascia, and make it easier to free restrictions in the web. In general, breathe in as you expand and breathe out as you contract or fold in on yourself.

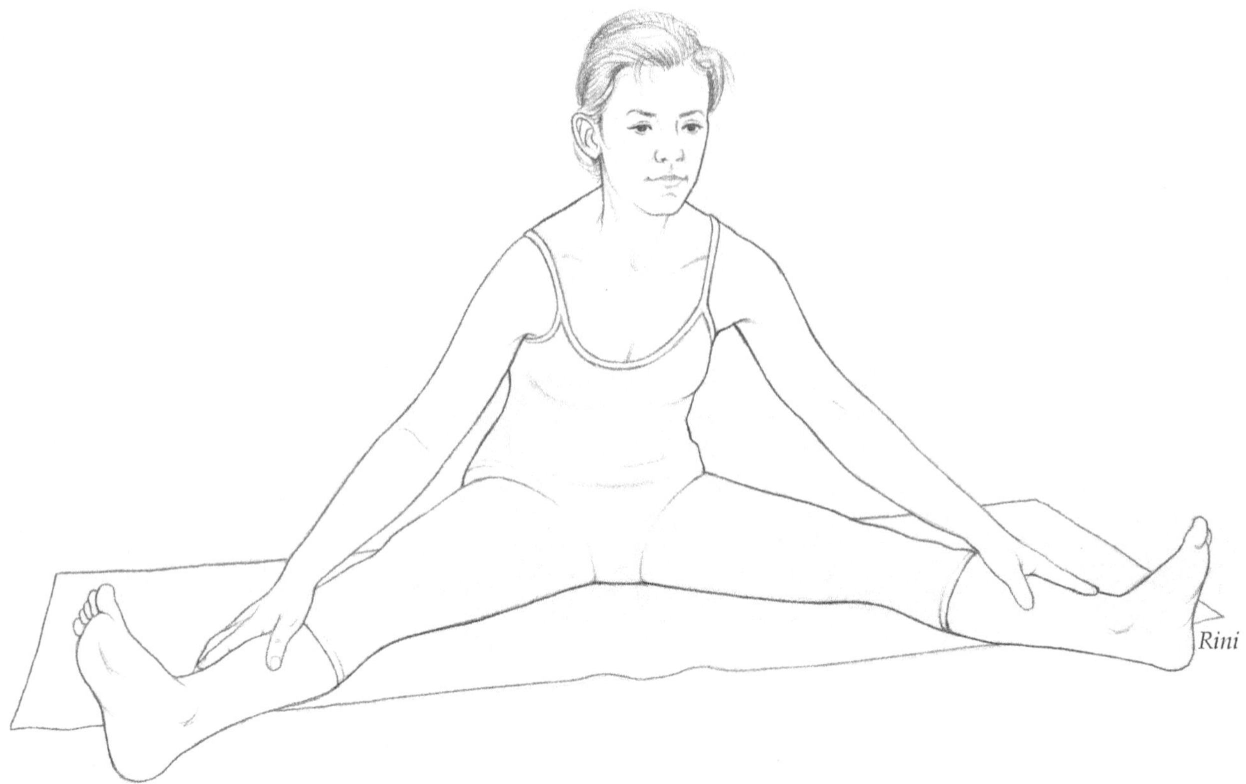

FIGURE 7-9 Adapted thigh stretch. Sit with your legs extended out to the sides to stretch the long adductors of the hip.

7. Remember that you are the expert when it comes to determining your body's needs. You know better than anyone does exactly when, where, and just how much resistance your body has. No one else can feel this as well as you can.
8. Practice your asanas when your body is warm. They will be easier to do, feel better, and be better for your body. Cold stretching hurts more and creates a greater opportunity to tear muscles.
9. Stretch only a little each time you practice, but practice more often. The effects of hatha yoga are cumulative. Five minutes of relaxed stretching twice every day is more effective that an hour spent grinding and groaning on the weekends.
10. Don't bounce! Pushing a stretch past the point where it hurts or bouncing up and down (ballistic stretching) will strain your muscles and activate the stretch reflex. These harmful procedures cause pain and physical damage because of microscopic tearing of muscle fibers. Tearing leads to the formation of scar tissue in the muscles and soft tissues, with a gradual loss of elasticity. Scarred muscles become even more torn and tender.
11. Try to follow forward-moving poses (e.g., sun pose) with backward-moving poses (e.g., cobra pose), right-sideways–moving poses with poses to the left, and so on.

Lessons to Learn from Hatha Yoga Practice

Although regular yoga practice improves body awareness, it requires some initial level of sensitivity to pain. Make sure clients understand that they should not push past a point where they feel a comfortable tension. This is the point of mild resistance and is the place where stretching has the most impact. When stretching correctly, after about 10 seconds have elapsed, the tension of the stretch should start to fade (Anderson, 1980). If the feeling does not subside or grows in intensity, the client is overstretching.

Muscles are protected by an internal mechanism called the "stretch reflex." As described in Chapter 2, any time muscle fibers are pulled too far or too fast (e.g., by bouncing or overextending), the stretch reflex is activated. A signal is sent to the muscles involved, telling them to contract. This prevents injury to the muscles. It is similar to the involuntary reaction that occurs when you accidentally touch a hot stove; without thinking, your body pulls away from the heat. When you stretch too far, the end result tightens the very muscles you are attempting to lengthen.

The major barriers to a continued practice of hatha yoga are working too hard and associating physical activity with

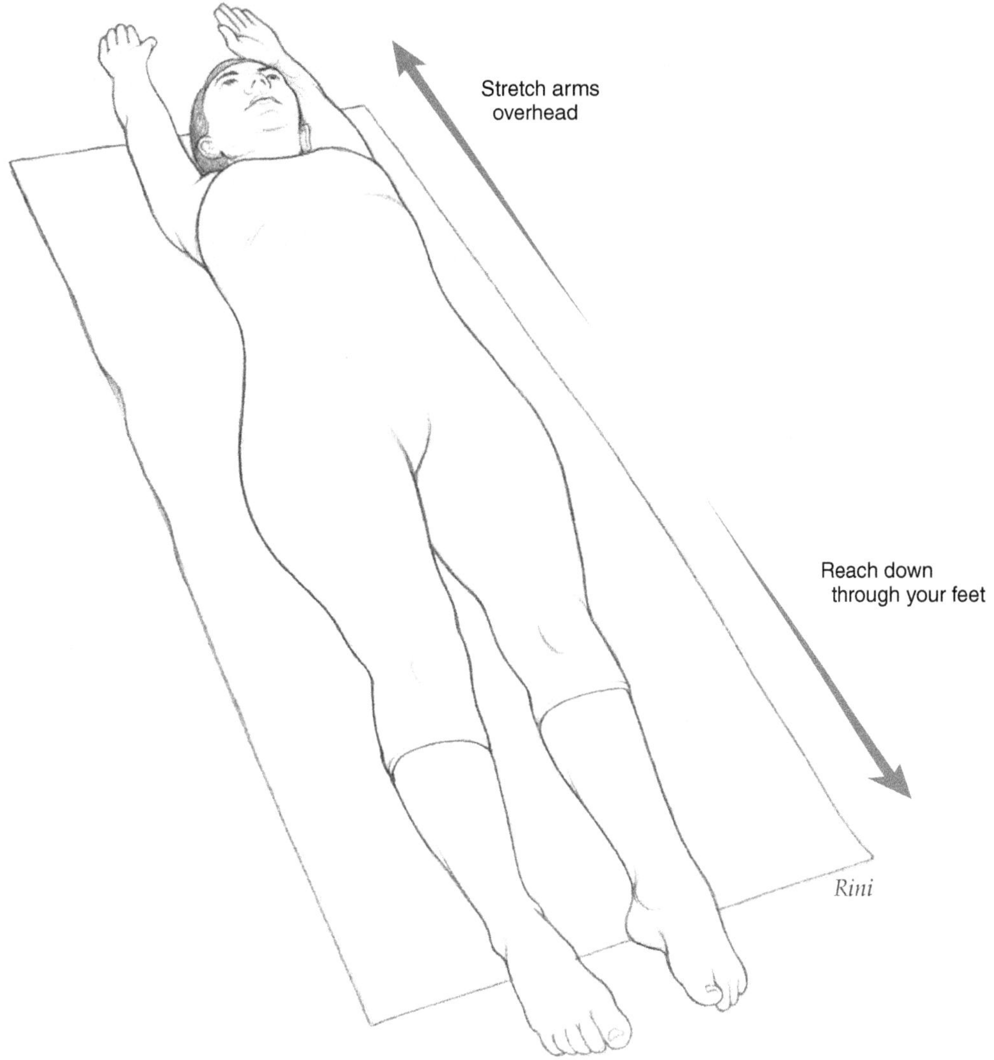

A

FIGURE 7-10 **Intense floor stretch (*Uttibitisan*).** Lie down and let your arms and legs extend out in an X shape. Alternate stretching each arm and leg in turn and then stretch in all four directions at once. (**A**) Starting position.

pain. Some clients may want to practice until it hurts or think practicing will not do any good without pain. This is not the way to reinforce the direct CT approaches to myofascial massage. Indeed, effort and strain can damage muscles and CT. When clients stretch to assume a posture, make sure they do so only to the limits of reasonable comfort. Help clients understand the importance of staying balanced and maintaining easy breaths.

A sample protocol for hatha yoga is provided at right for your reference.

Remember that any yoga protocol can only serve as a starting point for client education and self-care. It is better to suggest fewer exercises (asanas) and have your client actually perform those few than to overwhelm your client with too much homework. Based on the outcome of your myofascial session, you and your client may wish to choose two or three strategic poses to practice between ses-

HATHA YOGA PROTOCOL: SAMPLE WORKOUT

Here is an all-over workout that uses asanas described in this chapter. Remember to return to the resting pose (e.g., corpse pose) after every few poses or after each asana, if you wish. In addition, a yoga session should always conclude with a resting pose.

1. Salutation to the sun
2. Mountain pose
3. Adapted hands over head
4. Sidebends or adapted sidebends
5. Spinal twist
6. Knee squeeze
7. Intense floor stretch
8. Corpse pose

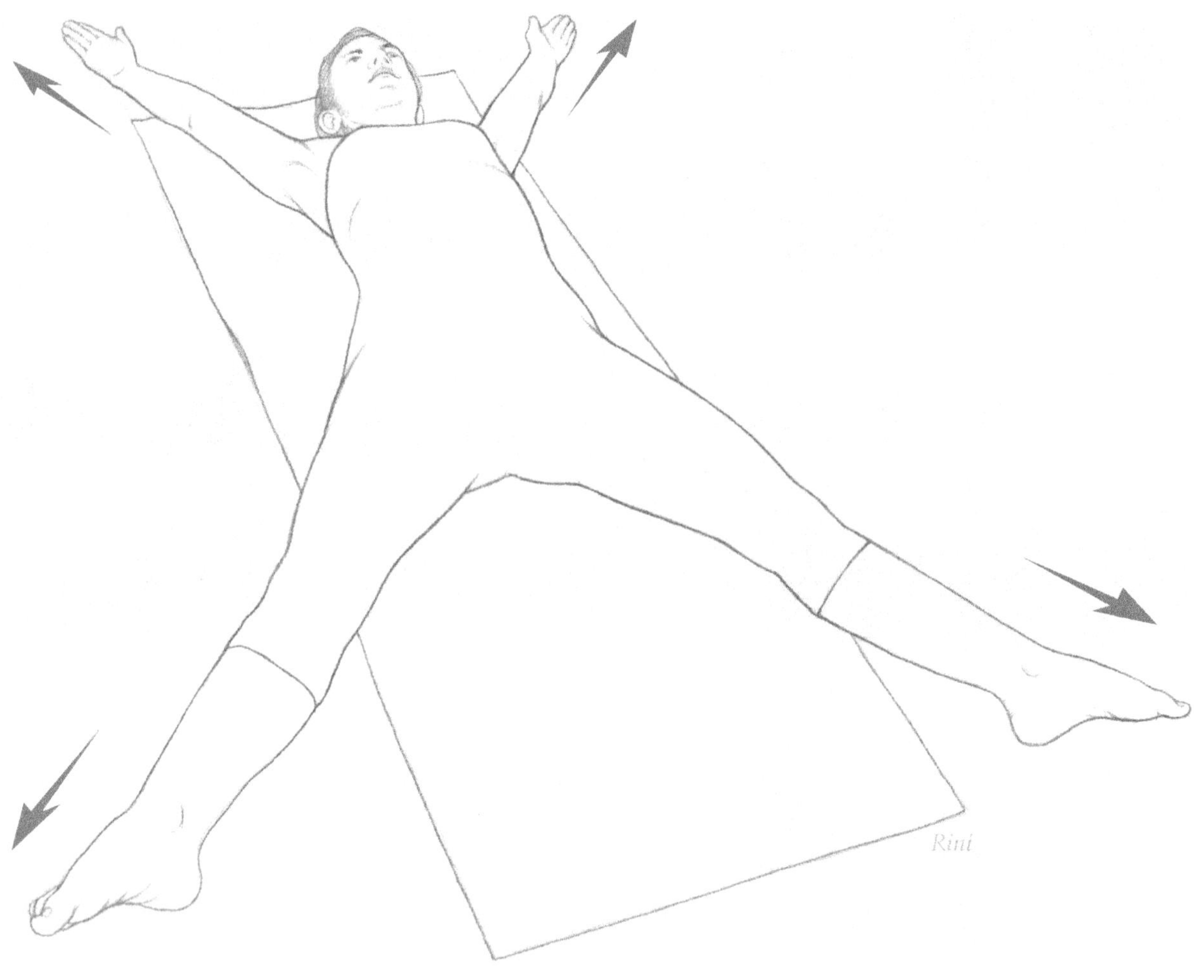

B

FIGURE 7-10 Intense floor stretch (*Uttibitisan*) (continued). (**B**) End position.

sions. You and your client may also wish to adapt poses to target areas of resistance in the soft tissues that were discovered during the myofascial session. Adapting body position is key for the effective administration of neuromuscular and direct CT approaches, and this is no different in the practice of hatha yoga. Your client's body awareness (which will also be developing in tablework sessions) will help him to modify movements for optimum efficiency. The more your client practices, the more he will build body awareness. This improved body awareness will, in turn, make it more desirable to practice, creating a positive feedback cycle that empowers your client to bring about healthy change.

SUMMARY

This chapter presents hatha yoga as the preferred adjunctive practice to complement and enhance direct methods of myofascial massage. Hatha yoga is both movement and self-care.

Hatha yoga is part of an ancient system of healing that focuses on asanas (physical postures) and pranayama (conscious breathing). Research supports the use of hatha yoga and provides some possible mechanisms of action.

The direct myofascial massage practitioner may suggest specific asanas. Salutation to the sun can be used by itself as a whole-body lengthener and toner. Other asanas can be used to supplement the salutation to the sun or can support healing of a particular body region.

Suggestions to optimize the use of hatha yoga include making sure not to work past mild resistance, incorporating breathing into the movements, and balancing the practice of asanas symmetrically.

Hatha yoga, when practiced in accordance with the precepts that have been profiled in this chapter and under the guidance of a qualified teacher, provides a supplement to direct methods of myofascial massage. It does this by reinforcing and enhancing the client's recognition and release of myofascial restrictions, work that has been initiated through direct myofascial methods.

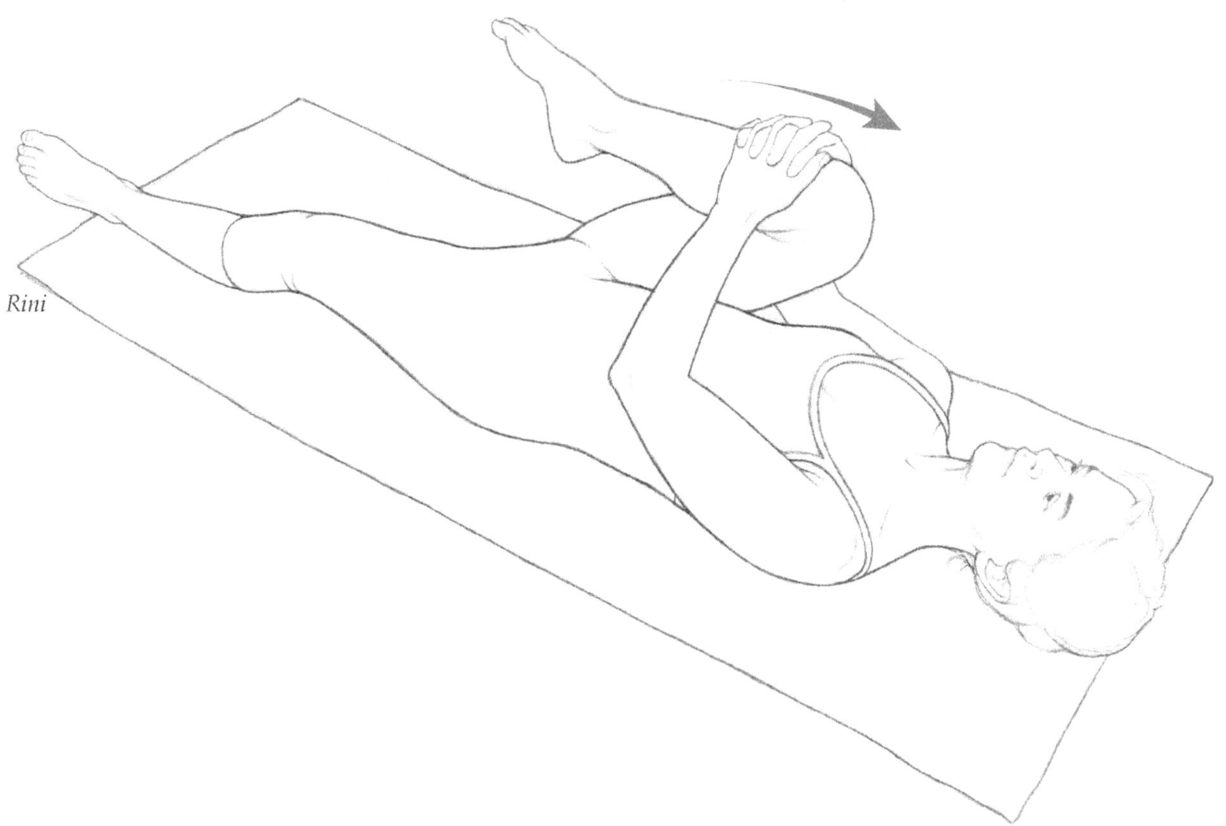

FIGURE 7-11 Knee squeeze (*Pavanamuktasana*). Squeeze one knee to your chest as you breathe in. Extend the leg when breathing out. Repeat on the opposite side.

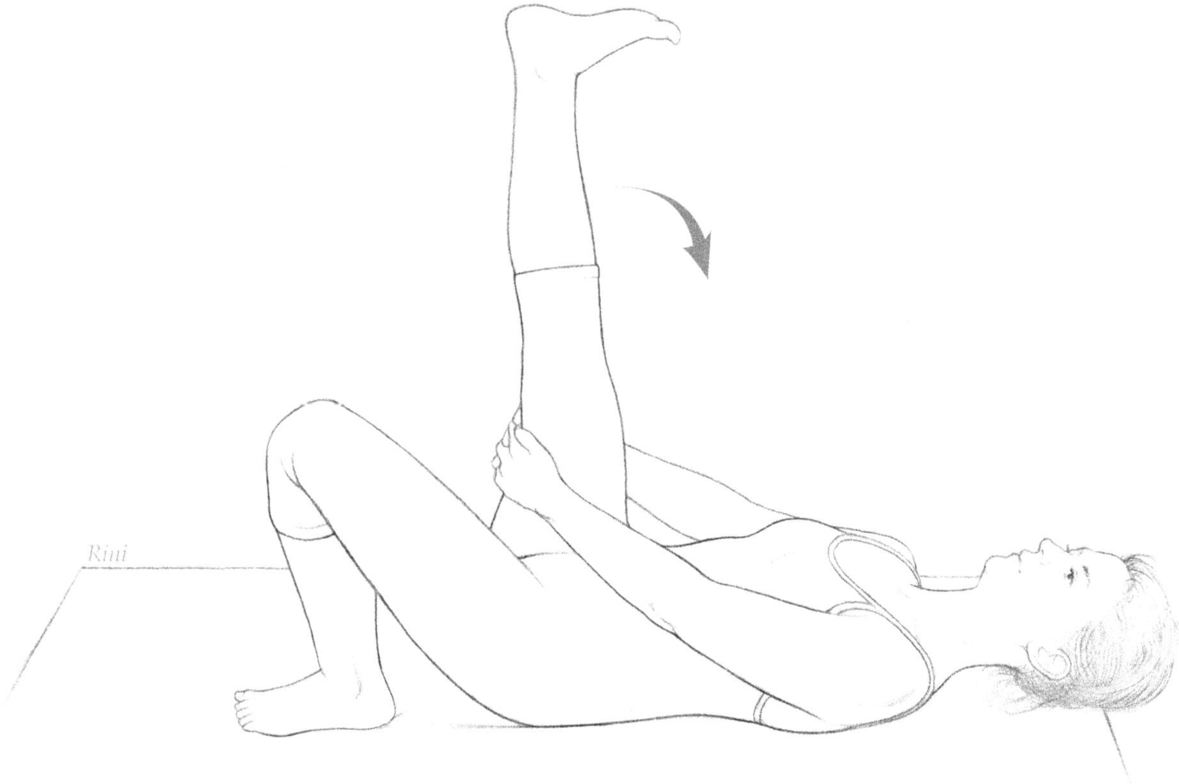

FIGURE 7-12 Adapted sun pose (reclining; *Pasdhimottanasan*). While lying on a mat, straighten the leg and breath out as you stretch the back of your thigh. Hooking a towel across your foot may make it easier to straighten your leg.

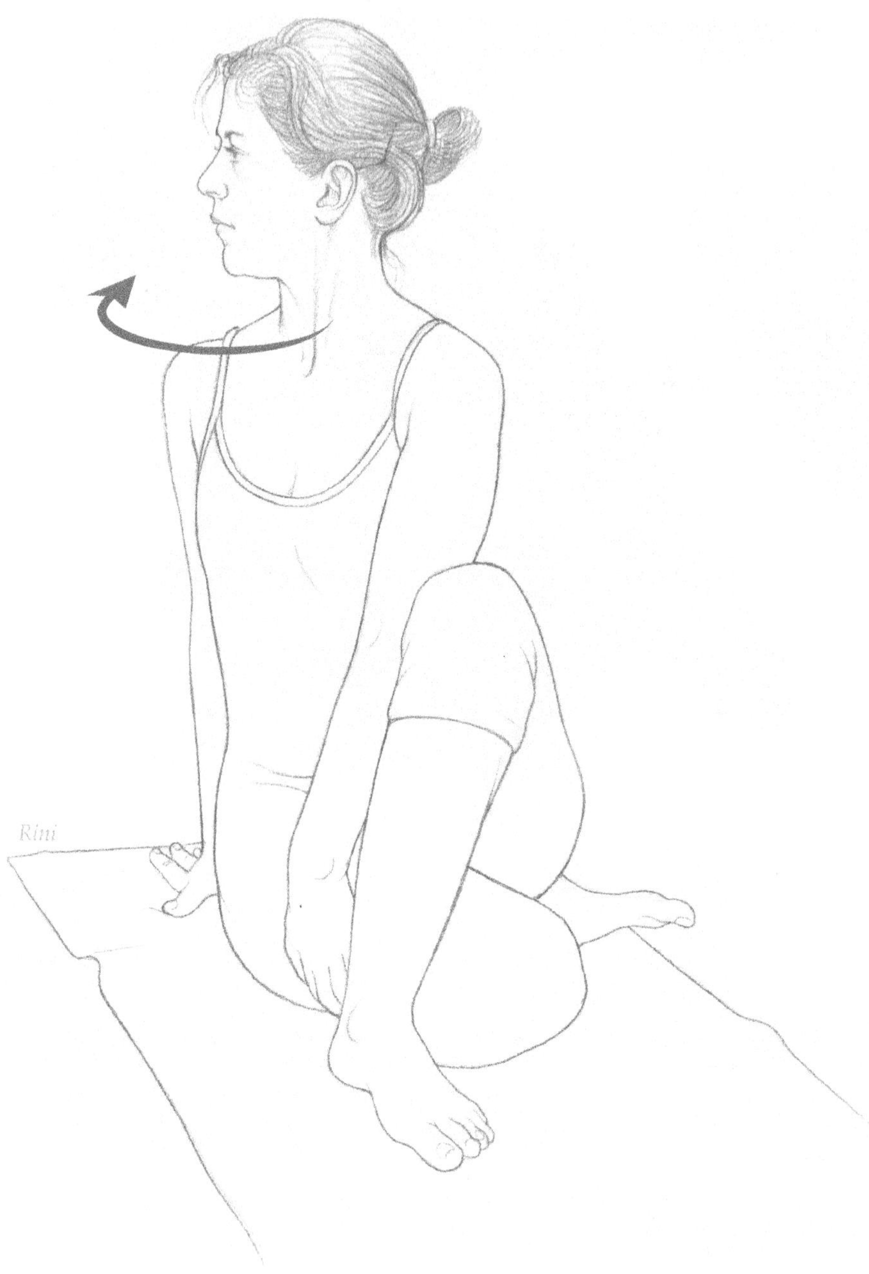

FIGURE 7-13 Adapted spinal twist (*Ardha Matsyendrasan*). From a sitting position, weave your right leg under your left so that your right knee rests on the floor. Reach over your left leg with your left arm so that your left hand can hold on to your right thigh or leg. Twist to the right as you exhale. Breathe gently while holding the pose. Repeat on the other side.

Review Questions

1. Pranayama refers to __________ exercises.
   a. religious
   b. deep
   c. breathing
   d. active
2. __________ refers to the postures or poses one moves into in hatha yoga.
   a. Prana
   b. Asanas
   c. Kripalu
   d. Kundalini
3. __________ is a series of poses designed to stretch and tone the whole body, especially the legs and spine.
   a. Salutation to the sun
   b. Corpse pose
   c. Easy spinal twist
   d. Reclining sun pose
4. True or false: In general, it is best to breathe in when you move into a pose.
5. True or false: The corpse pose is a resting pose.
6. True or false: In general, it is best to take a pose past the point of mild resistance.
7. __________ is the basic meditative posture.
8. __________ is a healthcare system that uses herbs, foods, lifestyle changes, on asanas (postures), pranayama (breathing practices), and mantras (sacred sounds) specific to a patient's unique constitution to maintain health.
9. Hatha yoga seeks to meet and follow resistances in the soft tissues with a counterforce, similar to the __________ method of myofascial massage.
10. Describe the benefit of hatha yoga practice for myofascial massage clients.

REFERENCES

Achterberg J, Dossey L, Gordon JS, et al. Mind-body interventions. In: Alternative Medicine: Expanding Medical Horizons. A Report to the National Institutes of Health on Alternative Medical Systems and Practices in the United States. NIH Pub No. 94-066, 1994(December): 3–43. Rockville, MD: National Institutes of Health.

Anderson B. Stretching. Bolinas, CA: Shelter Publications, 1980.

Baldwin MC. Psychological and physiological influences of hatha yoga training on healthy, exercising adults. Diss Abstracts Intl 1999; 60(suppl 4-A):1031.

Ernst E. Breathing techniques—Adjunctive treatment modalities for asthma? A systematic review. Eur Respir J; 2000;15:969–972.

Farrell SJ, Marr Ross AD, Sehgal KV. Eastern movement therapies. Physical Med Rehab Clin North Am 1999;10:617–629.

Feuerstein G. Yoga and Yoga Therapy. Lower Lake, CA: International Association of Yoga Therapists, Yoga Research and Education Center, 2001.

Garfinkel MS, Schumacher HR, Husain A, et al. Evaluation of a yoga based regimen for treatment of osteoarthritis of the hand. J Rheumatol 1994;21:2341–2343.

Garfinkel MS, Singhal A, Katz WA, et al. Yoga-based intervention for carpal tunnel syndrome: a randomized trial. JAMA 1998;280:1601–1603.

Globus S. What yoga can do for you. Current Health 2000;27:30.

Holloway E, Ram FSF. Breathing exercises for asthma [Cochrane Review]. In: The Cochrane Library, Issue 2, 2001. Oxford: Update Software.

Jain SC, Uppal A, Bhatnagar So, Talukdar B. A study of response pattern of non-insulin dependent diabetics to yoga therapy. Diabetes Res Clin Pract 1993;19:69–74.

Kamei T, Toriumi Y, Kimur H, et al. Decrease in serum cortisol during yoga exercise is correlated with alpha wave activation. Percept Mot Skills 2000;90:1027–1032.

Kant S, Bhattacharya S, Pandey US, et al. Evaluation of effect of yogic breathing exercises on pulmonary functions, free radicals and antioxidant status on healthy individuals. Chest 2000;118(suppl):240.

Luskin, FM, Newell KA, Griffith M, et al. A review of mind/body therapies in the treatment of musculoskeletal disorders with implications for the elderly. Altern Ther Health Med 2000;6:46–56.

Mishra L, Singh BB, Dagenais S. Historical perspective and principles of the traditional healthcare system in India. Alternative Therapies in Health and Medicine 2001;7:36–42.

Ornish D, Scherwitz LW, Doody RS, et al. Effects of stress management training and dietary changes in treating ischemic heart disease. JAMA 1983;249:54–59.

Pandya DP, Vyas VH, Vyas SH. Mind-body therapy in the management and prevention of coronary disease. Compr Ther 1999;25:283–293.

Schell FJ, Allolio B, Schonecke OW. Physiological and psychological effects of hatha-yoga exercise in healthy women. Int J Psychosom 1994;41:46–52.

Sovik R. The science of breathing—the yogic view. Progr Brain Res 2000; 122:491–505.

Swami Rama. Lectures on Yoga. Honesdale, PA: Himalayan International Institute of Yoga Science and Philosophy, 1979.

Telles S, Nagarathna R, Nagendra HR, Desiraju T. Physiologic changes in sports teachers following 3 months of training in yoga. Indian J Medical Sciences 1993;47:235–238.

Udupa KN, Singh RH. The scientific basis of yoga. JAMA 1972;220:1365.

Wood C. Mood change and perceptions of vitality: a comparison of the effects of relaxation, visualization and yoga. J R Soc Med 1993;86:254–258.

SUGGESTED READINGS

Christensen A. The American Yoga Association Beginner's Manual. New York: Simon & Schuster, 1987.

Christensen A, Rankin D. Easy Does It Yoga. Cleveland Heights, OH: The Light of Yoga Society, 1979.

Satchidananda YSS. Integral Yoga Hatha. New York: Holt, Rinehart and Winston, 1970.

Schatz MP. Back Care Basics: A Doctor's Gentle Yoga Program for Back and Neck Pain Relief. Berkeley, CA: Rodmell Press, 1992.

Part

III

Indirect Methods Used in Myofascial Massage

Chapter 8

Indirect Connective Tissue Approach

OBJECTIVES

- Describe the indirect connective tissue approach and its rationale.
- Identify origins and influences on the indirect connective tissue approach.
- Explain indirect connective tissue approach effects on thixotropy and interconnectivity.
- Describe indirect connective tissue techniques, including jostling, rocking, compression, traction, shaking, and flopping.
- Discuss positioning, draping, and support.
- Discuss treatment planning and decision making.

CHAPTER OUTLINE

KEY TERMS

Direction of ease: Moving in the direction that the body wants to move or moves most easily, or moving back from a point of restriction.

Movement reeducation: Any style of bodywork or active exercise that is used to reeducate the client's body to optimize functionality, increase range of motion, and make unconscious movement conscious. Some popular movement reeducation styles include Hanna Somatics Education, Trager, Feldenkrais Method, Alexander Technique, Rubenfeld Synergy, and Aston Patterning.

Trager Approach: Trademarked indirect connective tissue style that aims to release psychophysiological areas of holding or guarding.

Hanna Somatics Education (HSE): Indirect connective tissue style; hands-on method for teaching voluntary, conscious control of the neuromuscular system to clients suffering from involuntary, maladaptive reflex disorders.

Myofascial Release: Trademarked style of manual therapy that includes indirect connective tissue, direct connective tissue, and soft tissue mobilization techniques.

Fascial release: Indirect connective tissue technique that takes areas of horizontal stress on the superficial fascia into a direction of ease (the way it wants to move).

Jostling: Indirect connective tissue technique; a rhythmic type of vibration applied with the whole body that moves the client's body or body part as far as it can easily go, then allows it to return.

Rocking: Indirect connective tissue technique; can involve up and down, side to side, or circular motions.

Traction: Indirect connective tissue technique; longitudinal stretching that pulls connective tissue in the direction of the muscle fiber and follows tiny movements to achieve a release.

Shaking: Indirect connective tissue technique; a type of vibration, beginning with lifting and pulling and followed with a downward or sideways motion that warms joints and prepares muscle groups, joints, or limbs for more focused bodywork.

Flopping: Indirect CT technique; a type of shaking by which a limb is bounced in a controlled way onto the massage table.

Chapter 8 introduces the indirect connective tissue approach to myofascial massage. The indirect connective tissue (CT) approach allows bodyworkers to address difficulties or pain in the client's body indirectly or within a perspective of ease. The first section of this chapter describes the approach and some of the bodywork perspectives (Trager, Hanna, and Barnes) that have influenced its development.

The second section introduces basic indirect CT techniques, which can be adapted for use anywhere on the client's body. These techniques are used in a variety of bodywork and movement reeducation styles such as Trager, Hanna Somatics, Alexander, Feldenkrais, and Aston Patterning. To better visualize the correct application of indirect CT techniques, the chapter reviews the structure of fascia, with emphasis on the quality of its movement. This section also discusses the correct application of body mechanics, positioning and support, and the use of verbal cues to enhance the process of soft tissue release. Decision making about where and when to practice the indirect CT approach is discussed, along with guidelines for adapting indirect CT massage to specific conditions or client needs.

The chapter concludes with a protocol for applying the indirect CT approach. This protocol can benefit most clients regardless of chief complaints; however, the chapter also offers some general guidelines for modifying the basic session to meet specific needs.

Why Use an Indirect Connective Tissue Approach?

Wouldn't it be better to approach all client complaints directly? It seems logical to locate a shortened muscle group or a restricted range of motion (ROM) and use one of the direct approaches to manually stretch out the restriction. Sometimes an area is so painful or traumatized, however, that it can only respond to direct methods with pain and redoubled guarding. By allowing the body to go in its **direction of ease** (i.e., away from the position that causes pain and only where the body naturally moves), the client remains in a state of safety. This can be very helpful for clients who resist or are afraid of direct change because to them, the direct approach may seem like a confrontation. These clients may be fearful of further pain or convinced that their bodies cannot feel better. The indirect approach bypasses such resistance to go to the source of ease (i.e., what feels good). The perceived and actual danger of reinjured tissue is removed, pain receptors are not activated, and the guarding response is avoided. The neuromuscular proprioceptors are allowed to reset by experiencing movement through an arc painlessly and effortlessly.

This feeling of comfort and effortlessness affects the entire body. Areas distant from the trauma can be manipulated to promote healing in painful and even acutely inflamed regions. For example, it is likely that an indirect CT technique applied to the foot will transmit waves of comfortable movement to a pulled muscle located in the neck.

Description of the Indirect Connective Tissue Approach

The indirect CT approach uses movement alone to free up bound up CT. Thus, a working definition of the indirect CT approach to myofascial massage is releasing the muscle by using gentle movement of the CT.

PRESSURE

Obviously, *some* pressure is used to contact the client's tissues and to apply the impetus for movement; however, beyond initiating the movement, pressure serves no purpose. Pressure is not applied to release tissue. Instead, the movement that is generated by the pressure serves to release the fascia. Although contact in the indirect CT approach is gentle, it is not weak. In fact, many clients describe the touch as full and firm but yielding rather than hard. As with deep direct CT work, indirect CT pressure is applied by sinking through to an appropriate level of CT, not by powering your way in. The "appropriate" fascial level is generally less than what would be used with the deep direct CT approach.

APPLICATION OF MOVEMENT

Movement is applied by gently rocking, shaking, or tractioning the client's arms, legs, trunk, or skull. At regular intervals, the bodyworker takes a break from the movement to step back and cue the client to breathe, stretch, and consciously absorb the kinesthetic changes. Indirect CT movements concentrate on bringing ease to areas of "stuckness" and must be precisely applied so that the client does not feel pushed or overloaded by uninvited sensations.

Movements that are too forceful or jerky are counterproductive in that they tend to make the client feel dizzy and unsettled. It is possible for unfocused movements to feel relaxing, but often they do not. Unfocused movements also do not concentrate the client's awareness of a sense of ease on the restricted site.

Origins of and Influences on the Indirect Connective Tissue Approach

A variety of movement reeducation styles have spurred the development of indirect CT techniques, which emphasize ease of movement, lightness, and flow. Many originators of these bodywork styles have been athletes or creative movers (e.g., actors, dancers). This is significant because these professions develop a kinesthetic sense of the physical body in movement. Movement reeducators are, by and large, people who healed themselves or others through reeducating the body to find a greater sense of ease. Some of the prominent pioneers in movement reeducation include Milton Trager, Thomas Hanna, F. M. Alexander, Moshe Feldenkrais, Irmgaard Bartinieff, Judith Aston, and Ilana Rosenfeld. This is only a partial list of the many contributors to this important field; for further study of movement reeducation, see the suggested reading list at the end of this chapter.

TRAGER APPROACH

Trager Approach consists of two components: the hands-on work, known as Psychophysical Integration, and the movement exercises, known as Mentastics. Psychophysical Integration refers to the presupposition that Trager bodywork harmonizes or integrates the mind and the body. The word Mentastics is derived from the phrase "mental gymnastics."

As a young man, Milton Trager was a boxer. When he first tried out his unique bodywork style on his boxing trainer, the response was extremely positive. He was encouraged to practice the modality on his father, who had suffered with sciatic pain for about 2 years. After one session, his father's discomfort was greatly decreased, and after two sessions, his pain never returned. Trager continued to practice with clients complaining of pain and dysfunction, later earning a doctorate in physical therapy. In his 40s, he also became a medical doctor.

Trager Psychophysical Integration uses rhythmic nonintrusive movements (e.g., jostling, rocking, traction, easy compression, and flopping) to transmit an experience of movement without effort. The passive movements transmit information about the tissues to the client's "functional mind" (Griffin, 1989). The "functional mind" uses the sensory data to relieve unnecessary tension and decrease pain related to tension. Voluntary protective responses (often a secondary cause of pain) can let go, so the client experiences a more peaceful and relaxed mental state, known as "*hook-up*." In performing the activities that lead a client to "hook-up," the therapist shares in this relaxed and peaceful state.

Tablework sessions last from 60 to 90 minutes. No oils or lotions are used. Clients wear underwear and lie under a drape or may remain fully clothed if they prefer.

Mentastics are light, simple ways of moving the body to create awareness, improve body function, and recall the lightness and freedom that are experienced on the table. Mentastics, which each practitioner is trained to teach, help the client build habits of relaxed movement. With practice, the feeling of release and ease can be recalled during periods of stress that occur in daily life. These "mental gymnastics" are also mentioned in Chapter 9 as good activities to supplement indirect CT tablework.

HANNA SOMATICS EDUCATION

The work of Thomas Hanna gives more structure to the concept of using therapist-applied and coached movements to activate the body to "self-correct." Hanna coined the term "autonomous human being" to emphasize that people are capable of self-correcting and self-regulating. This principle is shared among prominent movement reeducators, including Milton Trager, Moshe Feldenkrais, and F. M. Alexander. Hanna Somatics Education (HSE) is the hands-on procedure for teaching voluntary, conscious control of the neuromuscular system. HSE is targeted to clients suffering from involuntary muscular disorders (i.e., basically anyone with musculoskeletal pain or discomfort).

Hanna's theory is that many cases of chronic pain are caused by *sensory-motor amnesia (SMA)*, a condition in which certain neurons of the cerebral cortex lose their memory of how certain muscle groups feel and how it feels to control them. SMA is not an organic lesion of the brain or musculoskeletal system, but rather a functional deficit whereby the ability to contract a muscle has been surrendered to subcortical (involuntary) reflexes. SMA involves unconscious holding patterns that once were useful (probably protective) but now are habitual and maladaptive. For example, SMA can manifest as habitually holding the body in an old pattern (e.g., locking the knees) that wears on the joints.

Hanna identifies three reflexes with emotional undercurrents that may lead to SMA pathology. These are the trauma reflex, the startle (red light) reflex, and the Landau (green light) reflex. Each carries a characteristically identifiable posture that leads to holding on to muscle tension and subsequent discomfort and pain.

The *trauma reflex* is a protective response to avoid pain. It may be portrayed in a client's reactive pattern to a fall or a surgery that happened many years ago. The characteristic pattern is to double over the area of the injury so as to enfold and shield it from further harm.

The *startle (red light) reflex* is a stress response to real or imaginary threat or worry. In the startle reflex, most of the contraction is in the front of the body and is characterized by high shoulders, a forward-jutting head, and a caved-in chest. It is sometimes known as the turtle response because it is reminiscent of a startled turtle. This habit creates shallow breathing and contributes to high blood pressure, rapid pulse, constipation, bladder problems, and other stress-related conditions (Welch-Baril and Baril, 1994).

In the *Landau (green light) reflex*, the reticular activating system signals the body to get ready for action (Welch-Baril and Baril, 1994). The phone ringing or the sound of a doorbell or alarm causes the body to contract into a military-type posture, with the shoulders thrown back and the posterior muscles tensed for a quick response.

Hanna Somatics Education promotes several techniques to gain conscious control over these and other maladaptive reflexes. These include *pandiculation*, a type of active resistive stretching in which the client's resistance to a stretch is gradually lessened, and the technique of manually pushing the origin and insertion of a muscle closer together, to turn off stretch receptors that are firing in error. Such techniques are based on neurological principles, discussed in Chapter 4.

A second HSE technique is *kinetic mirroring*, which Hanna (1994) describes as "the principle of going with another person's resistance and never going against it." In kinetic mirroring, the therapist brings the origin and insertion of a muscle together. To do this, the therapist can manually push the ends of the muscle toward the muscle belly, as described in the paragraph above, or can strategically apply gentle rocking and jostling movements. The object is not to achieve maximum ROM but to find the maximum ease in ROM. Hanna uses Feldenkrais' explanation of kinetic mirroring: "If you do the work of a muscle, it ceases to do its own work, that is, it relaxes." This principle also helps describe how Trager Psychophysical Integration works.

Hanna's third technique, *means-whereby*, emphasizes the *process* of moving through a pain-free ROM exercise, *rather than the goal*. Hanna observed how German physical education teacher Elsa Gindler implemented the Alexander technique and saw that Gindler's students gained greater self-control by means of greater sensory awareness. By focusing conscious attention on the proprioceptive sensations accompanying an outward movement, the quality of their movement began to improve (Hanna, 1994).

Oliver Sacks, the distinguished neurologist who writes about people suffering with neurological disorders, tells a story that helps explicate the significance of kinetic mirroring and means-whereby. The incident concerns Sacks himself, who tore his quadriceps tendon completely off the bone while running from a bull. The prognosis was not good for regaining full function to extend the knee. During his recuperation, he first was able to make involuntary jerks of his leg into extension, but he could not make his leg extend by willing it to do so. This showed that the motor neurons could carry messages but were still functionally impaired. A clear conception of the goal alone could not return function. After a care provider repetitively took his leg into extension and back many times on many occasions, Sacks began slowly to regain voluntary control of his quad muscles. My theory is that it was necessary to feel the quads moving through all the intermediate steps of an action before Sacks could duplicate the complexity of "simple" extension. Functioning is a matter of process and involves the entire sequence of a motion, not just the end result.

Hanna Somatics Education also instructs therapists to reinforce easy movement with questions and images. Kinetic mirroring and means-whereby provide sensory feedback to the client. When the therapist incorporates pauses and suggests that the client voluntarily move during pauses, it encourages the client's conscious sense of the ease. Thus, when the bodywork is applied in conjunction with communications that reinforce success, indirect CT techniques can better reprogram the sensory-motor feedback loop for healthy change.

BARNES MYOFASCIAL RELEASE

John Barnes has grouped a number of techniques to access the myofascia into a trademarked modality, which he calls Myofascial Release. Barnes (1995) defines Myofascial Release as "a whole-body, hands-on approach for the evaluation and treatment of the human structure. Its focus is the fascial system." The Barnes system does not neatly fit into any one approach to myofascial massage. Some Myofascial Release soft tissue mobilization techniques are discussed in Chapter 5 because they focus on the neuromuscular aspect of the myofascia. Other techniques, which Barnes himself refers to as craniosacral, are covered in Chapter 10. Still other techniques seem to have an indirect orientation. Barnes calls these "fascial releases"; they are also taught by Upledger as diaphragm and sacral releases. I classify fascial release as a technique of indirect CT, insofar as it requires following the fascia—not the dura or cerebrospinal fluid movement—into a direction of ease. Fascial release applies the same fundamental technique to different regions of the body in the same way that the basic deep direct CT stroke can be applied to different body regions.

Fascial Release

As just noted, Barnes' fascial release and Upledger's diaphragm and sacral release are essentially the same technique. The basic fascial release combines two directions of pressure. First, the therapist sinks down to locate the landmark bone. Then, the therapist eases up until her hands "float" up to the superficial fascia layer; the second direction varies according to the client and body region. It is found by "testing the fascial waters" along the surface to see which way the tissue most easily moves.

Initially, bodyworkers may have difficulty figuring out where the fascia "wants to go." To help them, Iris Wolf, a physical therapy educator in Portland, Oregon, teaches the "stacking" technique. In stacking, the therapist first exaggerates a resistance (e.g., stretches the fascia) in the client's body to feel the tension and encourage resolution. Stacking involves choosing one of three spatial dimensions (superficial–deep, side–side, up–down) and taking the tissue into slight resistance along the chosen dimension, then holding and feeling that resistance, then letting it go. Novices are taught to find each resistance and release in that dimension sequentially. More experienced therapists may stack all three resistances and then allow the whole matrix to unwind (twist and turn) through all three dimensions simultaneously. Table 8-1 identifies specific fascial releases with suggestions for regional applications.

Guidelines for the Basic Fascial Release Technique

Gentle pressure (what Barnes terms "low load") applied steadily and slowly will stimulate a viscous medium such as CT to flow to a greater extent than a strong pressure that is quickly released. The viscosity of the ground substance in CT is believed to control the ease with which collagen fibers can rearrange to form more aligned CT. Viscoelasticity causes CT to resist a suddenly applied force but results in gradual elongation to a constantly applied force over time. "Creep" is the progressive deformation of soft tissues resulting from constant low loading over time (Twomely and Taylor, 1982). The indirect CT approach follows the motion of the fascia, from barrier to barrier, until freedom from restriction is felt. The Arndt-Schultz law offers a rationale for using gentle, sustained pressure to loosen myofascial restrictions. This law states that "weak stimuli increases physiologic activity and very strong stimuli inhibit or abolish activity" (Thomas, 1997).

The therapist should identify the restriction, either with stacking or palpation alone, and then establish a level of hand contact that just reaches the barrier. Wait a few

TABLE 8-1 Specific Fascial and Diaphragm Releases

Technique	Description	Application
Pelvic diaphragm release	Supine client; therapist at side. The palm that is closest to the client's head is placed under the sacrum. The top palm covers the pubic bone, with both thumbs oriented superiorly.	Low back, sacral, lower abdomen, and urogenital conditions (Upledger and Vredevoogd, 1983)
Respiratory diaphragm release	Supine client; therapist at side. The palm that is closest to client's head is placed underneath. The bottom hand is placed on T12. The top hand covers the xiphoid process (from the lower edge of the sternum down to the abdomen).	Midthoracic organ conditions (e.g., liver, gallbladder, stomach, lower lung); also some low back pain, psoas muscles (Upledger and Vredevoogd, 1983)
Thoracic outlet*	The bottom hand is placed on C7. The top hand covers the place where the clavicle meets the sternum and reaches down the sternum toward the heart.	Lung conditions, neck, shoulder, and upper extremity musculoskeletal conditions; to promote lymph flow (Upledger and Vredevoogd, 1983)
Hyoid diaphragm release	The bottom hand spans C2 and C3. The top hand covers the hyoid bone (ask the client to swallow and observe where the Adam's apple moves to locate hyoid).	Neck conditions, headaches, throat conditions, temporomandibular joint disorder (Upledger and Vredevoogd, 1983)

*Called thoracic inlet release in Upledger (1983).

minutes for the release to begin. Although a few minutes can seem like an eternity, be patient and do not try to force through the barrier. Allow the fascia to move back from the barrier into a direction of ease. There may be several barriers (e.g., the different dimensions), so this technique may take up to 5 minutes to complete. It is also possible that the fascia may unwind and complete the release rapidly, so do not feel as though you have to stay in an area when movement has clearly stopped. The pressure you use to engage the tissue is very gentle—5 g of pressure or less, less pressure than the weight of a nickel. Feel the weight of a nickel and do not use more than this force. In fact, if you do not feel the fascial release, ease up on your pressure. It is one of the strange paradoxes of this work that less can sometimes be more. Depending on where you are contacting the body, following the moving fascia may feel to the client like you are instigating the movement, and to you like the client is initiating the movement. Barnes refers to this phenomenon as "unwinding," and Upledger calls it "regional positional release." No matter what you call the technique, you are essentially just listening to and following the fascia to its greatest ease (until it stops moving).

Physiological Effects of the Indirect Connective Tissue Approach

Indirect CT massage has two primary physiological effects.

HOW THE INDIRECT CONNECTIVE TISSUE APPROACH AFFECTS THIXOTROPY

As discussed in Chapter 3, the term *thixotropy* describes the way fascia can vary in viscosity. The effects of thixotropy are demonstrated when you sit through a 3-hour movie and find at the end that it is difficult to get up out of your seat. Thixotropy occurs because CT solidifies into a "suit of armor" whenever we stay in one position for a long time (e.g., after we break an arm and do not move it to avoid pain). In simple terms, CT stiffens very well on its own but is not so good at softening by itself. That is where exercise and massage can be very helpful. Moving fascia around is like stirring molasses or a thick soup: movement helps the mixture to become more pliable and less congealed. Specifically, the passive movements applied in the indirect CT approach promote softening of the myofascia.

HOW THE INDIRECT CONNECTIVE TISSUE APPROACH AFFECTS INTERCONNECTIVITY

Review the figure of musculoskeletal anatomy in Chapter 3 (see Figure 3-6), noticing how the white areas next to and around the bones denote fascia. Observe how the fascial network is really one unit that stretches throughout the entire body. This is why a tug on the foot can pull the shoul-

One Therapist's Experience: The Experience of Performing an Indirect Connective Tissue Session

One of my standard classroom assignments is to have students complete a case study report that includes client feedback and what it actually feels like to be a massage therapist administering the techniques. The following is an excerpt from one of these student reports. This account provides a reflection of what it might be like to perform indirect CT massage.

"Going about (the session) with an explorer's sense of curiosity, wonder, and attention, I started at the feet. Pulling gently at the ankles then resting them on my belly and rocking back and forth, I scanned the body that lay before me, just paying attention to how it moved but careful not to label anything as stiff or not moving. I paused for a moment. Then resumed rocking. A bit more pull of light traction, then walked up to the head. After turning my volunteer over, I started with some of the techniques. . . . Cat paws, the wave thing under the neck, and so on. I felt timid. But I did enjoy what I was doing. As long as I kept reminding myself that I was an explorer. "How does this part move?" I kept asking myself. "What about this way? What if I move like this, or stand this way? How does this affect who I'm working on?" I completed about 35 minutes of this type of "playing." I finished by going back to the feet to add some closure and completeness. I have to say that I was surprised. I think I did better than I expected. I felt much more comfortable than I did in class working under limited amounts of time. I enjoyed having an explorer attitude. I think that helped me learn a lot and not be critical of my movements. . . .

[After two more sessions] I'm getting to enjoy this method. It makes me feel much freer to be instinctual with the body rather than so protocol oriented. I like very much that the people I work on also report feeling freer. It's so much better than having them only feel where they are tense and knotted up and me digging in to try and force the tension out of them."

der. This is exactly what happens when you traction the foot with indirect CT massage. Other kinds of movement ripple through the fascial network, and this is why rocking the hip moves up through the spine.

You may also want to review the horizontal lines of stress in the superficial fascia, the "body straps" or retinacula, where the skin shows visible horizontal folds, such as the belt strap at the pelvic floor (Barnes, 1995; Upledger and Vredevoogd, 1983). These are depicted in Figure 6-1. Barnes and Upledger recommend that massage therapists address these areas as a prelude to most sessions because the straps of tension seem to act as a barrier to ease. Thus, when performing an indirect CT session, it would be appropriate to begin with fascial release in these areas.

Indirect Connective Tissue Techniques

Indirect CT techniques focus on the fascial web as a whole. The direction of the movements is not especially determined by the direction of specific muscles because the fascia is a network. It is common, for instance, to clang the client's leg like a bell to release a fascial restriction in the neck.

Indirect CT strokes can be applied in any direction. When you are jostling, pushing, or pulling, it is a good idea to face the direction of your impetus. In this way, the impetus to move can originate from your whole body, not just your arms and hands. Fine tune your alignment to the client's body as it rocks back to you. It is also a good idea to keep clearly in mind a sense of the areas that could be targeted for more ease. By doing so, your body will be aligned toward the area of restriction, and your intent will be set on moving that area within its range of ease.

A variety of techniques are used to release CT in the indirect approach. Those include jostling, compression, traction, and flopping and shaking. Some indirect CT techniques may seem similar to procedures you have already learned in Swedish, Shiatsu, or sports massage classes. To apply these proficiently as indirect strokes, keep in mind that you are attempting to mirror the client's own body rhythm and convey a sense of ease with underlying support.

With all of the indirect CT techniques, avoid bearing down or working harder to try to soften stiffened limbs or hardened tissue. Indeed, through the motions of your hands and body, ask yourself, "What could be lighter or freer right here? And what could be lighter and freer still?" Anchor the feeling of letting go in the client's conscious mind with strategically timed questions (e.g., "How does this side that we've worked on feel different from the other side?"). These questions will enable your client to recall the sensation of letting go, easily and effortlessly, and instill the idea that living with ease is the natural way to be.

JOSTLING AND ROCKING

Jostling and **rocking** are types of vibration. Jostling is rhythmic and should be applied with the whole body. Rocking can involve up and down, side to side, or circular motions (Figure 8-1). Many practitioners combine directions in "around the world" or "hula hoop" strokes in which one body region is moved in two directions at once (the therapist activates each direction with a separate hand).

Jostling and rocking actions move the body as far as it will go easily, then allow it to return. They do not push past the edge of resistance but instead go right up to that point. The nonverbal message to the body is "look at what you are capable of doing, and don't focus on what you cannot do." After two or three returns, the client's natural rhythm emerges. At this point, the massage therapist can fine tune the jostling or rocking rhythm to focus all the way up to, but not beyond, the point of resistance. Also at this point, the client's tissues may relax spontaneously, and you will notice that his body naturally rocks a little farther. Nothing is abrupt, there is an even ebb and flow to the method like an easy porch swing or gentle tropical breeze (Fritz, 2000). Jostling and rocking act on the joint receptors (proprioceptors) but are also extremely effective in activating the parasympathetic nervous system for rest and repose. Thus, stimulation of the nervous system occurs both at the individual joint level and the whole body.

COMPRESSION

Compression is an easily tolerated stroke that you can use at the beginning of an indirect massage to warm the tissues without lubricant or requiring the client to undress. It simply means pumping the muscle (and surrounding

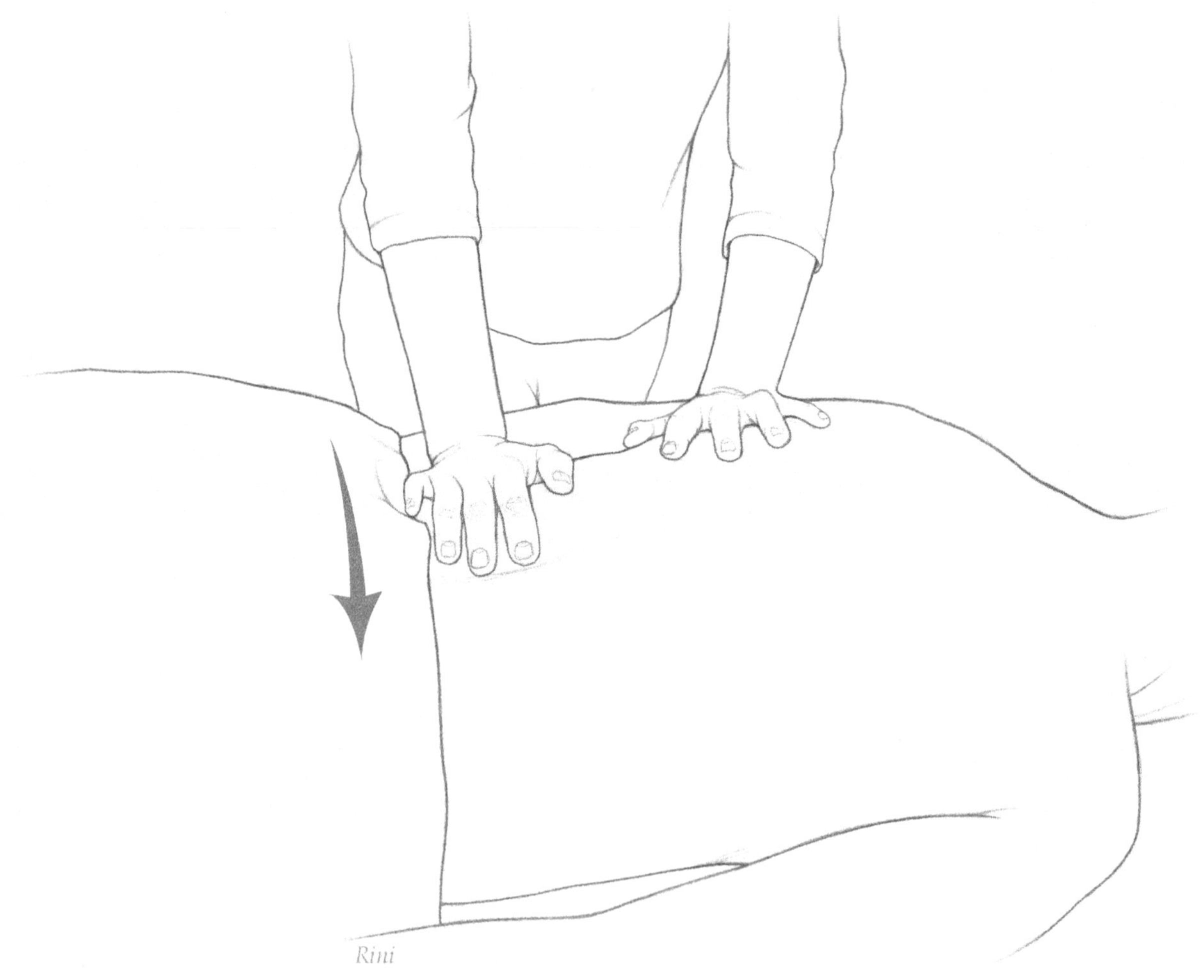

FIGURE 8-1 Rocking. (**A**) The impetus for rocking can be a push away from the massage therapist.

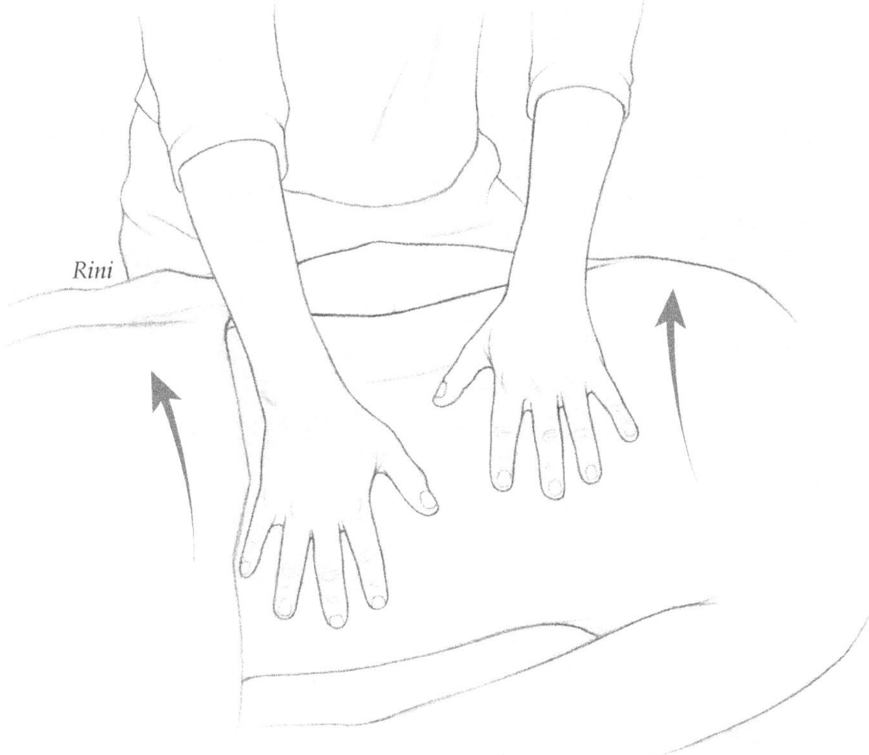

B

FIGURE 8-1 **Rocking (continued).** (**B**) The impetus for rocking can be a pull toward the massage therapist.

fascial layer) against the bone (Figure 8-2). It is not mashing, compacting, squeezing, or punching. If you use compression as a means to listen to and follow the fascia, compression becomes more than just pushing and sequentially letting go of the push. There is a quality of listening to the natural rhythm of your client's body and releasing when the body is ready, not before or after. "Following the natural rhythm" in compression does not mean pressing down on the client, but rather sinking with her and following her lead.

Compression has two special advantages that make it especially useful at the start of a myofascial massage. Compression can be used for warming the tissues all over the body as a substitute for effleurage; compression strokes can also be performed through a sheet, so that the client can remain covered.

TRACTION

The traction that we use in the indirect CT approach is a form of longitudinal stretching, and therefore, is a way of pulling tissue that reduces tensile stress (Fritz, 2000). In longitudinal stretching, the therapist pulls the CT in the direction of the fiber configuration and listens to and follows tiny joint movements to achieve a release. Indirect CT traction is not like simple stretching. In traction, you do not try to move past the body's resistance to lengthening. Instead, pull gently and slowly, waiting for movement. Wait for the client's body to release its resistance rather than overpowering its natural resistance with a manual force. It may help to imagine that you are pulling on the line of a boat in the water (Figure 8-3). If you pull on the rope too hard or too fast, you will get knocked into the sea. If you maintain a slow and steady pull that waits for the water to transmit your impetus to the boat, you will be rewarded with the boat coming toward you (and not falling into the sea).

Traction allows you to use tiny ebb-and-flow movements that accompany the client's breathing to lengthen the myofascia. Lengthening is achieved in conjunction with the exhale so that muscles of the area do not form protective spasms. The tensile stress from stretching warms the CT and increases the water-binding properties of its ground matrix (the gelatin or Silly Putty-like base). The result is softer and more pliable fascia.

SHAKING AND FLOPPING

Shaking is often classified as a vibrational technique, although the application of shaking begins with lifting and

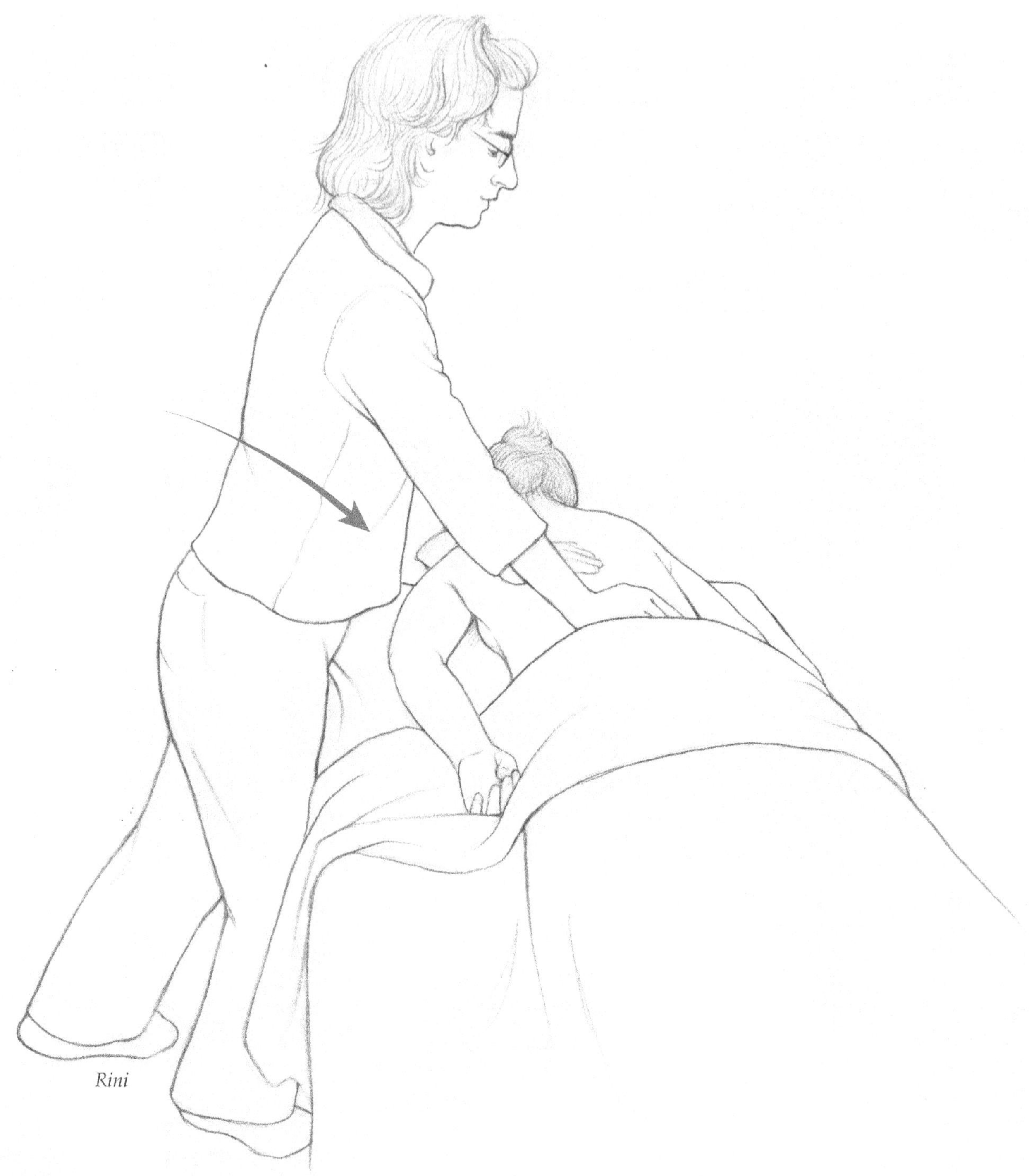

FIGURE 8-2 Compression. In indirect connective tissue massage, compression does not mean pressing down on the client; rather, it means following and sinking down in conjunction with the client's natural rhythm.

pulling rather than a compressive motion (Figure 8-4). According to Fritz (2000), shaking manipulations confuse the client's positional proprioceptors so that the muscles can relax. Fritz states that going limp is the natural response to the sensory input that is too unorganized for the integrating systems of the brain to interpret. Thus, shaking acts on the nervous system, but also has a mechanical effect on the CT from the lifting and pulling. Fritz advises bodyworkers to think of a dog shaking her favorite toy to get it away from you. The intensity may vary, but the basic steps are first to lift and then make a downward or sideways motion as if you are throwing something off.

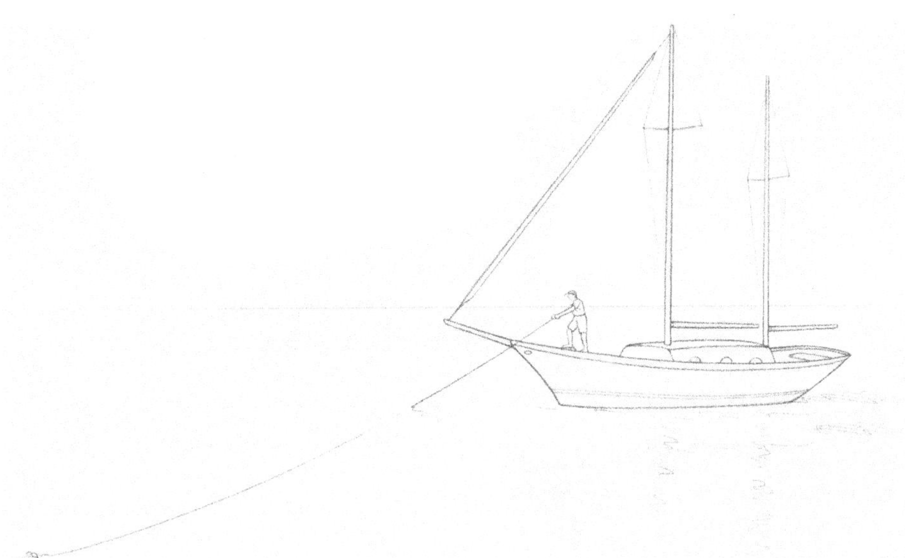

FIGURE 8-3 **Traction.** Use gentle pressure distributed slowly to soften and move connective tissue, just like the pressure you would exert on a boat's towline to pull it into shore.

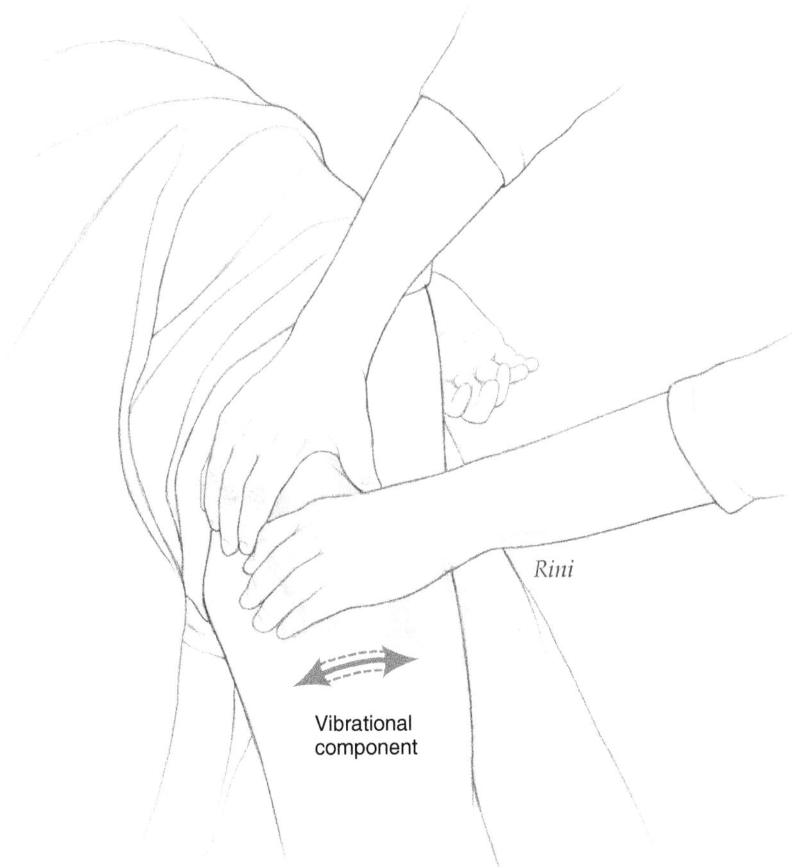

FIGURE 8-4 **Shaking.** Shaking begins with lifting and pulling before the vibrational component is added.

Shaking warms joints in a nonspecific manner and prepares muscle groups, synovial joints, or an entire limb for more focused bodywork. The joints of the shoulders, hips, and extremities respond well to shaking, as do the upper trapezius muscles, any muscle in the arms or legs, the abdominal muscles, and the pectoralis muscles close to the axilla. Always stay within the "give" of the tissue and its easy ROM. The larger the muscle or joint, the bigger the movements. As your intent to focus on a particular area of discomfort becomes more specific, the movements become smaller.

Flopping is a special type of shaking that is usually performed on the arms or legs (Figure 8-5). The limb is bounced in a controlled way onto the massage table. The nonverbal message is "feel the weight" or "feel the support," not "I'm going to let you bounce willy-nilly." Flopped limbs learn how to let go and feel some freedom within an atmosphere of safety.

Table 8-2 provides a quick reference for the indirect CT techniques discussed here.

RECOMMENDATIONS FOR OPTIMAL USE OF INDIRECT CONNECTIVE TISSUE TECHNIQUES

1. Do *not* poke, push, or shove. For fascial releases, locate bony landmarks and then allow your hands to rise to the level of superficial fascia. Use less than a nickel's weight of pressure for this. Note: The level of superficial fascia may differ widely for different clients.
2. Know the anatomical structures that you are palpating (i.e., muscles, fascial coverings, ligaments, tendons, vessels, bones) and use that knowledge to guide pressure and movement as you free the fascia.
3. If you think that you feel a release in the tissue (i.e., a movement in a certain direction), give yourself permission to believe in and follow that change.
4. You are looking for a softening in the area where you are working. As the tissue softens, it will feel as if the client's body is moving more easily.
5. If your body feels out of line, stop and readjust your position. As you take your hands off the client, ask her to breathe and move the area in a comfortable way. Use this time to stretch and breathe for yourself as well. When you reconnect, you will be fully present with your client rather than halfway there.
6. Breath cues (i.e., telling your client to continue to breathe easily) will increase your client's (and your own) awareness, engage the stuck layer, and make it easier to free restrictions.
7. Cues to move ("stretch," "take a deep breath") during pauses maintain interaction between the bodyworker and client and increase the client's sense of control. Asking for voluntary movement helps create conscious awareness of the changes that are occurring in

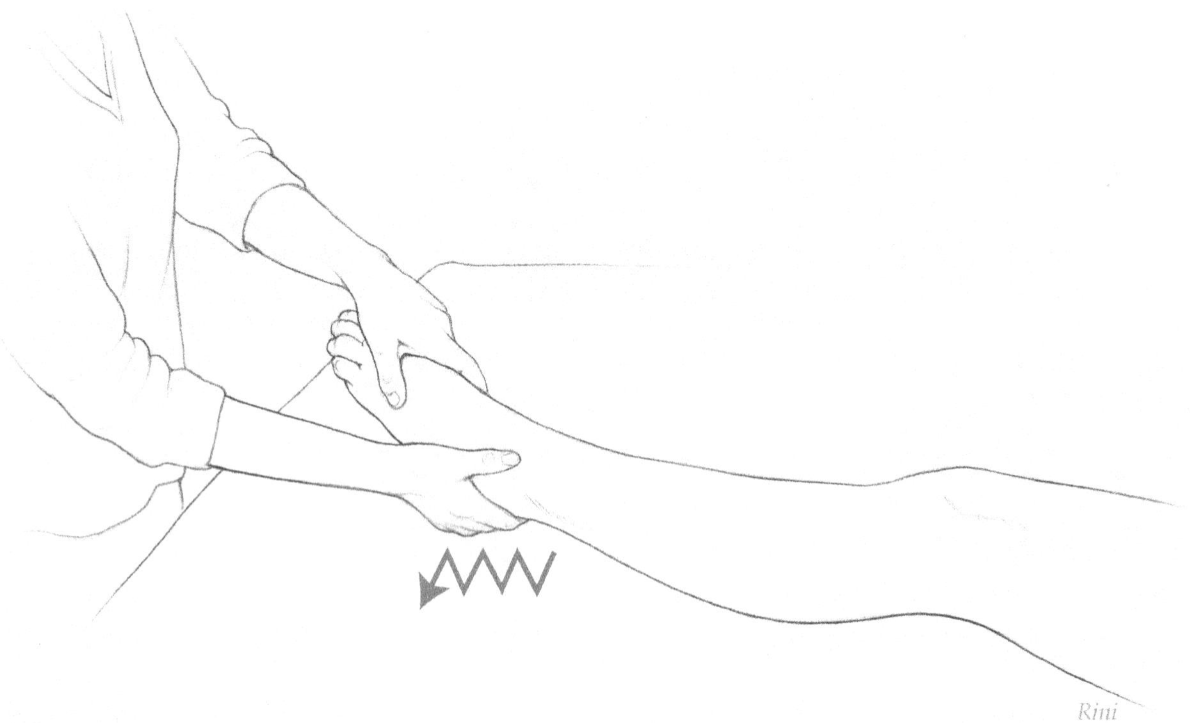

FIGURE 8-5 Flopping. In flopping, a limb is bounced in a controlled way onto the massage table. This tells the sensory receptors that "the limb is supported by the table."

TABLE 8-2 Indirect Connective Tissue Techniques

Technique	Description	Application
Compression	Pressing the muscle against the bone	Can be used for warming tissues, rather than effleurage, all over the body; can be performed through a sheet
Jostling (or rocking)	A type of vibration; jostling is rhythmic and applied with the whole body. Rocking can involve up-and-down, side-to side, or circular motions or any combination of these.	Whole body, often used on the back, at the hips; especially effective for deep relaxation through access of the parasympathetic nervous system; can be performed through a sheet
Traction	A mechanical method of longitudinal stretching or pulling tissue to reduce tensile stress. The therapist holds the skull or limb and steps back with the whole body into a lunge.	Used for neck or on limbs for spine, hip, or shoulder joint, akin to pulling on the rope of a boat in water; can be performed through a sheet
Shaking (including flopping)	Often classified as vibration, although shaking begins with lifting and pulling rather than a compression. First lift, then make a motion as if you are throwing something off (as flopping); applied to arms, legs, and neck by controlled bouncing on the massage table.	Shaking warms joints and prepares muscle groups, synovial joints, or limbs for more focused bodywork; the joints of the shoulders, hips and extremities respond well to shaking as do upper trapezius muscle, arm or leg muscles, abdominal muscles, and pectoralis muscles

the fascial network and facilitates the utilization of self-help exercises that help maintain more lasting change. See the specific suggestions below.

8. If you cannot follow a movement, change the placement of your hands (even if only by a half inch), and try again. If you cannot find a good orientation to the tissue after several tries, move to a different area.
9. For fascial releases, after you have accessed the right depth, follow the way the tissue moves most easily.
10. For fascial releases, if you cannot find the line of ease, try stacking or initially increasing the restriction you feel from the tissue. Do this systematically in different directions (e.g., up–down, side–side, twisting).
11. When stacking, take time to position your body behind each of the restricted planes of fascial tissue. Keep your pelvis, shoulder girdle, wrists, and hands in the same line. This will allow all of your body efforts to work in unison.

RECOMMENDATIONS FOR COACHING MOVEMENTS AND OPTIMIZING BODY AWARENESS

Asking the client to move during strategic pauses in the indirect CT approach helps engage the tissue beneath your hands (or elbow, knuckles, or forearm). When the client moves, it helps you to better sense the ease in the CT. You can see at once what the client instinctively wants to do to stretch. In addition, asking for movement maintains interaction between you and your client and can thereby increase the client's sense of control. Asking for voluntary movement also helps the client become consciously aware of the changes that are occurring in his fascial network and makes him more inclined to use self-help exercises to maintain more lasting change.

The following are recommendations for optimizing the client's body awareness with movement cues:

1. Stop every so often to let the client integrate changes that are happening.
2. Ask the client to stop and feel how movements affect a given area.
3. Ask the client to describe how a given area feels after you have worked there. When the client has to put her sensations into words, it makes the sensations more real and memorable.
4. Use questions to help the client visualize and reinforce movements or sensations. Some queries that enhance safety and ease beneficial movements include:
   - What would be easier?
   - What would be lighter?
   - Can you feel the support of the table (or my hand)?
5. Use imagery to help the client visualize and reinforce movements or sensations. The best images come from clients themselves. For instance, it would not be helpful to suggest the feeling of floating over a mountaintop if your client were afraid of heights.
6. Focus on areas that are ratchety or discontinuous in their movement. Do not shy away from these areas, but select small movements that are easy for the body to make. Focus on finding the easy range so that the movements become more smooth and continuous.

7. Another good instruction for movement is to guide the client into breathing comfortably at her own pace. Guided easy breathing is particularly beneficial when addressing the fascia that surrounds muscles that move in inspiration or expiration (e.g., over the chest, neck, and upper and lower back).
8. Another good cue is to guide the patient to alternately push into and away from your hands with very tiny movements. You could effectively coach this movement by saying "move into my hands, then release."
9. Help the client visualize the area you are working on. Show her a picture of the region from an anatomy chart or text. This engages conscious and voluntary aspects of healing into your session. Clients will better understand where you are working and actually see the unobstructed direction of the muscle and fascia that lie in that area.
10. Use a mirror to show the client how her fascial web holds and displays tensions before and after a session and to point out and reinforce improvements that she has made during the session.
11. Ask the client to walk and notice how easy (or difficult) it is to move both before and after a session. It is better to emphasize what clients can do as opposed to what they cannot. Words of encouragement are more empowering when they focus on ease of movement rather than stuck points or difficulties. This does not mean ignoring difficulties but rather looking to see the freedom that can be achieved within the boundaries that exist.

Indirect CT techniques are suitable for every region of the body. The key is to know what lies beneath your hands because the technique that you choose and the part of your body (your contact tool) that you use to contact the client's body are determined by the target zone and the tissue condition. You can adjust your contact to be very broad by using an outspread palm or very pointed and focused by using a knuckle or single finger. You can adapt through a continuum of focus by shifting from the radial (fleshy) side of the forearm for a wide, diffuse focus to the ulnar (bony) side of the forearm for a wider but more focused contact. You can concentrate the locus of movement more and more specifically by bending your arm through a more acute angle until the elbow becomes the point of contact. The elbow can apply the easy movement with a very precise touch.

Positioning, Draping, and Support

In general, because the intention is to convey a sense of movement across the fascial network and to let reverberations ripple through the web, the less propping you use, the better. Although propping tends to stop movement, the client's comfort takes priority, and if she needs support under her legs to relieve tension on her back, you should definitely place a pillow or bolster there. When the client is lying prone, you do not typically use a face rest in the indirect CT approach. Again, this is because you do not want to stop the ripple of movement at the neck, nor do you want to jar the client's face against the rest as she is rocked. Typically, the client is cued to turn her head to the other side as you complete work on one leg. You can also cue the client to turn her head to the opposite side as you complete indirect CT on the second leg and to turn at least twice more as you jostle her upper body and torso on one side and then the other. Use common sense. If holding the head to one side is uncomfortable for the client, use a face rest.

You can complete an entire indirect CT session with the client fully clothed, and in that case, draping is not necessary for modesty. The client should be reminded to wear loose-fitting and comfortable clothes for the session. It is also common to have clients undress down to their underwear; a drape is then required. If you are combining indirect CT techniques with direct CT or neuromuscular massage or with Swedish-style massage, it would be more convenient to have the client undress to her level of comfort; of course, a drape is then required.

I like to have a top sheet and a blanket over the client for warmth, regardless. The additional weight of the covers sends a signal of support and safety. Draping is performed with client supine and prone as in Swedish massage, with the use only of the diaper (Buddha) drape on the legs (which can be clothes pinned to keep it in place). This is to ensure modesty when flopping the client's legs and rotating them at the hip.

Treatment Planning and Decision Making

When designing a session or series of indirect CT sessions for a client, always begin with the needs of the individual and a thorough history-taking and intake procedure. Based on this information, identify a locus of attention (e.g., spending most of the treatment session on jostling the lower legs because of a low back complaint), which is then modified as you work and feel how the tissues respond to applications of movement and ease. If an area moves continuously and easily through the entire ROM at the outset, this region does not need additional work.

The indirect CT approach is effective for reducing all types of inflammation (chronic, subacute, and even acute) from both recent and past injuries that have not healed correctly. Let pain be a sign for caution. In this gentle approach, it is never appropriate to cause pain because pain causes a guarding response that is contrary to a sense of ease. If you inadvertently exceed the arc of comfortable movement, as signaled by a grimace or "ouch" from your client, reduce the movement range through a smaller arc that does not cause pain. You can safely target areas that are restricted as long as you stay within the arc of pain-free gentle movement (e.g., with rocking). You can even use the indirect CT approach for an acutely inflamed and painful site. Remember that you can move a painful area from a distant fulcrum (e.g., vibrating a painful back by means of rocking the belly), as long as it does not cause pain to the site.

Remember to attend not only to targeted areas of focus but also to the body as a whole. The indirect CT approach requires curiosity and interest, and you may want to devote more of your time and attention to areas that initially do not move easily. Furthermore, it takes time to tap into the fascial network and listen to where the movements stop or flow. Clients report that directed attention feels more complete than a superficial session that glides over all parts of the body but does not pay real attention to any distinct region.

Follow the protocol on page 151 if your goal is to affect the client's whole body. Alternately, you could use Tables 8-2 and 8-3 to find options for applying indirect CT techniques to a given region. These tables will also help you identify how to position yourself and your client to optimally work each area with indirect CT techniques. My

TABLE 8-3 Protocol for an Indirect Connective Tissue Session

Region	Therapist' Body Tools	Description of Movement
Client is supine:		
Head and neck		Push down on client's shoulders: • On the tops of shoulders down to the feet. • On the chest near the axilla down to the table.
	Palm of one hand	Rock the client's neck from side to side.
	Radial edges of the index fingers	Circle the neck up and toward you to extend and traction the client's neck.
	Cupping the client's head with your palm	With the client's head held on the diagonal, rock her head in your hand.
Upper extremities	Grasping (with a gentle but full hold) just above the client's wrist joint	Traction client's whole arm *slowly* from the shoulder.
	One hand holding the client's palm and the other grasping (as above) each digit in turn	Traction each digit *slowly*, visualizing sequentially all phalangeal, metacarpal, and carpal joints.
	Hold the client's hand in an L shape up from table	Jostle the arm with focus on movement at the shoulder joint.
Chest and abdomen	Full hand contacting sides of client's torso	Pull up and into center, moving sequentially down from above the client's hip bones to the ribs (upper torso).
	Full hand contact	Jostle with hands holding on to: • Both hips. • One hip and the opposite rib. • Then reverse the diagonal. • Ribs on both sides.
	Grasping between fingers and thumbs	Lift and shake the belly, starting at the client's hip.
	Ulnar side of hand	Compress along the sternum, moving superiorly.
	Full hands with outstretched fingers	Compress around the client's chest (avoiding the nipples), expanding outward three times.
	Cupped hands	Push down at the shoulders to the feet.
Legs	At the foot of table, reaching to shake hands with the ball of the foot	Traction and then flop the leg: "Hello, leg."
	At the foot of table, heel of the client cupped in your hand	Jiggle the heel side to side; heel is saying "Hello" back to you.
	From side, full hand contact	Jostle the leg medially: • Superior direction. • Inferior direction. Can repeat the entire sequence.
	Sitting on the table, facing out, grasping the foot in your two hands	"Clang the bell."

(continued)

TABLE 8-3 Protocol for an Indirect Connective Tissue Session (Continued)

Region	Therapist' Body Tools	Description of Movement
Legs (continued)	Sitting on the table, facing away toward the feet	Lengthen and widen the foot. Traction the leg from the hip joint.
	Facing the head of table	Jiggle the thigh.
	At the foot of table, cradling the lower leg in your arms	Bounce the thigh and calf.
Client is prone:		
Legs	At the foot of table, reaching out to shake hands with the ball of foot	Compress the ball of the foot. Traction the leg from the hip joint. Flop the leg. Shake the bent leg.
	Therapist at side of table, ball of the foot between the thumb and fingers	Traction the foot as you shake and reduce the angle of the leg. Set the bent leg on the table and use the other hand to roll the tissue around the calf.
	Hands on either side of the thigh	Jiggle the thigh.
Gluteals	Knuckles, backs of hands, or forearm or elbow	Compress and jostle at the: Sacrum Greater trochanter Ischial tuberosities
Back	Full hands	"Hula hoop" at the hip.
	Heels of hands, then knuckles	Jostling on either side of the spine.
Upper back or shoulders	Full hands with outstretched fingers	Compress around the shoulder blades, expanding outward.
	Cupped hands	Push down at the shoulders to the feet.
Neck or shoulders	Client's arm to side bent off the table; therapist sitting on the table facing the head with the leg underneath as a bolster.	Lift and roll the triceps like making bread.
	Inner hand on the medial shoulder; outer hand cups under the client's arm where it meets the scapula.	Flop the scapula with the outward hand and hold at several points with the inner hand. Rotate the arm at the shoulder.
	Stand to the side of the shoulder	Swing the arm like a pendulum. Pull the arm down and flop on the table.

hope with all myofascial massage, especially with the indirect CT approach, is that you use the protocol as a jumping-off point to begin to express the rhythms you seek and find in each individual body. See the protocol as an ingredient list and feel free to embellish with creativity and joy as you move your clients into greater freedom and lightness with the indirect CT approach.

SUMMARY

Indirect CT massage is especially useful for dealing with acutely painful and inflamed areas by working with them indirectly, gently, and often offsite. The indirect CT approach allows bodyworkers to address resistances in the client's body from the perspective of ease, which can be very helpful for patients who resist direct change. Indirect CT work involves the application of movements to stir up the fascia and soften it like stirring up thick soup. Important influences on the indirect myofascial massage approach can be found in Trager work, HSE, the Feldenkrais method, the Alexander technique, other movement reeducation styles, and Barnes' Myofascial Release.

Indirect CT strokes include jostling, rocking, compression, traction, flopping and shaking, and fascial releases.

The therapist should keep his or her body moving in rhythm with the jostling, rocking, traction, shaking and flopping, and compressive movements to optimize the effectiveness of indirect CT massage. Taking time to pause from the rhythm and let it sink in to the client's consciousness is essential. The fascial release requires gentle and slow pressure to listen for and follow a fluid CT movement into the

PROTOCOL: SAMPLE SESSION OF INDIRECT CONNECTIVE TISSUE MASSAGE

The following list and Table 8-3 provide a reminder of a good ordering and procedure for working through the full body in a general indirect CT session. Such lists, however, can really only give a starting orientation for the application of the indirect CT approach. Keeping your body relaxed as you work is the only way that you can effectively flow with and follow the rhythms of your client. Body awareness of your own discomfort will help you to modify your hand positions so that they are most effective. Keep your breath flowing, and when you become aware of tensions, let them go. If you cannot shift your body to be more relaxed, take a break from the position. Coach your client to do the same as you breathe deeply and shake off tensions. Then, when you reconnect, you will be more fully present for your client and more available to identify natural rhythms and your client's easy ROM. Shifting out of uncomfortable body positions will help you with your ability to sense shifts in the fascial movement. If your body is tense, you will be braced against the movements and unable to register them. Moving with the flow of the CT allows you to listen to (and follow) the movements of a client's body in the most effective way:

1. Head and neck (supine)
2. Upper extremities, belly, and chest (supine)
3. Lower extremities (supine)
4. Lower extremities (prone)
5. Buttocks and back, going up the spine (prone)
6. Shoulders, neck and upper extremities (prone)
7. Head and neck (supine)

Table 8-3 below identifies in more detail this way of ordering an individual session, how to position your client, and what part of your body to use as the contact tool. It is important to remember that the protocol can really only serve as a starting point for your application of the indirect CT approach. Keeping your body moving as you work is the key to effectively freeing the client's body rhythms. Awareness of your own discomfort (or lack of ease) will help you to modify your movements for optimum efficiency. "Fiddling" around with body position is at the heart of all CT massage. "Fiddling" means moving your body into positions that match the flow of the CT to better follow the direction of ease.

direction of ease. This direction is palpable as the way the CT moves most easily.

When administering indirect CT techniques, the therapist needs to follow the slow fascial releases in his own body and incorporate breaks for the client's body to integrate the change. It is essential to encourage breathing and questions and cue the client to perform active stretches of his own choosing to reinforce conscious awareness.

Therapists can customize indirect CT techniques to any part of the body and can also customize massage sessions to incorporate indirect CT strokes as needed, in conjunction with other styles, for an eclectic massage.

Review Questions

1. Psychophysical Integration is a component of which of the following approaches?
   a. Feldenkrais
   b. HSE
   c. Trager
   d. Upledger
2. In HSE, the stress response to a real or imaginary threat or worry is called the __________.
   a. Landau reflex
   b. startle reflex
   c. spinal reflex
   d. trauma reflex
3. An indirect CT technique by which the client's limb is bounced in a controlled way onto the massage table is called __________.
   a. flopping
   b. shaking
   c. jostling
   d. rocking
4. True or false: Indirect CT techniques can help areas that were recently injured and are red, hot, swollen, or sore.
5. True or false: The indirect CT approach to myofascial massage involves applying movement to the client's body without excess pressure.
6. True or false: SMA is a functional deficit whereby the ability to contract a muscle has been surrendered to subcortical (involuntary) reflexes.
7. When using the indirect CT approach to work with a client, a primary question to ask yourself is, "What could be easier or __________?"

8. ________ is one principle of HSE. It allows clients to focus on the process and to feel the entire sequence of a movement with all of the intermediate steps, rather than just focusing on the end result of an exercise or stretch.

9. HSE teaches people to take ________ control of their muscles so they can bypass automatic (autonomic) responses that may not be helpful.

10. Name and describe four indirect CT techniques.

REFERENCES

Barnes JF. Myofascial Release Handbook. Paoli, PA: MFR Seminars, 1995.

Fritz S. Mosby's Fundamentals of Therapeutic Massage. 2nd Ed. St. Louis: Mosby Lifeline, 2000.

Griffin JL. How Anybody Can Learn to Swim Well. Silver Spring, MD: Manifest Press, 1989.

Hanna T. Clinical somatic education. Somatics 1990/1991, 1994:4–10.

Thomas CL, ed. Taber's Encyclopedic Medical Dictionary. 18th Ed. Philadelphia: FA Davis Company, 1997.

Twomely L, Taylor J. Flexion, creep, dysfunction and hysteresis in the lumbar vertebral column. Spine 1982;7:116–122.

Upledger JE. Class Notes—Craniosacral I and II. Portland OR, 1996.

Upledger JE, Vredevoogd JD. Craniosacral Therapy. Seattle, WA: Eastland Press, 1983.

Welch-Baril C, Baril R. Movement as medicine: an interview with Carol Welch-Baril. Massage Therapy Journal 1994(Winter):69–80.

SUGGESTED READINGS

Hanna T. Somatics: Reawakening the Mind's Control of Movement, Flexibility, and Health. 4th Ed. Reading, MA: Addison-Wesley Publishing Co, 1991.

Juhan D. Job's Body: A Handbook for Bodywork. Barrytown, NY: Barrytown, Ltd., 1998.

Sacks O. A Leg to Stand On. New York: Simon and Schuster, 1984.

Schultz RL, Feitis R. The Endless Web: Fascial Anatomy and Physical Reality. Berkeley, CA: North Atlantic Books, 1996.

Schwartz D. What could be lighter? The work of Milton Trager. Massage Magazine 1997(May/June):56–63.

Chapter

9

Exercises to Supplement Indirect Methods

OBJECTIVES

- Explain why exercise is an important supplement to indirect myofascial massage methods.
- Discuss the research on, goals of, and benefits of exercise.
- Discuss reinforcing indirect myofascial massage with recommendations that encourage safe exercise.

CHAPTER OUTLINE

KEY TERMS

Exercise: Purposeful movement or physical activity, including formal activities such as team sports, dance, and games, and less formal activities, such as walking, jogging, and swimming. Can refer to large muscle activities or nontaxing, specific small muscle movements.

Warm-up: A session of light to moderate activity, including stretching, done before serious exercise or, in some cases, as a stand-alone exercise period.

Stimulus period: The core of the exercise workout or period of most intense activity.

Cool down: A session of light to moderate tapering-off activity after more vigorous exercise, often consisting of the same exercises used in the warm-up.

Chapter 8 introduced the hands-on indirect connective tissue (CT) approach, by which the therapist responds to resistance in the tissues by shifting back toward the direction of ease. In such indirect methods, myofascial therapists kinesthetically teach clients to replace difficult, jerky, and painful reactions with easy, smooth and continuous, painless movement. These lessons can be enhanced with self-care activities that reinforce letting go, feeling the support of the body's weight and gravity, and searching for movements that create ease.

Because the direct method is designed to maximize the client's ability to sense resistance in the soft tissues, self-care for clients receiving the direct method could be supported through just one practice (hatha yoga). In contrast, indirect methods seek to enhance the client's ability to move without pain and to experience easy, supported, comfortable movement. These methods are best supplemented by a client-oriented, multi-option approach. Some activities may be comfortable and supportive for one client (e.g., swimming) but frightening and stress laden for another. Therefore, it is important for the myofascial therapist to provide ground rules for supportive indirect method self-care without endorsing only one discipline or training.

The word exercise *can convey a sense of rigidity and obligation, but at its most basic, the term simply means purposeful movement. In this chapter, the terms* exercise, physical activity, *and* movement *are used interchangeably and do not imply obligation or adherence to any one protocol.*

This chapter discusses exercise performed in support of indirect myofascial massage. Therefore, it describes the goals and benefits of exercise and provides recommendations for using exercise to supplement indirect methods. The chapter is not intended to cover all aspects of exercise. Please consult the chapter references and suggested readings for more information.

Additionally, keep in mind that diagnosis and prescription are outside the scope of practice for massage therapists. Thus, any exercise routine should be prescribed by a licensed and qualified professional (i.e., a sports therapist, physical therapist, physical trainer, or exercise physiologist). Knowledge of the goals and benefits of exercise, and ways to recommend and inspire its appropriate use, however, will greatly improve the clinical practice of indirect myofascial massage methods.

Research on Exercise and Health

In an Internet search of the scientific literature using MEDLINE (key words: exercise and health benefit), over 2,000 entries were displayed for the last 5 years alone. These studies looked at a vast array of disease conditions, including diabetes (Castaneda, 2003), cancer (Schneider et al, 2002), arthritis (Da Costa et al, 2003) and coronary heart disease (The Vestfold Heartcare Study Group, 2003); and physiological changes such as lowering blood glucose and contributing to weight loss (Castaneda, 2003).

Exercise improves the health of numerous physiological and psychological systems in the human body. Studies have found that exercise decreases fatigue, improves functional capacity, increases immune function, and leads to perceived improved quality of life (Schneider et al, 2002). One review showed that exercise, particularly walking, increases muscle strength and aerobic capacity and reduces functional musculoskeletal limitations (Keysor, 2003). Exercise appears to help the digestive system to function more efficiently, contributing to weight loss, lowered blood glucose levels, and increased insulin action (Castaneda, 2003). Physical activity can also reliably lower triglyceride levels and favorably affect both low-density lipoprotein (LDL) and high-density lipoprotein (HDL) counts (Szapary et al, 2003). Through these mechanisms, exercise contributes to increased endurance and aerobic power, improved blood flow, and reduced risk for cardiovascular disease.

Several studies link exercise to stress reduction. Based on the previous work of Sutton (1978), Tharp (1975), and Winder et al (1982), Seaward (1994) theorizes the effects of exercise on reducing stress as threefold. One, a single session of aerobic exercise appears to "burn off" existing stress hormones by directing them out of the bloodstream and toward intended metabolic functions. Two, the training effect of repeated exercise sessions may prepare the body for future stressful episodes by decreasing the level of hormonal secretions in connection with feelings of anger or fear. Three, in the long term, exercise appears to reduce susceptibility to stress by improving the functioning of several physiological systems, including the heart, lungs, blood vessels, kidneys, and muscle and skeletal tissue.

Principles of Exercise Therapy

All people, regardless of age, gender, or ability, can enjoy movement if they carefully choose their activities and follow basic guidelines that promote ease and a sense of fun. Exercise therapy can provide a number of goals and benefits.

SYNERGISTIC GOALS

Easy, comfortable movements have a synergistic relationship with the indirect CT and craniosacral approaches. Letting go of a physical barrier with easy movements mirrors the experience of an indirect CT release on the massage table. (This is also true for craniosacral recipients but in a subtler, less detectable way.) The experiences of jostling, rocking, and rolling can be likened to mindfully and kinesthetically experiencing the full sequence of an easy, comfortable exercise activity.

BENEFITS OF EXERCISE THERAPY

Because motivation is a major factor for determining whether an exercise program is faithfully followed or abandoned, it is especially important to help clients with physical challenges understand the benefits of exercise and its role in rehabilitation. Being educated on specific benefits that can be reasonably expected is more helpful than hearing that "exercise is good for you." Understanding these benefits will help you to clearly communicate to clients how exercise can help them.

1. **Improved posture and body mechanics:** Easy, comfortable exercise can promote new musculoskeletal patterns that no longer create conditions for a second injury. Improved ways of sitting, standing, and moving reduce the probability of new or recurrent injury in vulnerable areas.
2. **Strengthened muscles:** Strengthening muscles is especially important if your client has become weak and debilitated. For example, if the leg muscles on one side have become weak from disuse, the client must work to strengthen both that side and the contralateral leg, which will be required to provide support during healing.
3. **Increased flexibility:** Flexibility allows the spine to rotate properly and ensures that the client can use all of the muscle groups. When the muscles work together, movements become easier.
4. **Pain relief:** The body produces its own internal analgesics, known as endorphins ("inner morphines"). Spinal fluid endorphins can be increased by exercise that activates large muscle groups (Schatz, 1992). An increase in endorphins decreases pain sensitivity and may also contribute to a positive mental outlook.
5. **Increased body awareness:** Becoming more aware of the warning signs of an injury may help prevent injury recurrence. Early warning signals may vary greatly between people but are often fairly consistent for each individual. Help your client to become sensitized to these kinds of signals:
   - A feeling of strain
   - General discomfort
   - A localized sensation of muscle soreness or tenderness
   - A diffuse, dull ache

Clients can learn to rest at the first signals of prepain and avoid the incapacity that could accompany a full-blown attack.

Psychological benefits also accrue from establishing exercise as a lifestyle change. Reported psychological benefits of habitual exercise (particularly from walking and jogging) include the following (Seaward, 1994):

1. Improved self-esteem. Feeling good about the steps you are taking to improve your health can help you to feel better about yourself.
2. Improved sense of self-reliance and self-efficacy. Clients who successfully perform exercise get an experience of "I can do it!"
3. Improved mental alertness, perception, and information processing.
4. Increased perception of acceptance by others.
5. Decreased feelings of depression and anxiety.
6. Decreased overall sense of stress and tension. Exercise metabolizes the body's activities at a higher rate, thereby ridding the body of many byproducts of the stress response.

Recommendations for Using Exercise to Supplement Indirect Methods

When practicing indirect myofascial methods, you need to be prepared to discuss how to make successful activity choices so that you and your client can arrive jointly at the most supportive adjunct to hands-on treatment. Thus, this section discusses ways to approach exercising that reinforce the ease, comfort, and support of indirect myofascial tablework.

Of course, it is always prudent to consult with a physician before beginning any exercise program. Although physical exercise may improve many aspects of physiological and psychological health, it can pose a threat to physical well-being if adequate precautions are not observed. Therefore, it is important for you to instruct clients to consult with their primary physician or healthcare provider before beginning any exercise program that you suggest as a supplement to myofascial work.

HELPING CLIENTS WORK WITH THEIR PAIN

Many people who are recovering from injuries, especially multiple injuries, are afraid to exercise. They may have had unpleasant experiences with exercising and do not realize that exercise can be adapted so that there is little or no pain. Those who "hurt all over" may believe that any physical activity will increase the pain. It is helpful for clients to realize that pain is not constant, to become aware of the conditions existing when they hurt, and to be able to pinpoint exactly where and how they hurt. With this knowledge, they can modify exercises to prevent additional injury.

Clients who have had injuries or surgery must learn to distinguish among the various types of sensations that may be perceived as pain. These include muscle stretch

One Therapist's Experience: The Experience of Purposeful Movement

My first book, *Bodylessons* (Dixon, 1992, republished by Findhorn Press, 2005), explored the effects of movement upon thoughts, emotions, and the experience of life. To provide a first-hand account of the significance of purposeful movement, an excerpt from the introduction follows:

"Something in young adulthood made many of my friends become self-conscious and embarrassed about the body and convinced that its actions were awkward and ugly. I know that nothing could be further from the truth, having danced with three and four and eighty-year olds, patients recovering from strokes, and people who could not see the ground in front of them. From these experiences, I know that everyone can move and everyone can dance—they do not need to talk or to see, they don't even need to walk. I have seen people confined to wheelchairs spin and dip and express sheer joy from purposeful movement. Experience has convinced me that not only can everyone dance . . . but what is more, everyone needs to.

Moving my own body has been a source of wonder and of joy. Purposeful movement has cheered my soul so many times and has made even the sad times worth living. Physical activity is like life, in that it becomes meaningful when we participate in it. It is not enough to sit back and watch someone else. Physical activity has helped me at times when I could not talk about my feelings. Movement (for me—exercise with the fitness ball, swimming and dancing, especially) has been a comfort when other sources of light seemed to dim. When I am feeling confused and not trusting my thoughts or emotions, my body has been an anchor. I trust my body. It tells me the truth. It tells me when I am stiff and need to move, or when I am hungry and need to be fed. The process of moving can be a teacher about so many things in life . . . about all that I do."

sensation, muscle overstretch pain, radiating nerve pain (shooting, burning pain like an electric shock), scar stretch pain, and postexercise pain (Schatz, 1992).

Any movement or position that creates numbness or a sharp "electric shock" (nerve pain) should be modified so that the basic movement can be performed without causing either of these sensations. This is not quite the same as ceasing completely whenever some kind of discomfort arises. According to Schatz (1992), a physician and author who specializes in chronic pain, stopping all exercise that causes any pain can eliminate some exercises that could be the most effective when properly modified. Persisting in an exercise and hoping to work through pain, however, is counterproductive. Numbness, shooting, and burning pain like an electric shock, and muscle overstretch pain, are signals that something is wrong. The body reacts to these sensations by tensing the muscles, which can create more pain, as well as the potential for injury.

If clients report that an exercise feels painful, advise them to decrease the intensity to a level at which they can relax into the movement and still feel at "ease." Radiating nerve pain is caused by nerve compression, often by a herniated intervertebral disc. Scar stretch pain is caused by stretching of shortened CTs around a previously injured vertebral segment. The pain does not radiate but is confined to the scarred tissues around the injury. Scar stretch pain is not constant but appears in body positions that stretch the scar and disappears when the position is released. Schatz (1992) claims this is a necessary pain that patients must gauge so tearing of soft tissue does not occur, yet sufficient stretch is placed on the shortened fascia to lengthen it. Scar stretch pain, nerve pain, and muscle overstretch pain are of short duration and end as soon as the incorrect action (or correct action in the first instance) is altered.

In contrast, postexercise pain begins after the exercise session is over and persists for several hours, usually as a dull ache. Schatz's (1992) basic rule is that if pain persists more than 2 or 3 hours after exercise, the amount, intensity, or alignment of activity should be altered. A consultation with a personal trainer, physical therapist, or other professional may be needed to modify the exercise at this point. Additional recommendations (adapted from Corbin and Lindsay, 1988) are provided in the next section.

LAYING THE GROUNDWORK

You may wish to lay the groundwork for clients' success by compiling the following suggestions into a self-care handout for clients. Handouts can be especially useful for reinforcing specific exercises that were identified in the course of an indirect CT (or craniosacral) session.

1. Prepare for exercise by including warm-up and cool-down periods. Exercise without proper warm-up and cool-down periods promotes injury to soft tissue and

causes pain. Preparation makes exercise easier and, therefore, more fun.

2. Give clients time to succeed with an exercise plan. This also means factoring in time for activity check-ins and encouragement during bodywork sessions. During your check-ins, make sure the client has had enough time to establish an exercise habit.
3. Psychological benefits enhance exercise enjoyment. For example, exercise makes patients feel "normal" and empowered, that "I can do it!"
4. A positive attitude helps clients to enjoy exercise. If there is a problem, acknowledge it and help the client find ways to meet the challenge and change what is not working.
5. When pursuing a competitive sport, it is more enjoyable to play with a partner of similar ability and to build some proficiency in the skills needed for the sport.

MAKING EXERCISE ENJOYABLE

Clients are more likely to follow through on a physical activity program when they find it enjoyable. Everyone, no matter what his or her circumstances, can enjoy some form of activity. I have had the privilege of enjoying movement with stroke recovery patients, children who use wheelchairs, and older adults with impaired vision. The trick is tailoring exercise to individual needs.

It is not uncommon to prescribe three or four self-care exercises, only to find during later bodywork sessions that the client has failed to implement any of the suggestions. Individually customizing exercises so that they are easier to remember and perform may be more beneficial than pointing out that the client was wrong not to exercise.

Do not overlook participation in sports as a way of making exercise enjoyable for your clients. Regular participation in sports can improve cardiovascular fitness, muscular endurance, strength, and flexibility, and provide valuable psychological and social benefits as well. Participants may also derive personal satisfaction and meaning from the social interactions of team sports or individual sports practiced in a group (e.g., fitness walking).

Sports activities that best support the indirect method include swimming, walking, bicycling, jogging, and running (Corbin and Lindsay, 1988). Other group activities that support the indirect CT approach (and the craniosacral approach, presented in the next chapter) are *tai chi* and *qi gong*, disciplines of traditional Chinese medicine that promote fitness, vitality, and balance. Gentle activities that nurture the continuous, flowing, easy, and supportive movements of the indirect method include bellydancing, Trager Mentastics (introduced in the previous chapter), Feldenkrais Awareness through Movement, exercise with a fitness (therapy) ball, and the Alexander Technique.

Tai chi chuan is a sequence of martial arts postures connected by slow, flowing, transitional movements (Figure 9-1). Tai chi gives a dynamic stretch to all the muscles and joints; generates muscle growth in the legs; stimulates acupuncture points; and encourages deep, rhythmic breathing (Seaward, 1994). Qi gong has been practiced for thousands of years. Its gentle, flowing movements encourage a balance of mind and body and are said to increase longevity.

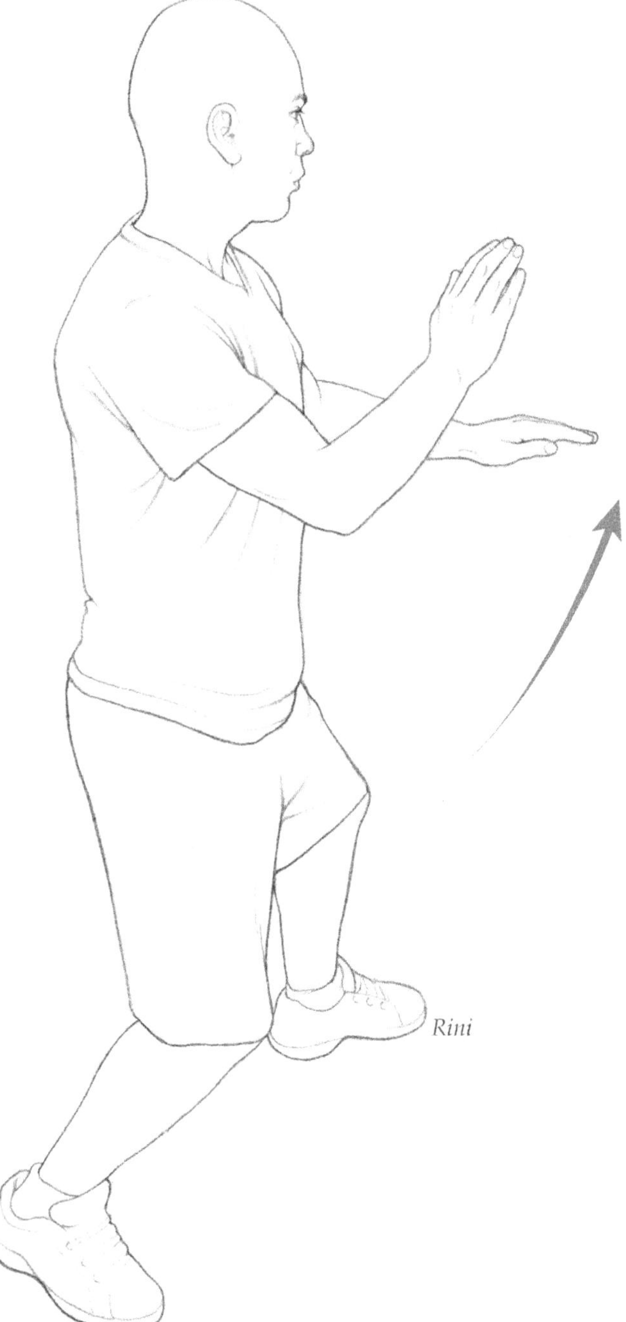

FIGURE 9-1 Tai chi chuan. Tai chi chuan emphasizes the flow from one martial arts stance to another.

Bellydancing helps to awaken energy throughout the body while lengthening and strengthening the muscle groups of the torso (Figure 9-2). It also trains the body to

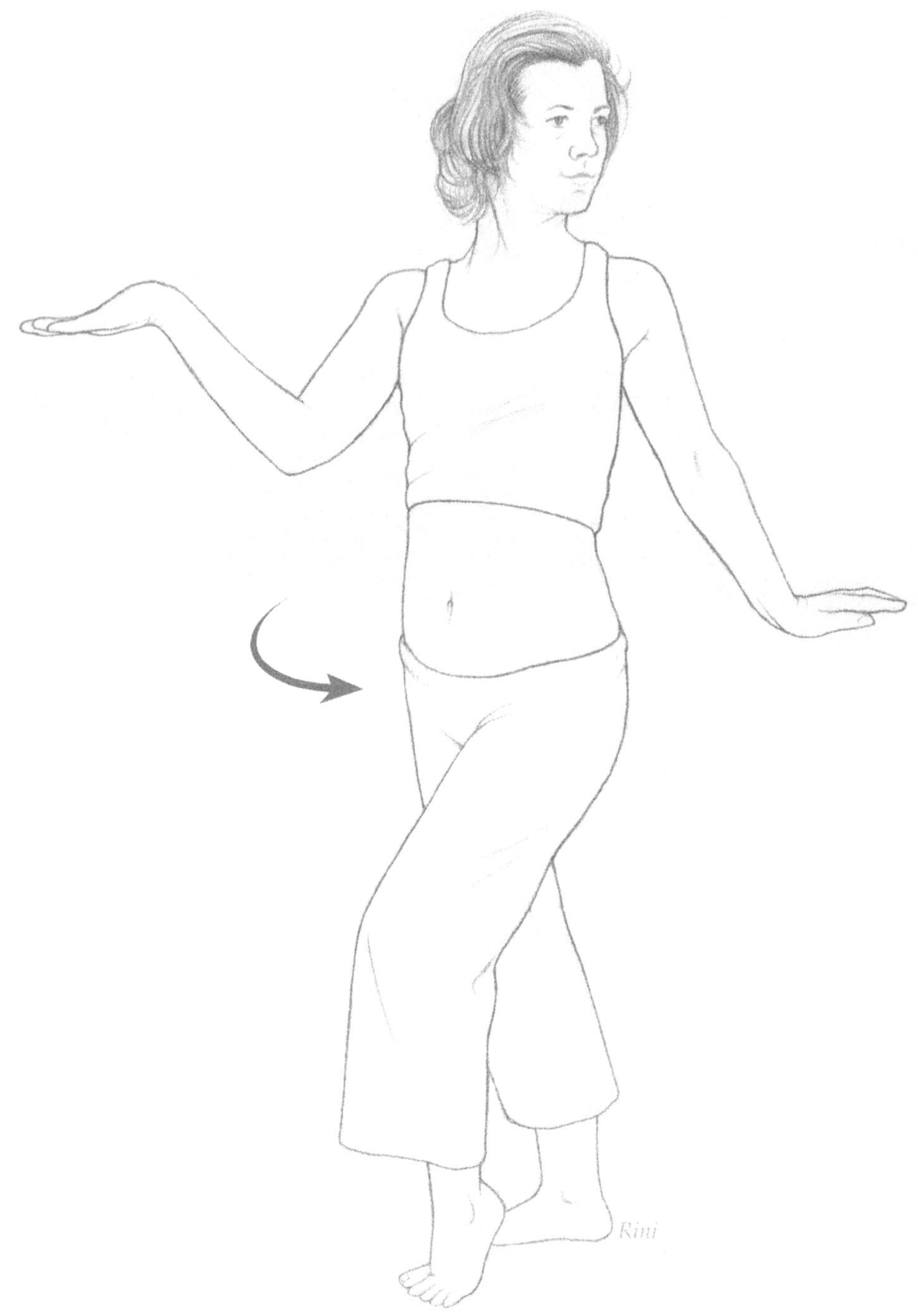

FIGURE 9-2 Bellydancing. Bellydancing emphasizes freedom of the torso and pelvis, which can be very helpful for clients with low back pain.

release holding through the pelvis (a common source of back pain).

Fitness ball exercise is used for stretching, toning, or a low-impact aerobic workout (Figure 9-3). Exercise with a fitness ball can relieve tension, increase circulation, and strengthen the back muscles.

Mentastics exercise relaxes the body, particularly the antagonists to a target movement. Because the object of Mentastics is to be light and playful and to feel good, there is little resistance to the new sensations of ease. Feldenkrais' tiny Awareness through Movement exercises help you find the easiest way of making a larger motion. The Alexander Technique aims to change movement habits by teaching the appropriate use of effort and the release of unnecessary tension for particular activities such as sitting, lying down, standing, walking, or lifting.

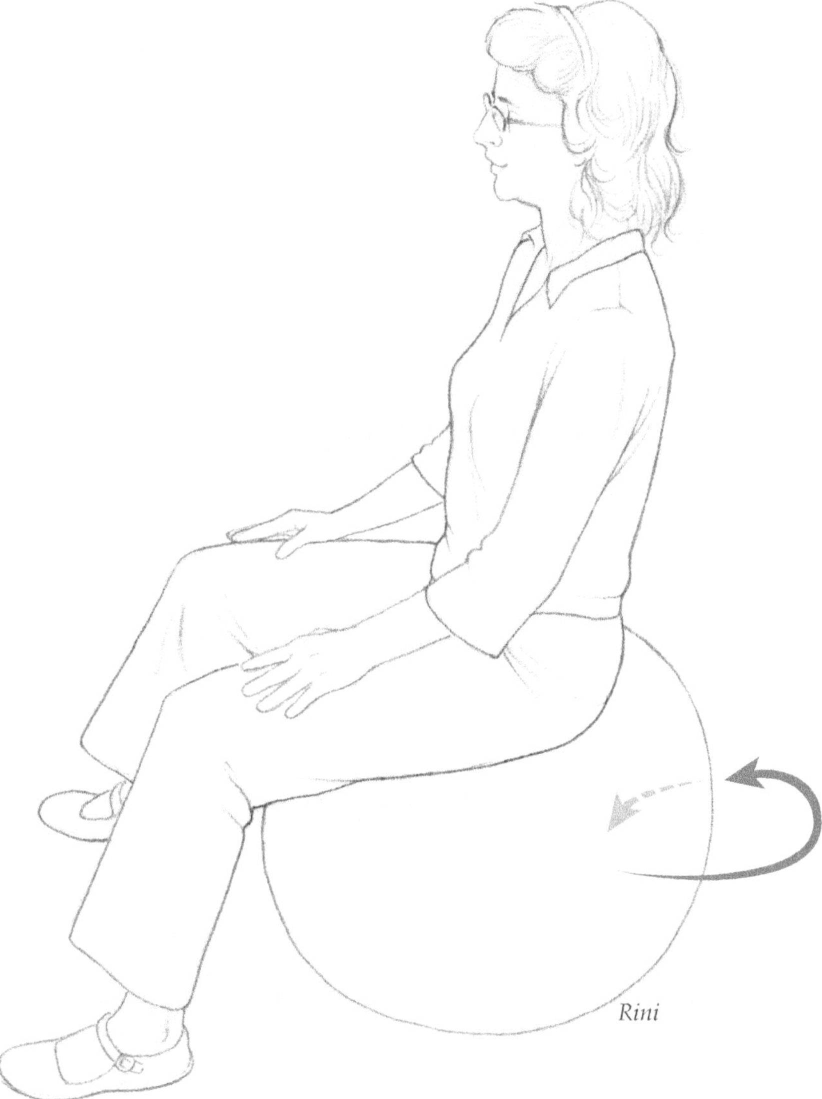

FIGURE 9-3 **Fitness ball.** Exercising with the fitness ball can build strength in the abdomen without excessive strain.

PREPARING FOR EXERCISE

If clients are sore, injured, or afraid of irritating a medical problem, exercise can become something to fear rather than something to enjoy. Dressing appropriately and including warm-up and cool-down periods makes the activity safer and less likely to cause stress.

Dressing Appropriately

Clothing worn for exercise should be comfortable and not too tight. Exercise apparel should not restrict movement or bind the joints. Clothing that is worn next to the skin should be porous to allow sweat evaporation. Some of the new microfibers are designed specifically to wick perspiration away from the body. Women may want to wear a sports bra to provide extra support for the breasts during exercise, and men may want to use an athletic supporter. A warm-up suit worn over other exercise apparel can be removed if the client becomes too warm during the session. If participating in outdoors activities, clients should wear apparel that is warm or cool enough for the season. For winter sports, this calls for dressing in layers.

Many types of exercise footwear are available. Shoes designed specifically for jogging and running have a high back to support the Achilles tendon; a wide, cushioned, and elevated heel; good arch support; and adequate room for the toes. Regardless of the type of shoe, it is important to try on shoes before making a purchase to ensure a comfortable fit. It is better to replace shoes too soon than risk injury (Corbin and Lindsay, 1988). If shoes are run down to the inside or the outside, the client's gait will be thrown off. Breakdown of the heel is the cardinal sign that shoes need replacing.

Warming Up

One reason to warm up before exercise is to stretch the skeletal muscles, thereby helping to prevent muscle soreness and injury. Another reason is to prepare the heart muscle for exercise.

A skeletal muscle warm-up includes static stretching of the major muscle groups that will be involved in the exercise to follow. Although warming up before an activity may help reduce the chance of muscle injury, warm-ups do not substitute for a regular exercise program designed to improve flexibility.

Adults who include a cardiovascular warm-up do not experience electrocardiographic abnormalities that can occur when exercise is begun too abruptly (Corbin and Lindsay, 1988). Approximately 2 minutes of slower, less-intense exercise (e.g., walking) prepares the heart muscle for more vigorous exercise.

A warm-up suitable for jogging or running would minimally include the following stretches: static calf stretch (part of the downward dog as described in the salutation to the sun in Chapter 7), adapted sidebend, sidebend, adapted sun pose (hamstring stretch), and knee squeeze (all described in Chapter 7). The cardiovascular warm-up should be 2 minutes of a slow walk or jog. Cardiovascular warm-ups can be adapted to most activities by simply performing 2 minutes of the target exercise in a gentle fashion. For example, a slow, 2-minute swim for swimmers or a slow, 2-minute bicycle ride (stationary or moving) for cyclists would be excellent cardiovascular warm-ups for those sports.

Warm-up stretches can be performed before or after the cardiovascular warm-up (Corbin and Lindsay, 1988). Some experts believe that a cardiovascular warm-up should always precede stretching because warm muscles stretch more easily and are less likely to be injured.

Your client's target activity may very well not require the heart to beat faster or harder. A reasonable goal may be just to get the arm to move easily and comfortably above shoulder height. Even for clients engaging in such limited exercise, it is helpful to perform a warm-up before the stimulus period. Use the rule prescribed above: clients should perform the target exercise in a gentler fashion a few times before they practice the full movement. Warm-up stretches may be omitted (and may even be contraindicated for severe or acute injury).

Stimulus Period

The stimulus period is the core of the workout and the period of greatest intensity. If the stimulus period is meant to provide a cardiovascular workout, Seaward (1994) suggests that it should be 20 minutes at a minimum. For low-intensity indirect method goals, a sensible guideline is to perform the target activity for the same amount of time it takes to complete both the warm-up and cool-down periods together.

Adopting a new activity regimen requires clients to maintain sensitivity to their pain level. Some clients may want to practice until it hurts or think practicing will not do any good without pain (e.g., "No pain, no gain."). This directly contradicts the principle of the indirect CT approach, which is to find the ease and comfort in a movement. Undue effort and strain can damage muscle and CT. Do not let your clients go past a point where they feel easy movement because physical activities have the most impact when performed within the client's pain-free range of motion. When your clients exercise, help them to understand the importance of staying comfortable and supported in movement.

Cooling Down

A cool-down period after exercise is also important. As with the warm-up, static muscle stretching and a cardiovascular component are the two principal parts. Some experts believe that static muscle stretching is more important *after* rather than before the workout because it can help reduce delayed-onset muscle soreness (i.e., muscle pain felt the day after exercise), as well as prevent shortening of muscles in general.

A cardiovascular cool-down is important when the target activity significantly elevates heart and breathing rate. During vigorous exercise, the heart pumps a large amount of blood to the working skeletal muscles to supply the oxygen necessary to keep moving. The action of the muscles squeezes the veins and forces blood back into the heart. Valves in the veins prevent the blood from flowing backward. As long as exercise continues, the muscles push blood back to the heart, where it reoxygenates for circulation. If exercise is halted abruptly, blood is left in the skeletal muscles with no way to return to the heart. For example, for runners, stopping short causes blood to pool in the legs. With less blood for the heart to pump, the blood pressure may drop precipitously. This can cause dizziness or fainting. The best way to prevent this complication is to gradually taper off the activity. A healthful cardiovascular cool-down includes approximately 2 minutes of a nonvigorous activity that uses the same muscles activated in the primary workout.

CUSTOMIZING ACTIVITIES

Preparing for activity also includes continually adjusting the movements that are practiced, as well as their timing and duration. Environmental factors such as cold, heat, or humidity could motivate a change in routine, as could the client's present condition (e.g., just recovering from the flu). Not taking account of these circumstances can make movement less enjoyable, less effective, or even unsafe.

Do not encourage your clients to push past their comfort level. If a client cannot distinguish signs of pre-pain from actual pain, teach the client to err on the conservative side and do less rather than more. Many people have incorrectly learned to associate pain with physical improvement and were taught that the more it hurts, the better. Remind clients that a sharp, acute pain is a warning to immediately stop what they are doing. Pain that does not go away after 4 or 5 days is an indication to seek medical attention.

Encourage your clients to notice when their body feels out of line and to take the time to readjust by breathing slowly and deeply and moving in a gentle fashion. When they return to their target activity slowly and gently, they will be more in synch and find more ease and support within.

GIVING EXERCISE ENOUGH TIME

Clients may unreasonably expect to see great increases in muscle strength or flexibility in just a few days. Although some people may report feeling better and a have sense of personal accomplishment at the outset, most physiological benefits take time to become apparent. Habits are difficult to shift in less than 3 weeks. Improvements in health may take several weeks or even longer to be noticed (Corbin and Lindsay, 1988). A typical mistake people make is exercising "too much and too soon." This causes disappointment and possible muscle and tendon damage, which may be the chief complaints that you have been asked to treat with myofascial massage. Myofascial therapists can serve a crucial role in teaching clients not to "expect" or "do" too much too soon.

Even though some clients may report feeling better and having a sense of personal accomplishment immediately, not all benefits are apparent at the start. Because of this delay, myofascial therapists should take some time during each session to review the client's activity level for the previous week. This review is done without judgement for the purpose of encouraging the client to continue with what is working well and to modify what is not working.

EXERCISE PROTOCOL: SWIMMING AS A MODEL ACTIVITY

Swimming provides an excellent example of how an activity can enhance indirect myofascial methods (Figure 9-4). How does swimming support ease in movement? Bodyworker Edward Pierrakos provides one answer:

> Harmony with life . . . can be compared to a swimmer. The swimmer floats on the water. The water carries him. And yet he moves, he is not passive. If he were entirely passive, he could not be sustained by the water. . . . The more rhythmic, relaxed and harmonious his movements are, the less strenuous moving is . . . (Pierrakos, 1978).

Principles of indirect myofascial massage that are supported by swimming include:

- **Relaxation:** In the water, only the relaxed are safe. Someone who thrashes around uncontrollably will sink. To remain buoyant, you need to let go of fear and relax.
- **Breath:** When swimming, the goal is to inhale fully to contribute to flotation, to exhale fully to make room to inhale fully, and to increase your awareness of how your breath can complement this rhythmic, whole-body activity. Expansion of the breath while swimming gives the reassuring signal to your body that you can open to take in energy, even when pushing against a force that resists you.

  When the lungs are full, you displace more water and are lifted more than if your lungs are not full. This also lengthens your body, exposes your sides, brings your head back, activates the extensor muscles of your back, lengthens the flexor muscles of your front, and draws in fresh air.

  Match your swimming rhythm to the rhythm of your breathing to feel safe and able to breathe

(continued)

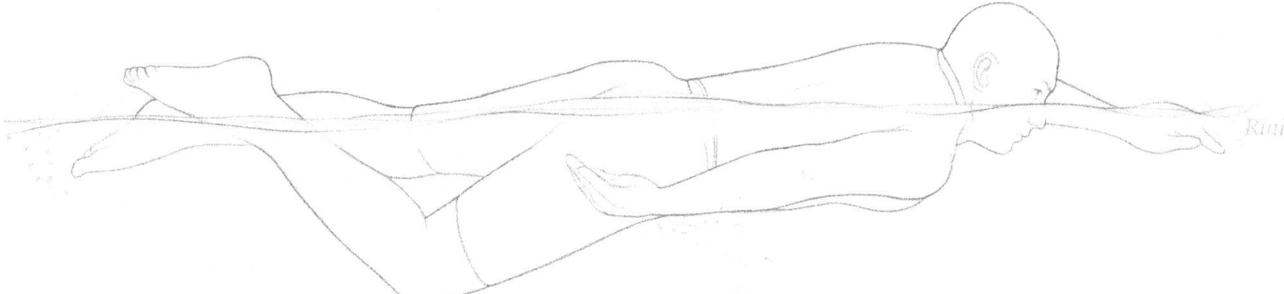

FIGURE 9-4 Swimming. Swimming can be an excellent exercise for those who feel comfortable in the water.

EXERCISE PROTOCOL (continued): SWIMMING AS A MODEL ACTIVITY

in the water. When you turn your face to breathe while swimming, your unconscious learns that you are still lifted by the water when you are tilted, just as when you are flat.

- **Alignment:** Body position in the water determines how easy movement through the water will be. Keeping your body in a straight line will cut down the resistance of your body as it glides through the water. Head position directly affects the balance of the body. Keeping the hands with the palms facing in to the body axis also cuts down resistance during strokes.
- **Mobility:** Arm movements in swimming require shoulder mobility. Reaching movements, full extension of the arm into the water, and the lift of the arm above the water during recovery all need freedom and mobility that come from the shoulders. Freeing up your shoulders may release unneeded tension and help old burdens that no longer need to be carried to slide off.
- **Centering:** Swimming improves when the center of the body becomes the fulcrum for movement. The concept of operating from center is basic to many forms of exercise. The largest muscles are found close to the center of the body, in the legs (quadriceps, hamstrings), the back and down into the thighs (gluteals and erector spinae), and the gut (abdominals and psoas), attaching on or near the pelvis.
- **Support:** Water supports and lifts you. The weight of water attempting to flow down presses on and lifts anything contained in the water. Archimedes' famous cry of "Eureka!" (or "I have found it!") was uttered when he discovered that water presses on any object immersed in water and lifts that portion of it that is equal in weight to the weight of the water that would fill the hole the object displaces.

  Not only does water lift you, but the more of you that is in the water, the more you are lifted. Floating and swimming involve accepting the support of the water to keep you afloat. The experience of swimming through the water provides a "kinesthetic understanding" that you can pull yourself along while accepting support.
- **Grounding:** On land, contact of your feet with the ground creates security through conscious (and unconscious) awareness of a connection with the earth. In the water, grounding comes from the "felt sense" of the water lifting you every time. To get a grounded feeling in the water, you have to be willing to play in the water with a childlike attitude of exploring with interest, without goals, without self-criticism. This is much akin to the attitude of going with the flow or moving in the direction of ease that is so essential to the indirect method.
- **Resistance:** Water's resistance can be used (e.g., in kicking or hand movements) to propel you forward in the water. Swimming teaches you that you can be active while being horizontal. In general, the goal in swimming is to decrease resistance to full-body movement and to increase resistance to hand and foot propulsion.
- **Kinesthetic learning:** Once you have learned to swim, it stays with you, like riding a bicycle. As you focus on a familiar task, the body automatically organizes and you need not consciously decide the details of how to perform each movement and which muscle to contract. For example, breathing while doing the crawl stroke is a complicated process that involves closing the mouth briefly just before you inhale, as your face comes out of the water, and just before you exhale, as your face goes back under. For the interval of the exhale, the mouth is open, so air can come out. This difficult stroke is mastered when you no longer need to consciously decide when to breathe.

SUMMARY

When performed in accordance with the precepts outlined in this chapter and under the guidance of a qualified teacher, exercise provides an approach to self-care that can support normalcy, empowerment, freedom, and ease. In this way, it can reinforce and enhance the healthful changes that are initiated with indirect myofascial methods.

Research supports the use of exercise and explores a variety of possible mechanisms of action. The benefits of exercise include improved posture and body mechanics, strengthened muscles, increased flexibility, pain relief, increased body awareness, and psychological benefits.

You can help your clients optimize exercise as a self-care strategy by helping them understand and work with their pain. Also suggest ways of making exercise more enjoyable, such as by doing it with others. Advise clients to prepare for exercise with appropriate clothing, engage in adequate warm-up and cool-down sessions, avoid pushing past pain barriers, customize exercise to their individual needs, and keep a positive attitude.

Swimming is a model activity that can reinforce relaxing, support, alignment, mobility, centering, grounding, the right use of resistance, and kinesthetic learning for indirect method clients.

Review Questions

1. __________ is physical activity or human movement.
   a. Dance
   b. Swimming
   c. Exercise
   d. Yoga
2. Pain that results from __________ is harmless and should be tolerated.
   a. nerve damage
   b. scar stretch
   c. muscle overstretch
   d. exercise overload
3. Which of the following would *not* contribute to enjoying exercise?
   a. preparing for exercise
   b. fitting in with a winning team
   c. wearing proper clothing
   d. a positive attitude
4. True or false: Two components of a good warm-up are static stretching of the skeletal muscles and a slower, less-intense version of the exercise to follow.
5. True or false: Psychological benefits are most likely to appear immediately and then disappear gradually with continued exercise.
6. True or false: Research on exercise has shown it to be beneficial for those suffering from diabetes, cancer, and coronary heart disease.
7. Exercise is most like the indirect method of myofascial massage when it is used to __________.
   a. let go of physical barriers
   b. find ease and support in movement
   c. train for competitive sports
   d. a and b
8. Swimming is an exercise activity that can help clients learn about resistance, breath, relaxation, and __________.
9. The __________ period is the core of the workout.
10. Dressing appropriately for exercise involves replacing __________ when they get old and worn.

REFERENCES

Castaneda C. Diabetes control with physical activity and exercise. Nutr Clin Care 2003;2:89–96.

Corbin CB, Lindsey R. Concepts of Physical Fitness with Laboratories. Dubuque, IA: Wm. C. Brown Publishers, 1988.

Da Costa D, Lowenstyn I, Dritsa M. Leisure time physical activity patterns and relationship to generalized distress among Canadians with arthritis or rheumatism. J Rheumatol 2003;30:2476–2484.

Dixon MW. Bodylessons. Findhorn Forres, Scotland: Findhorn Press, 2005.

Keysor JJ. Does late-life physical activity or exercise prevent or minimize disablement? A critical review of the scientific evidence. Am J Prev Med 2003;25(suppl 2):129–136.

Pierrakos E. Pathwork Lecture #160—Conciliation of Inner Split. Phoenicia, NY: CLF Publications, 1978.

Schatz MP. Back Care Basics. Berkeley, CA: Rodmell Press, 1992.

Schneider CM, Dennehy CA, Rooseboom M, Carter SD. A model program: exercise intervention for cancer rehabilitation. Integ Cancer Ther 2002;1:76–82.

Seaward BL. Managing Stress. Boston: Jones and Bartlett Publishers, 1994.

Sutton JR. Hormonal and metabolic responses to exercise in subjects of high and low work capacity. Med Sci Sport 1978;10:1–6.

Szapary PO, Bloedon LT, Foster GD. Physical activity and its effects on lipids. Curr Cardiol Rep 2003;5:488–492.

Tharp GD. The role of glucocorticoids in exercise. Med Sci Sport 1975; 7:6–11.

The Vestfold Heartcare Study Group. Influence on lifestyle measures and five-year coronary risk by a comprehensive lifestyle intervention programme in patients with coronary heart disease. J Cardiovasc Risk 2003;10:429–437.

Winder WW, Beattie MA, Holman RT. Endurance training attenuates stress-hormone responses to exercise in fasted rats. Am J of Physiol 1982;243(suppl R):179–184.

SUGGESTED READINGS

Dixon MW. Bodylessons. Findhorn Forres, Scotland: Findhorn Press, 2005.

Dixon MW. Body Mechanics and Self Care Manual. Englewood Cliffs, NJ: Prentice Hall Health, 2001.

Feldenkrais M. Awareness Through Movement. New York: Harper & Row Publishers, 1977.

Griffin JL. How Anybody Can Learn to Swim Well. Silver Spring, MD: Manifest Press, 1989.

Soo C. The Chinese Art of Tai Chi Chuan. Northhamptonshire, England: The Aquarian Press, 1984.

Chapter 10

Craniosacral Approach

OBJECTIVES

- Describe the craniosacral approach and its rationale.
- Identify the origins of and influences on the craniosacral approach.
- Describe craniosacral techniques, including diaphragm and sacral releases, dural tube release, listening to and following the craniosacral rhythm, inducing a still point, using direction of energy, and sutural releases.
- Discuss positioning, draping, and support.
- Discuss treatment planning and decision making.

CHAPTER OUTLINE

KEY TERMS

Dural tube (dura): The outer layer of connective tissue that surrounds the brain, spinal cord, and cerebrospinal fluid; sometimes (incorrectly) used synonymously with meninges.

Cerebrospinal fluid (CSF): An extract from the blood that circulates around, cushions, and provides nutrients for the brain and spinal column.

Choroid plexi: Braids of capillaries located in spaces (ventricles) within the brain where blood is filtered and refined into cerebrospinal fluid.

Arachnoid villi: Outpouchings located throughout the cerebral cortex where cerebrospinal fluid is reabsorbed back into the bloodstream.

Pressurestat theory: Upledger's explanation of how movement of the cranial bones is necessary to accommodate the cerebrospinal fluid pulsations as the fluid is filtered into the system and then reabsorbed.

Flexion: Filling, widening, expansion, or outward rotation of the body corresponding with an increased amount of cerebrospinal fluid filtering into the system.

Extension: Emptying, contraction, narrowing, or inward rotation of the body corresponding with a decreased amount of cerebrospinal fluid filtering into the system.

Craniosacral rhythm (CSR): One complete cycle of flexion and extension.

Still point: When the cranial wave stops; still points can occur spontaneously without intervention or can be induced in response to specific craniosacral techniques.

When you place your fingers . . . they must think, feel, see and know the anatomical picture that lies beneath them. . . . Fingers should be like detectives, skillful in the art of locating things hidden. . . . The fingers should not only feel while diagnosing, but also while treating.

SUTHERLAND (1962)

As you know, the organization of the hands-on therapies in this text progressed from the most direct and tangible to the more indirect and subtle techniques. In Chapter 8, you learned about the sensitivity and specificity needed to sense and return from the resistances to movement encountered with the indirect connective tissue (CT) approach. The craniosacral approach to myofascial massage requires an even more subtle level of palpation and technique. Craniosacral (CS) therapists must learn to listen to and follow the tiniest movements of the dural tube as they reflect the flow of the cerebrospinal fluid (CSF) around the brain and spinal cord.

This chapter explains the CS approach to myofascial massage. The CS approach uses indirect and sometimes direct manipulations of the dura mater, the outermost layer of the CT meninges that surround the central nervous system. Most CS techniques are unique and look very different from other myofascial approaches. Yet CS is similar to the other approaches in that it focuses on the fascial network that spans the human body. The first section of this chapter presents specific osteopathic principles as an underlying influence to CS theory and follows the development of cranial osteopathy into the CS approach.

Cranial techniques emphasize the therapist's subtle palpatory skills to assess and release tension associated with interrelated cranial and sacral oscillations. The oscillations are said to be transmitted through a complex combination of dural (covering) and ligamentous (dense CT or deep fascia) connections. The first section also examines the physiologic explanation for CS massage along with the need for more research showing a causal connection between the manual techniques, changes in the CS system, and therapeutic effects.

The second section introduces the basic categories of CS strokes. Basic categories include listening to and stopping the CS rhythm, fascial releases (which have been previously described in Chapter 8), and cranial releases that focus on the sutures between the cranial bones. The anatomy of the CS (brain and spinal cord, CSF, and the dural sac that envelops and penetrates the structures and fluid) system is discussed in brief and reviewed to help the therapist better visualize the correct application of CS strokes. This section also discusses the correct use of the therapist's body in CS work, propping and support, and the use of verbal imagery that reflects the listening process.

The chapter concludes with a formalized plan for applying the CS approach. The plan includes a 12-step protocol, adapted from the 10-step protocol popularized by John Upledger, which he claims can benefit most clients. Decision making about CS indications, contraindications, and modifications and applications are covered to address specific client needs.

Overview of the Craniosacral Approach

The CS approach seeks to improve the flow of CSF by using the cranial and sacral bones as "handles" to free restrictions in the CT or nervous system. Proponents of the CS approach maintain that it is especially useful for addressing pain and dysfunction in the head, spine, and pelvis, and that it can release physical and emotional trauma throughout the body. CS techniques are noninvasive and are performed with the client clothed.

The CS approach is unique in that it provides bodyworkers with access to both the nervous system and the CT network with a very gentle touch. Practitioners focus on the fascial (dural) tube that envelops the brain and spinal cord and the nourishing supply of CSF that bathes the system. This fascial tube protects and serves as the container for the innermost core of the body (the brain and spinal cord). CS practitioners aim toward helping clients get "to the core" of themselves and their healing process. The subtle hand holds on cranial or sacral bones that gently tug on the fascial tube also connect with the entire fascial network, extending outward to surround every bone, organ, muscle, nerve, and vessel in the body. Thus, areas distant to the area of trauma can access troubled and even acutely inflamed regions that are painful or otherwise sensitive to touch. For example, a cranial technique applied to the neck may have a beneficial effect on a pulled wrist muscle that is innervated by nerves originating in the cervical spine.

Very light pressure is used to contact the client's tissues. Upledger suggests 5 g of intentional pressure as the maximum load. Aim toward using less pressure than the weight of a nickel. One of the many paradoxes within CS work is that when the therapist meets resistance from the client's body, the best way to move past the resistance is to apply a lighter pressure. In fact, even when the hands are off the client's body but meeting resistance, the solution is still to work "lighter." How can this be achieved? You cannot work lighter than zero pressure—or can you? To use lighter pressure when the hands are not in physical contact means that you lighten your intent to heal the client's body. Pressure or intent serves only to meet the client's resistance and see where it needs to go, not to push past, change, or "fix." Although CS contact is very subtle, almost nonexistent, it is not tentative or weak. In fact, many clients describe CS "touch" as a full *presence.* As with both direct and indirect myofascial work, any CS pressure (or non-pressure) is applied by sinking the intention down to focus on the appropriate level of CT (either the dura or the CT between the sutures of the skull), not by powering your way in.

ORIGINS OF THE CRANIOSACRAL APPROACH

The CS concept was originally conceived by William Garner Sutherland, DO (doctor of osteopathy) as an extension of the osteopathic theories of Andrew Taylor Still, DO. The terms *sacrocranial* and *craniosacral* refer to the same body of knowledge and are interchangeable. Craniosacral Therapy is a trademarked term; however, sacrocranial or CS techniques and CS massage are not.

Basic principles of osteopathy help to clarify the perspective that gave birth to CS massage. The term *osteopathy* comes from the Greek words meaning bone (*osteon*) and disease (*pathos*) and means literally the treatment of bone disease. Three tenets of osteopathy have influenced the development of CS work:

1. **The body is a whole, not just the sum of many parts.** Uniting the body parts is CT, which surrounds every muscle, nerve, vessel, and organ. Collagen fibrils link the entire body in a matrix from head to toe. Thus, you cannot accurately classify or treat a client as a "psoas problem."
2. **Structure and function are interrelated.** If an anatomical structure exists in some area, that structure serves a physiological function. Conversely, if there is some abnormality in structure, it will adversely affect function. And if function is impaired, then the anatomical structure will be reshaped.
3. **The body has the potential, capacity, and inner wisdom to heal itself.** The body has an inherent force to return to homeostatic balance and toward organization. There is no need or benefit to "fixing" a client. Instead, focus on helping the natural process of healing oneself.

In the early 1900s, as a student at the American School of Osteopathy in Kirksville, Missouri, Sutherland became fascinated by the anatomical structure of the cranial bones and intrigued by the second principle of osteopathy, that structure and function are interrelated. Marzal (1993) recounts that Sutherland used the phrase "like the gills of a fish" to describe the suture lines where the parietal bones articulate with the temporal bones (Figure 10-1). He was examining a model of a disarticulated skull, with each part held in anatomical relationship but exaggerated separation. Sutherland thought this indicated that the structure of cranial bones supports the function of movement in the same way that a fish's gills are part of the respiratory system and designed to move. This was in direct contrast to the prevailing teaching of American and British anatomists, who taught that sutural ossification and cranial immobility normally occur early in life. The American and British interpretation, however, was not the accepted teaching worldwide. Even in the early 1900s, Italian anatomists taught that cranial suture ossification was pathological in adult humans. Sutherland also reported a synchronous pulsation felt at the cranium and sacrum and theorized that it reflected the continuity of the dura mater, which links the occiput to the sacrum with only a few attachments to bone in between.

Sutherland experimented for decades on himself and later on living clients. By around 1940, after extensive study of specimen skulls, cranial membranes, brains, spinal cords, and vertebrae, Sutherland began to publish and teach. His therapy consisted of manual correction of movement irregularities at the CT junctions between the cranial bones at their sutures or at the underlying CT membranes. He also taught the self-regulating power of the CSF, which, as an extract of the blood, is another type of CT.

Until the 1970s, cranial osteopathy was considered controversial, even in osteopathic medicine, because it was still widely assumed that the cranial bones did not move. In 1975, John Upledger, DO, with a research team at the College of Osteopathic Medicine at Michigan State University, attempted to clarify whether the cranial bones did indeed move. Through the study of fresh specimen skulls and their membranes, instead of chemically preserved ones, the team was able to demonstrate the existence of blood vessels, nerve fibers, collagen, and elastin fibers in

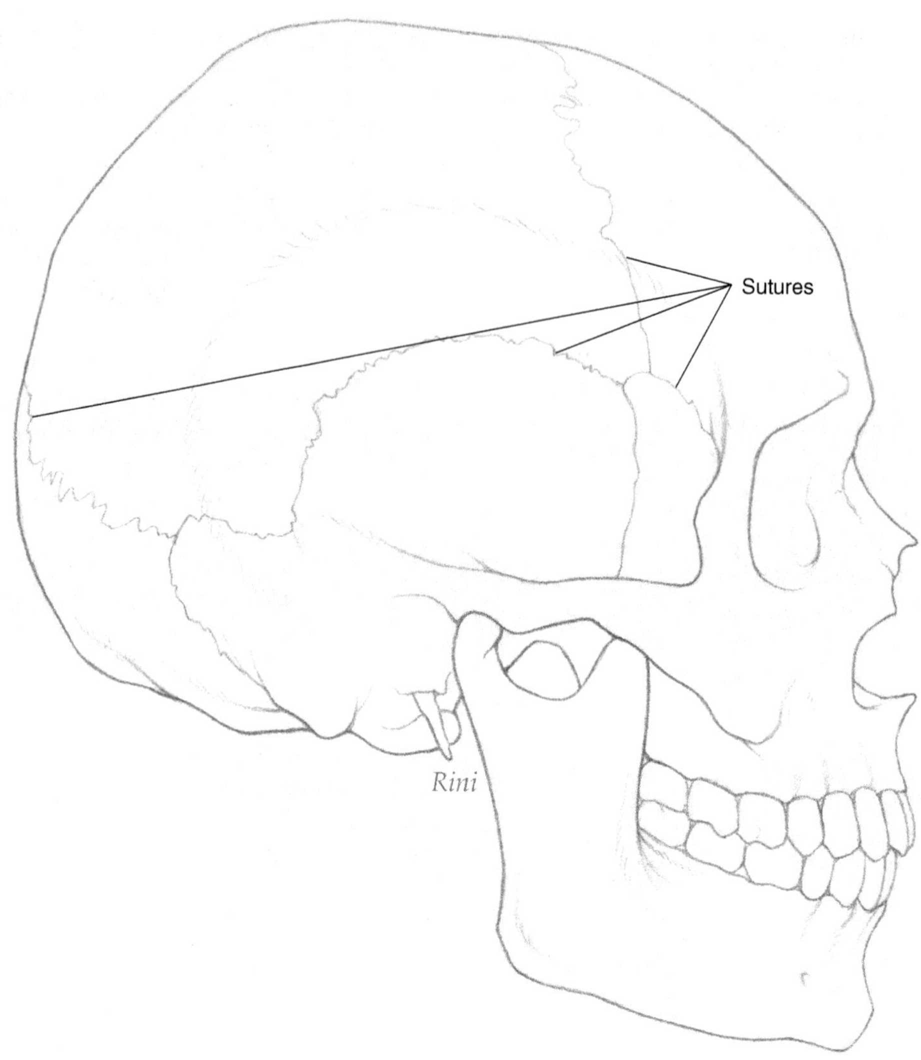

FIGURE 10-1 **Sutures of the skull.**

the sutures of the skull (in other words, CT). This group found no indication of ossification of the sutures, which was, until that time, the basis for the argument that the cranial bones had no movement. Other Michigan studies demonstrated a rhythmic movement in the cranial bones. Furthermore, the research team theorized the mechanism behind this movement with the "pressurestat theory" (described shortly). Upledger has contributed significantly to the circulation and popularity of CS techniques. In 1985, Upledger founded his own school and clinic of Craniosacral Therapy in Florida.

A variety of osteopathic and chiropractic methods for the treatment of dysfunctions of the CS system have become popular, using terms such as Craniology, Craniosacral Therapy, and Sacro-Occipital Technique. Various cranial schools have developed, each emphasizing different aspects of cranial technique.

One of these aspects is the indirect approach, in which a problem is first exaggerated to encourage resolution. This practice was developed by Sutherland and is referred to in European osteopathic schools as the Sutherland technique.

One contemporary school in San Francisco, founded by osteopath Hugh Milne, DO (1995), is known for emphasizing the "spirit" of CS work in the manner of Sutherland. Sutherland described the cerebrospinal pulse as the "breath of life." Milne (1995) describes the "breath" or spirit as both an electrical energy field and a field of information and intelligence that exists as feelings, images, aspirations, and "psyche" or soul.

PHYSIOLOGY OF THE CRANIOSACRAL SYSTEM

The head, or *cranium,* contains 27 separate bones (excluding the teeth) and 67 joints. Most of these joints are sutural joints that appear as the squiggly lines on a skull where two plates of bone fit together like a jigsaw puzzle (see

Figure 10-1). The cranial sutural joints are bound together with dense CT.

Movement between the sutural joints is not large like the elevation of the shoulder girdle or the rotation of a shoulder joint, but movement does occur. Thus, as with all other joints in the body, it is beneficial to keep the sutures open and mobile. **Craniosacral massage** practitioners believe that cranial sutures are designed to allow the cranium to adapt to the varying amount of CSF flow.

In the human body, the brain and spinal cord float in a stream of CSF. An extract from the blood, CSF is filtered and refined in braids of capillaries (called choroid plexi), located in the spaces (ventricles) within the brain. The CSF circulates, cushions, and provides nutrients as it moves through and around the brain and spinal column. It is then reabsorbed back into the bloodstream via arachnoid villi, located throughout the cerebral cortex. According to Upledger's (1983) pressurestat theory, the cranial bones expand and contract to accommodate the CSF, which moves in pulses as it is filtered into the system and then reabsorbed. Upledger likens the filtering process to a faucet in a bathtub that is rhythmically turned on and off. The reabsorption mechanism in the arachnoid villi is said to be similar to a slow drain that is always slightly open. The end result is a bathtub that has cycles of filling slowly, then emptying slowly, then filling again, and so on. As the internal pressure rises and falls, the CSF moves from one portion of the brain to another, and the surrounding bones are carried with it through a range of motion of expansion (which Upledger terms flexion) and contraction (which Upledger terms extension). Notice that, in CS massage, the terms *flexion* and *extension* have a different meaning from that understood in traditional muscle kinesiology. Flexion typically means "bending or folding in" the joints, and extension means "straightening, lengthening, or opening out." In CS massage, the meanings of *flexion* and *extension* are contradictory to these muscle kinesiology meanings (Figure 10-2).

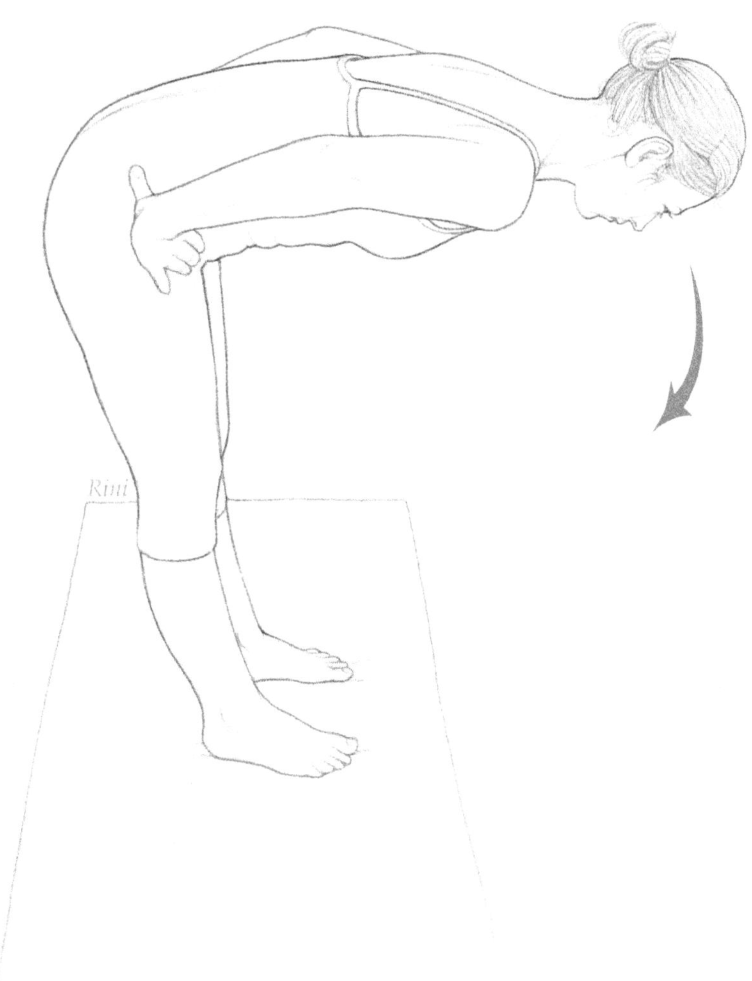

A

FIGURE 10-2 **Contrasting terminology.** (A) Flexion of the trunk in traditional muscle kinesiology.

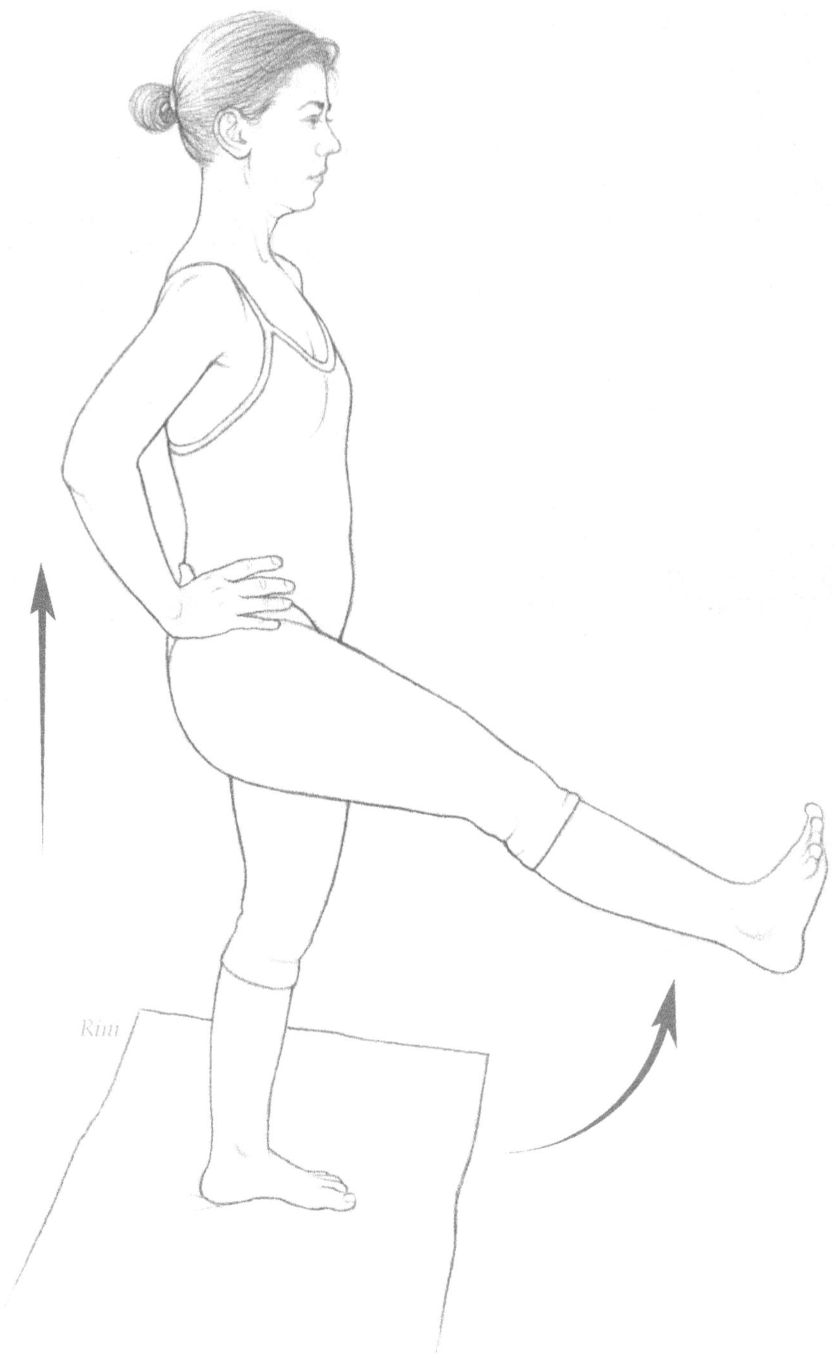

B

FIGURE 10-2 **Contrasting terminology (continued).** (**B**) Extension of the trunk and flexion at hip joint in traditional muscle kinesiology.

RESEARCH ON THE CRANIOSACRAL APPROACH

The craniosacral approach does not fare well with biomedical researchers. In a recent systematic review and critical appraisal of the scientific evidence on CS therapy (Green et al, 1999), the review panel judged that research showing benefits of CS therapies was based on weak study designs (retrospective case control, retrospective case series, before and after, and case reports) and did not meet the standards of randomized, controlled experimental trials. The available research on the effectiveness of CS techniques was criticized because studies did not include enough subjects or controls or because treatment subjects could guess which was the CS treatment and which was not. This criticism, however, can be applied to all massage because it is very difficult to create situations in which the therapist (or the client) does not know whether he is touching the client

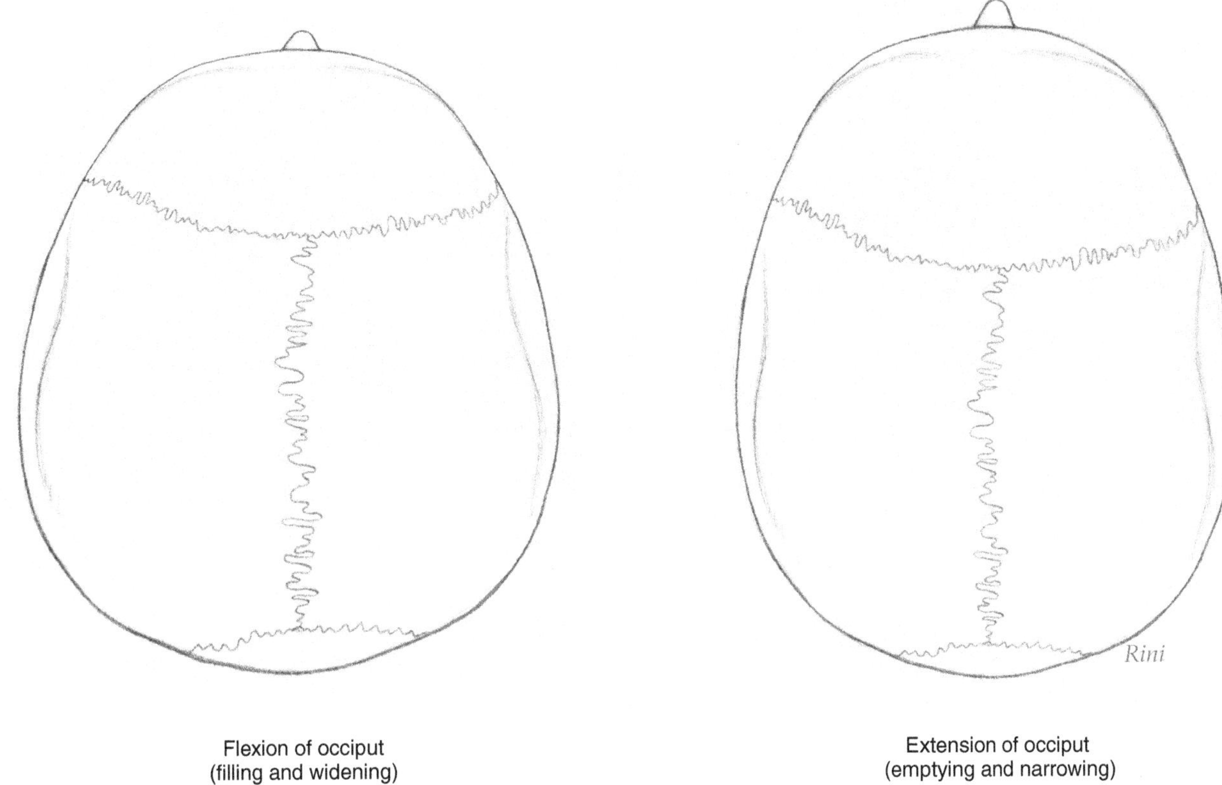

FIGURE 10-2 Contrasting terminology (continued). (C) Flexion and extension in the craniosacral approach to the occiput.

therapeutically. In fact, when phrased in this way, arguments for striving for research validity in bodywork become almost ridiculous.

Research studies have contributed evidence for causal links potentially connecting CS mobility restrictions to health outcomes. The existence of movement between the cranial bones and the existence of rhythmic flow patterns in CSF has been observed. Skeptics (including many in the medical profession) deny the existence of any significant bone movement or the influx of CS flow.

Seven studies have reported on mobility or fusion at cranial sutures in adults (Frymann, 1971; Greenman, 1970; Heifetz and Weiss, 1981; Hubbard et al, 1971; Kokich, 1976; Kostopoulos and Keramidas, 1992; and Pitlyk et al, 1985). Research evidence from these seven studies supports the theory that the adult cranium is not always solidly fused and that minute movements between the cranial bones may be possible. A set of nine retrieved studies (Avezaat and van Eijndhoven, 1986; Cardoso et al, 1983; Du Boulay et al, 1972; Enzmann et al, 1986, Feinberg and Mark, 1987; Li et al, 1996; O'Connell, 1943; Takizawa et al, 1983; and Zablotny et al, 1995) verify that CSF movement and pulsation is a clearly observable phenomenon by encephalogram, myogram, magnetic resonance imaging (MRI), and intracranial and intraspinal pressure monitoring. Furthermore, the body of research also supports the contention that a cranial pulse or rhythm exists, distinct from either cardiac or respiratory activity. The research, however, has not yet demonstrated whether or not movement at the cranial sutures can be achieved with manual manipulation such as CS techniques.

Craniosacral Techniques

Craniosacral techniques focus minimal or no pressure on the CT that surrounds the brain and spinal cord. Sometimes the point of focus may be a suture between two cranial bones; sometimes it may be another joint articulation such as the sacroiliac joint. Sometimes the focus is on the fascia that surrounds the dural tube. Sometimes the focus is on the CSF rhythm itself. Regardless of the targeted feature, the amount of pressure is always minimal.

GUIDELINES FOR CRANIOSACRAL TECHNIQUES

Very subtle pressure applied steadily and slowly encourages a viscous medium (e.g., the CT covering over the brain and spinal cord) to flow to a greater extent than does a stronger pressure. If you find a restriction, one of the strange paradoxes of CS bodywork is that less can sometimes be more.

One Therapist's Experience: The Experience of Performing Craniosacral Massage

One of my standard assignments in CS class is to have students complete a case study of what it feels like to both the client and student practitioner to use CS techniques. The following is an excerpt from one of the student reports. I hope these words will provide a glimpse into what it might be like to work with CS techniques.

"During the session I noticed that G's breath was pretty consistent as he moved in and out of sleep. I was not sure if I was actually feeling rhythms or if I was making them up. I also got a bit confused as to if they were his or my rhythms that I was feeling. I felt a little silly and stuck in my own effort at times. He told me that felt a lot more relaxed. I learned that I needed to relax a bit more and just have fun with it. The more effort I put in the more stuck I felt. . . .

My second session . . . I did a half-hour meditation. . . . I focused on relaxing my mind and body more, which enabled me to feel and sense more. . . . I could feel his sacrum release and flow. Throughout the whole session his body twitched. (I am not sure if it was because of the work or phasing in and out of sleep.) I felt that I could feel a little flexion and extension at the occipital atlas, which was really exciting. I also could tell when some of the tissue was resisting or flowing. I am still a bit confused as to what is his rhythm and what is mine, although I really thought that I was feeling his. I felt a lot of emotion come up in me during this session. I tried to use a lot of breath work to reground. G said that he felt a bit of an emotional release as well as his blood flowing more rapidly throughout his body. He also said that his body felt like it was growing and lengthening.

My third session was the best. . . ! Most of the time I began my holds on the skin, but ended up doing most of the work a little off his body. I realized that I could sense more (off the body) and did not feel as though I was constricting his flow. I did a lot of visualization of the tissue and sutures moving freely. G's breath rate and rhythm changed a lot during the session. At times I was a little confused about which way the rhythm was flowing but I realized that it is all right to be confused. After the session, G said that he felt relaxed and 'more free.' He said that he felt his blood moving throughout his body, and that this felt really strange to him. He also mentioned that his sinuses felt clearer. This last session gave me confidence and excitement. It's amazing what a difference there is when I feel free and relaxed within myself."

As noted earlier, the pressure you use to release the tissue is very gentle—5 g or less. Feel the weight of a nickel, and do not use more than this force. In fact, if you do not feel a release, use still *less* pressure to meet the resistance layer. Remember one of the strange paradoxes of this work is that less effort can actually be more effective in producing a therapeutic change. The therapist may actually have *no* skin contact and still need to reduce therapeutic force or intent. If the client's tissue is not shifting or moving in response to your work, lighten your touch. If you are not touching the client, lighten your intent, so that you are not trying to change or fix anything but rather are mentally inviting the client's permission to change. This adage goes back to the osteopathic principle that *every body has the potential, capacity, and inner wisdom to heal itself.* The body has an inherent force to return to homeostatic balance and toward organization. There is no need or benefit to "fixing" a client. Instead, focus on helping the client's own process of healing.

Identify the restriction, either with stacking (discussed in Chapter 8) or just with palpation, and create a contact that just meets the barrier. Wait a few minutes for the release to begin. (These few minutes of waiting can seem like an eternity. "Aren't I supposed to be *doing* something?") Allow the tissue to move to its direction of ease. There may be several barriers (i.e., in the three dimensions of space), so this technique may take up to 5 minutes to complete. CT *is* capable of completing its unwinding more rapidly, so do not feel as though you have to stay in an area when the movement has clearly stopped.

Following the moving fascia may feel to the client like you are applying the impetus to move, but you may feel like the area is moving all by itself. When this phenomenon happens on a limb or at the head and neck, it is known as "regional positional release" in Craniosacral Therapy and as "unwinding" in Barnes' system of Myofascial Release. The process still consists of just listening and following the fascia to its greatest ease (until it stops moving).

Here are some additional guidelines to keep in mind as you approach CS work:

1. Prepare yourself for the quiet and stillness necessary to listen to such subtle movements. This can take the form of meditation, tai chi, or a few yoga stretches. Or you may simply take a few breaths to relax your body before you touch your client.
2. Use less than a nickel's weight (5 g) of intentional pressure. Note: If a client says that you are using too much pressure, ease off even if you are using less than 5 g to begin with.
3. Sit on a height-adjustable rolling stool (preferable to a chair, which can be used in a pinch). (For certain techniques, you may need to take alternate positions such as standing or resting one foot on a chair.) Take the time to establish a comfortable body alignment and easy body mechanics. You will not be able to feel the very slight releases in client tension if your body is tight and tense.
4. Even though you are expending a very small amount of force to apply a light pressure, it is still a good idea to face the direction that you are working so that the tension is distributed throughout your entire body, not just your arms and hands. Orient your whole body to the client's rhythm even if you are just floating with the fascia in its direction of ease. It is also a good idea to clarify in your own mind which fascia, suture, or restriction in the rhythm you are trying to release, so that your body stays aligned with the area of restriction. This will also help keep your intent set on moving the area easily and continuously and allow you to follow the unraveling without forcing, pushing, or pulling the system.
5. If a restriction does not seem to ease under your touch, ask internally if you are finished at this time. If you cannot find a good orientation to the tissue, fluid, or suture, move to a different area.
6. Know the anatomical structures that you are palpating (i.e., bones, sutures, fascia) and use that knowledge to guide pressure and movement as you free the fascial, CSF, or sutural restrictions.
7. If you think that you feel a release in the tissue (i.e., a movement in a certain direction), give yourself permission to believe in and follow that change.
8. Signs of tissue release can include a softening or lengthening, heat, pulsations, magnetism, feelings of being done or repulsed, or other sensations such as colors, imagery, sounds, words, or music. Do not dismiss a sensation just because it does not make sense.
9. If your body feels out of line, stop and readjust your position. As you take your hands off the client's body, ask her to breathe and move the area in a comfortable way. Use this time to stretch and breathe for yourself as well. When you reconnect, you will be fully present with your client rather than halfway there.
10. Breath cues (i.e., asking your client to continue to breathe easily) increase your client's awareness after you complete a technique.
11. Cues to move ("stretch," "take a deep breath") during pauses also reduce tension in the client and help to free restrictions in the craniosacral system. Asking for voluntary movement helps create conscious awareness of the changes that are occurring in the client's CT and facilitates the use of self-help exercises that help maintain more lasting change.
12. Use direction of energy (described shortly) to help a blocked area to shift and relax.

DIAPHRAGM AND SACRAL RELEASES

Diaphragm and sacral releases are incorporated into the 10-step Craniosacral Therapy protocol taught by Upledger. As noted in Chapter 8, Barnes teaches these releases as Myofascial Release techniques. Because fascial release can be classified as an indirect CT approach, insofar as the manipulations aim to follow fascia (as opposed to the dura or cranial CT only) into its direction of ease, this text described diaphragm and sacral releases in Chapter 8. Fascial diaphragm releases are revisited here because they are so commonly used in CS styles and because they are included in the sample CS protocol provided at the end of this chapter.

Each diaphragm and sacral release is a variation on one fundamental technique adapted for several specific areas (fascial diaphragms) of the body. This variable use is similar to that of the basic deep direct CT stroke, which may look different when applied to different body regions. Diaphragm releases are summarized in Table 10-1.

DURAL TUBE RELEASE

Sit or stand comfortably at the side of the table. Facing the client's pelvic region, slip the hand that is closest to the client's feet under the sacrum to cradle it and place your other hand under the client's neck with your palm spanning C2 and C3. Follow the slide and tuck of the cranial wave as it rocks back and forth like a very slow pendulum (Figure 10-3). Focus attention on any area that seems discontinuous, not moving, or out of synch with the rest of the wave.

LISTENING TO AND FOLLOWING THE CRANIOSACRAL RHYTHM

Listening to and following the craniosacral rhythm (CSR) sounds so simple, yet I have found it to be the single most

TABLE 10-1 Diaphragm Releases

Technique	Description	Application
Pelvic diaphragm release	Supine client; therapist at side. The palm that is closest to the client's head is placed under the sacrum. The top palm covers the pubic bone, with both thumbs oriented superiorly.	Low back, sacral, lower abdomen, and urogenital conditions (Upledger and Vredevoogd, 1983)
Respiratory diaphragm release	Supine client; therapist at side. The palm that is closest to client's head is placed underneath. The bottom hand is placed on T12. The top hand covers the xiphoid process (from the lower edge of the sternum down to the abdomen).	Midthoracic organ conditions (e.g., liver, gallbladder, stomach, lower lung); also some low back pain, psoas muscles (Upledger and Vredevoogd, 1983)
Thoracic outlet*	The bottom hand is placed on C7. The top hand covers the place where the clavicle meets the sternum and reaches down the sternum toward the heart.	Lung conditions, neck, shoulder, and upper extremity musculoskeletal conditions; to promote lymph flow (Upledger and Vredevoogd, 1983)
Hyoid diaphragm release	The bottom hand spans C2 and C3. The top hand covers the hyoid bone (ask the client to swallow and observe where the Adam's apple moves to locate hyoid).	Neck conditions, headaches, throat conditions, temporomandibular joint disorder (Upledger and Vredevoogd, 1983)

*Called thoracic inlet release in Upledger (1983).

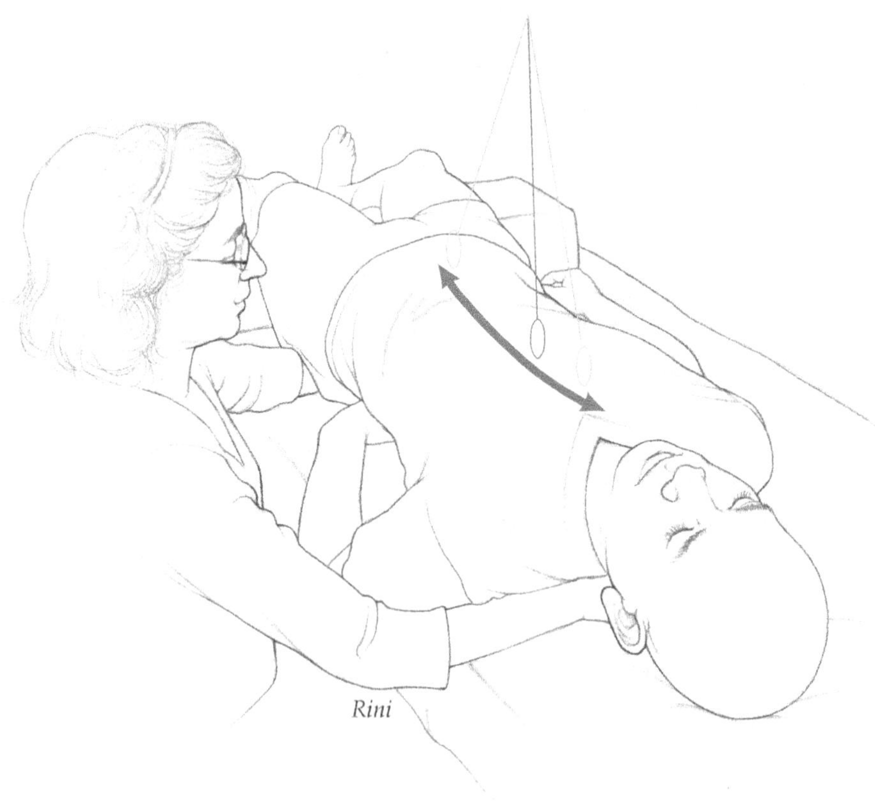

A

FIGURE 10-3 **Dural tube release.** Follow the dural tube as it moves like a slow pendulum between its cervical and sacral attachments. (**A**) Anterior view.

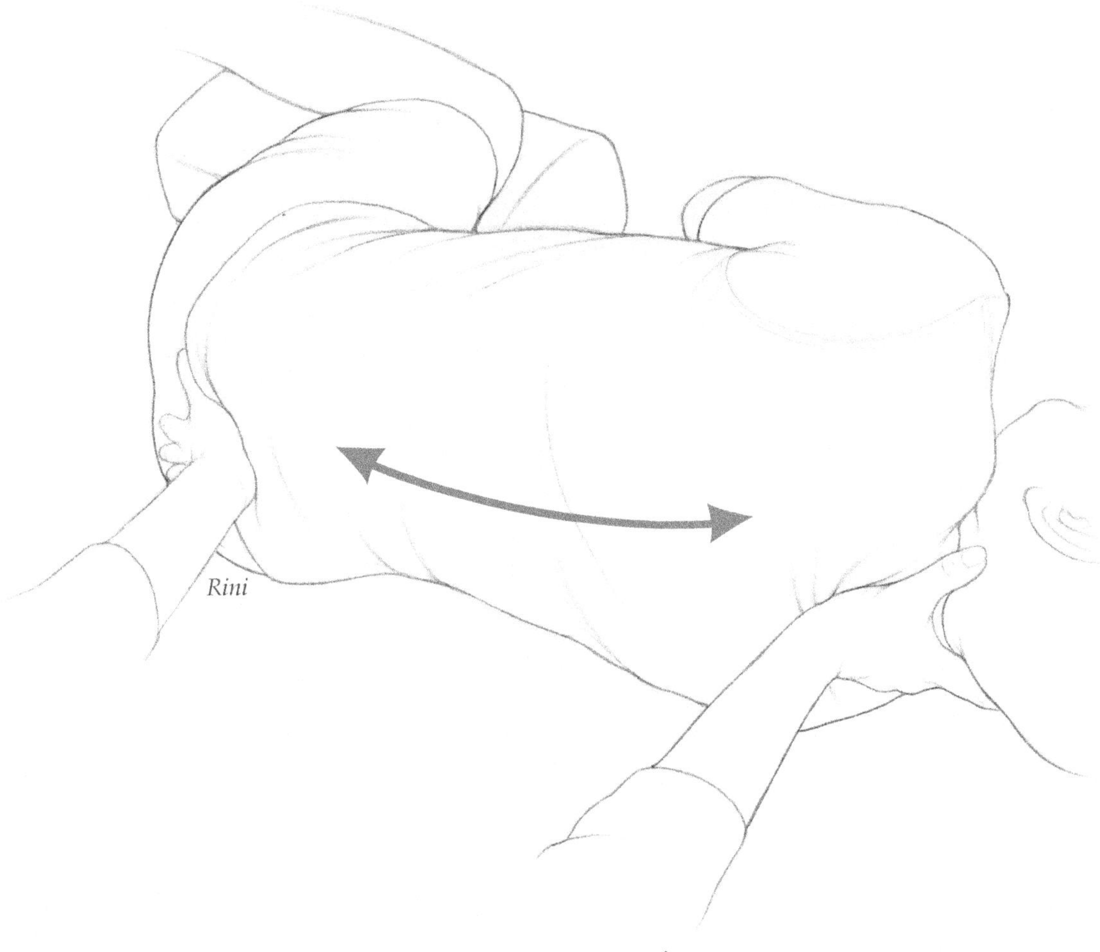

B

FIGURE 10-3 **Dural tube release (continued).** (**B**) Posterior view.

profound technique in the CS approach. It demonstrates so clearly the Heisenberg principle of physics, that the act of *observing something will change what is the object of your observation*. In other words, observing by listening to and following the cranial wave will, by itself, spark a change.

To practice listening to and following the CSR, sit on a height-adjustable rolling stool (preferable to a chair, which can be used in a pinch). The client should be lying supine on a massage table. Sit at the head of the table and cradle your client's head comfortably in your hands, with your thumbs behind the ears and hands draped comfortably down the client's neck (Figure 10-4). Allow your hands to meld with your client's cranium by letting your hands sink and soften into the table, relaxing enough to receive the weight of the client's skull. Listen for the feeling of a slight motion of filling or emptying transmitted into your own body. "Surf" this cranial wave (i.e., follow the subtle movement with a subtle moving of your own body) if you can feel a movement. If you do not feel a kinesthetic sensation, internally imagine when the wave is filling and when it is emptying. Allow yourself to follow that felt or imagined wave.

STILL POINT

A still point occurs when the cranial wave stops. Still points can occur spontaneously without any intervention, or they can be induced in response to subtle pressures applied at strategic points. Why stop the CSF wave? Upledger presents empirical data suggesting that when you stop the wave and then allow it to restart, the wave emerges as more balanced, symmetrical, and vital.

To induce a still point, gently resist one phase of the cranial flexion (filling) or extension (emptying). Whether you choose to resist flexion or extension will be based on the anatomy of the area. An excellent place to induce the still point is at the skull, where you have already been listening for the cerebrospinal pulse. Remember that as the cranium goes into flexion, it feels as if it is widening

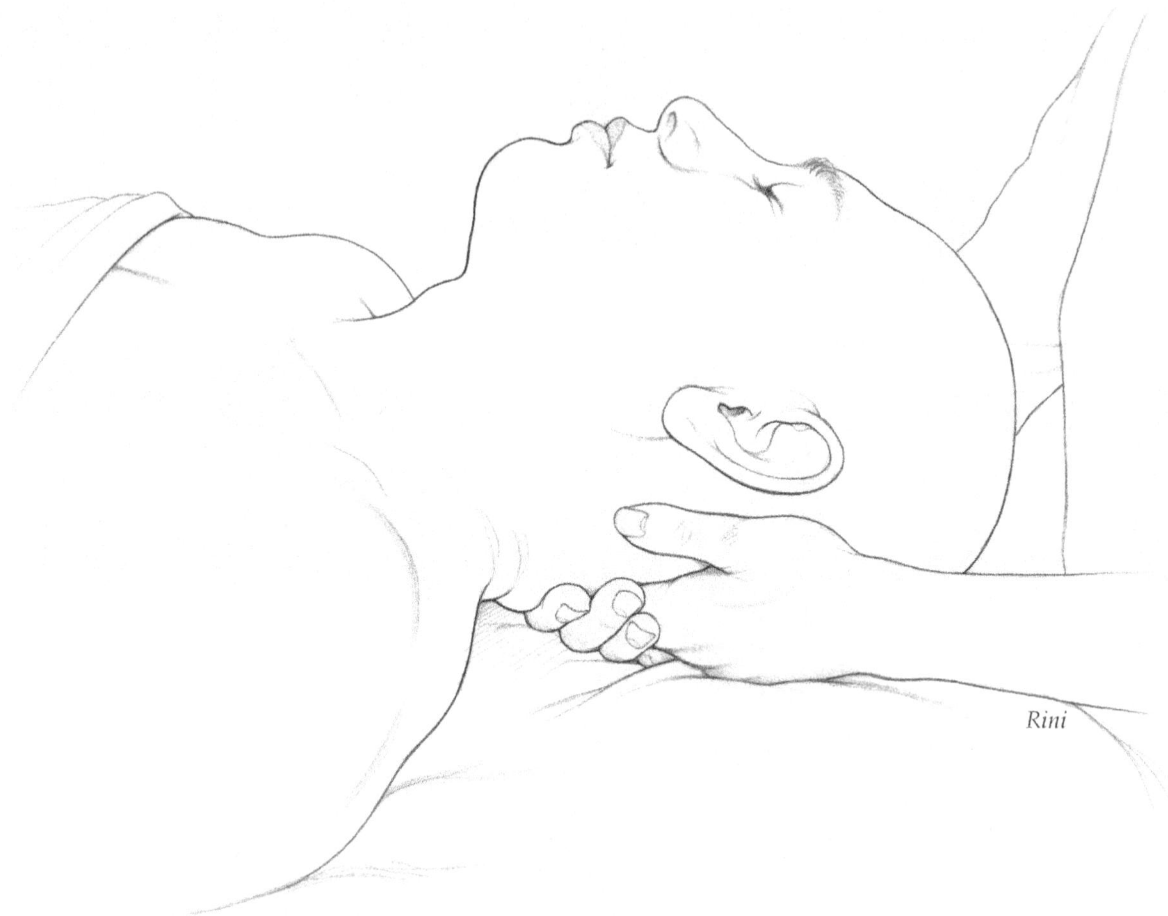

FIGURE 10-4 Listening to and following the craniosacral rhythm (CSR). Hand position for listening and following the CSR at the occiput.

slightly at the occiput. And as it goes into extension, the head feels as if it is narrowing at the occiput. Your hands cradled under the occiput will feel as if they are being pushed apart, then the resistance will lessen (Figure 10-5). Follow the lessening resistance in and, the next time it begins filling, resist that with the gentle 5 g or less of intentional pressure. Wait. In a few seconds to minutes, you may feel one of several things. One, the cranium may seem to narrow again—then you will follow that narrowing in and wait again. Two, you may feel the system begin to rhythmically disorganize and "wobble"—then you will just maintain your presence without the resistance. Three, you may feel nothing—if you feel this stillness, again do nothing. Just maintain your presence without the resistance.

After a few moments or as long as a few minutes, you will begin to feel the "knocking at the door" of the CS pulse as it begins to reemerge. It will feel like a pushing against your thumbs as the occiput begins to widen in flexion again. When you feel a clear impetus toward flexion, allow it to flow and just listen again. Usually, the rhythm will manifest as a more symmetrical, even, continuous, and balanced wave. If you do not feel the widening and narrowing ("the surf"), just imagine when the client's body seems to be filling and when it seems to be narrowing ("the swing"). Follow your inner impetus to time your induction of the still point. (Follow this impetus to allow the CSR to reemerge as well.)

DIRECTION OF ENERGY

In the CS approach, the direction of energy (called V-spread by Sutherland [1962]) refers to targeting a specific area (or areas) with more focused healing intent to help a blocked area to shift and relax. I believe the technique is best described as sending "love" to a targeted area. Aim for the actualization of the client's natural self-healing response. Many massage therapists are sending some type of directed energy ("love") whenever they work.

To practice direction of energy, simply place your hands on either side of a restricted tissue and imagine a current of healing energy running between them (Figure 10-6). Sutherland called the technique the V-spread because in his application of the technique, the index and second finger are spread apart in a V, with each finger contacting a

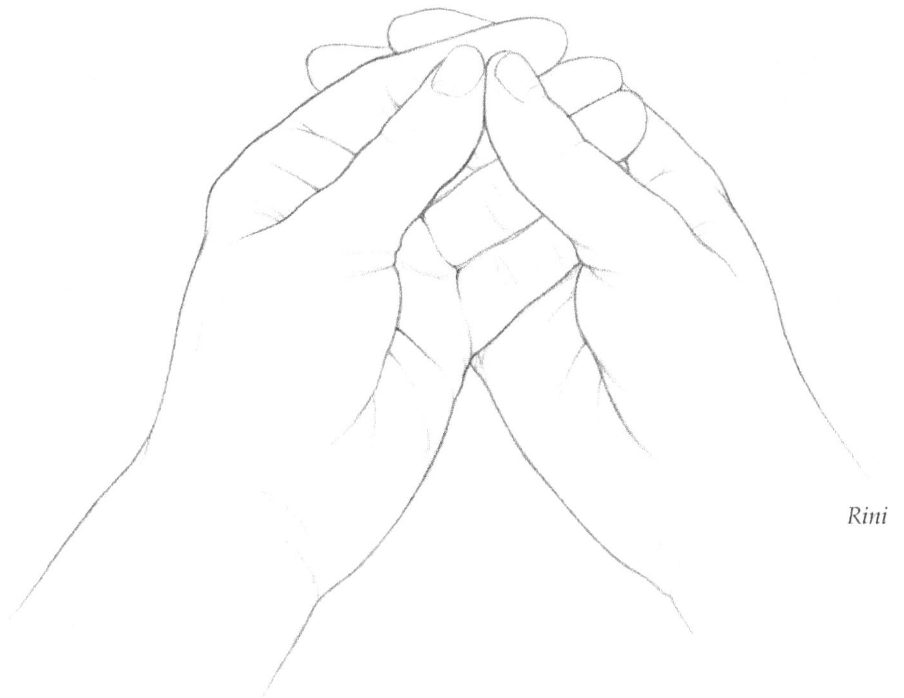

FIGURE 10-5 **Still point.** Hand position for inducing a still point at the occiput.

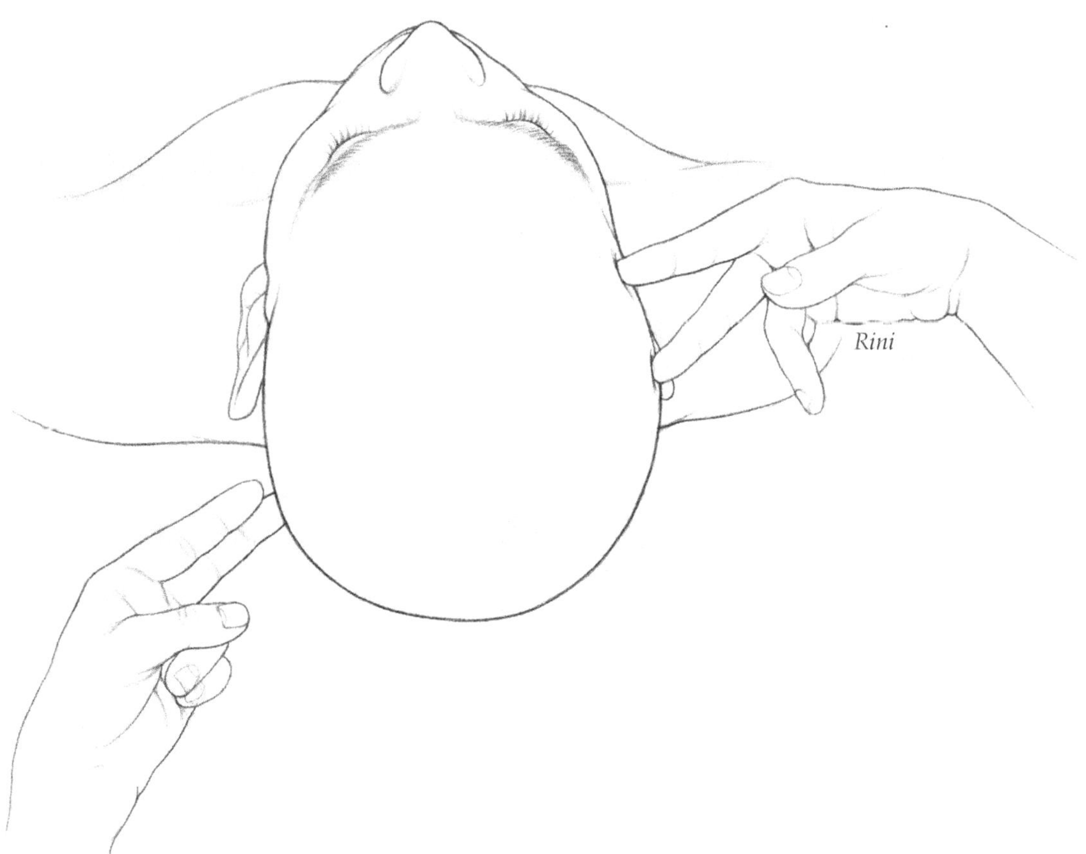

FIGURE 10-6 **Direction of energy.** In performing direction of energy, the hands are placed around the area that you want to release.

separate bone that is adjacent to a targeted suture. The direction of energy (including V-spread) can be applied to any area that feels restricted and can be directed toward a fascial, cerebrospinal rhythm, or sutural constraint.

SUTURAL RELEASES

It is possible to traction apart all of the sutures that zipper the skull. The joints do not move very much—but even a tiny bit more space allows for the self-healing rhythm of the cerebrospinal waves to more freely emerge. Upledger suggests that there are proprioceptive nerve endings within the sutures and a possible connection between the sagittal suture and the rate of production of CSF.

Before you begin, review the anatomy of the particular sutures and bones that adjoin sutures with which you intend to work. (For example, look at the orientation of the frontal bone to the parietal bones. The coronal suture that adjoins the frontal with the parietal bones can be widened with a vector of force directly anterior to the client or directly up to the ceiling, from the therapist's perspective, looking down at the client lying on a massage table; see Figure 10-6.) If you do not understand how to free up a particular suture, do not attempt a release.

To make more space within a suture (and at the same time, tug gently on the CT that binds the two bones and connects with the dural tube), meld your hand with your client's skull using 5 g or *less* of intentional pressure. Meet the CT's resistance within the sutures with very light traction using the fingers or thumbs. Make sure to position your hands so that you traction the targeted bone away from the adjoining bone (or bones) without compressing other sutures. At certain points, you may feel an impulse to hold the traction while the bones move slightly in different directions than your intentional pressure. Follow this movement, and when it settles down, continue your traction in the determined direction. Each sutural release is described and illustrated next. The five sutural releases are summarized in Table 10-2.

Frontal Release

Place your hands so that your third or fourth fingers (or both) catch on the indentation of the eyebrows, just above the orbits (Figure 10-7). Mentally imagine that you have magnets on your fingers to draw the bone upward. Apply gentle traction directly anterior (toward the ceiling) and wait for the CT between the sutures to soften. Three distinct stages can generally be palpated in a sutural release. The first is the osseous stage of release, when you feel as if you are trying to free cement. The second is the elastic stage (elastic fibers in the CT), when you feel some movement. At this point, it feels as if the tissue would spring back like a rubber band if you let go. The third osseous stage of release is the viscous stage, which can feel as if you are floating into the direction of release. You may or

TABLE 10-2 Sutural Releases

Sutural Technique	Hand Hold	Vector of Release
Frontal	Third finger (and/or fourth) contacts the eyebrows, hooking into a small indentation about three quarters of the way to the lateral side. The thumbs are held above the sagittal suture.	Client POV: Directly anterior Therapist POV with supine client: Straight up to ceiling
Parietal	Thumbs on the sagittal suture, rest of fingers draped down the sides of parietal (to ensure you are above the temporal bones, ask client to open and close mouth)	Client POV: Three steps—Medial pressure, pause, then directly superior Therapist POV with supine client: Three steps: Medial pressure, pause, then directly toward you
Temporal (ear pull)	Thumb in ear canal but not covering center or blocking sound, index finger behind elastic part of ear, as close to the bone as possible	Client POV: Diagonal made up of lateral, inferior, and dorsal forces Therapist POV with supine client: Diagonal made up of forces going lateral, down toward the client's feet, and down toward the table
Mandible	Four fingers (or three) on indentation at ramus of mandible.	Client POV: Directly inferior Therapist POV with supine client: Away from you, down toward the client's feet
Sphenoid	Thumbs on soft spots at the lateral corner of client's eyes, rest of fingers drape down to "magnetize" the occiput	Client POV: Directly anterior Therapist POV with supine client: Straight up to the ceiling

POV = point of view.

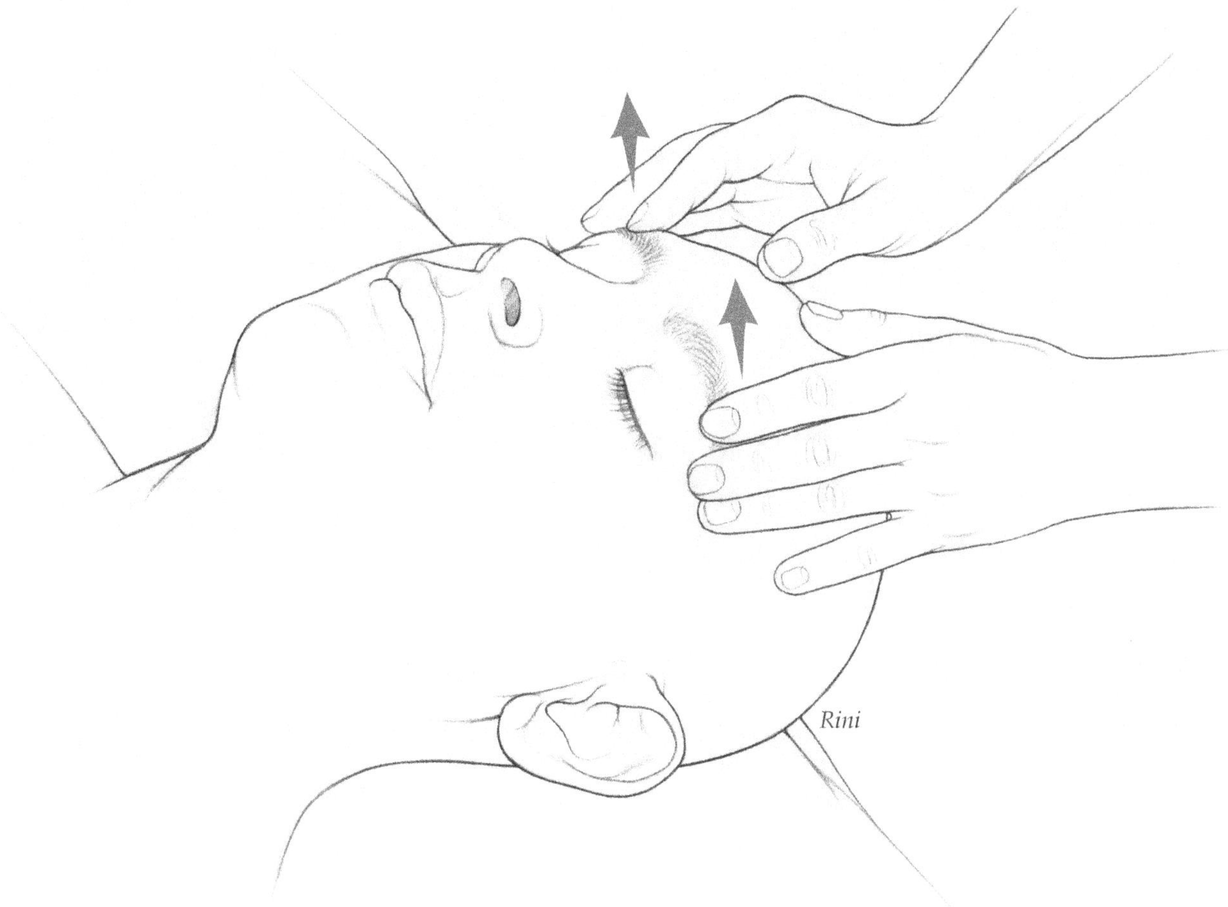

FIGURE 10-7 **Frontal release.** The hands are placed so that the third (and/or fourth) finger touch(es) the client's eyebrows. The thumbs are held above the sagittal suture and the direction of pressure is anterior.

may not progress through all the stages as you perform a sutural release.

Parietal Release

Begin with your thumbs on the sagittal suture and fingers spread above the temporoparietal suture (Figure 10-8). Because the temporal bones overlap the parietal bones like the gills of a fish, exert some medial pressure on the parietal bones to move them in from the grip of the temporal bones. Pause to allow the system to readjust. Then traction straight superiorly (directly toward you).

Temporal Release

Grasp the earlobes with the thumbs and forefingers, with the thumbs in the ear canal and the fingers behind and below the auditory meatus (Figure 10-9). Both the thumbs and the fingers are positioned as close as possible to the root of the ear at the temporal bone, away from the elastic cartilage of the ear. Traction down toward the back of your client's shoulders in a direction that is a composite of lateral, posterior, and inferior force.

Mandible Release

Sit or stand at the head of the table. Place four fingers (or three) on the indentation at the ramus of the mandible (Figure 10-10). Push away from you toward the client's feet. You can add a little anterior (i.e., toward the ceiling, for a supine client) motion at the end to mimic the protraction of the mouth.

Sphenoid Release

Sit or stand at the head of the table. Place your thumbs on the soft indentation just lateral to the corner of the client's eyes (Figure 10-11). Lift directly anteriorly (i.e., up toward the ceiling).

Table 10-3 summarizes and identifies the intentions that guide the CS techniques discussed in this chapter. For each technique, the table suggests what the myofascial therapist is hoping to accomplish.

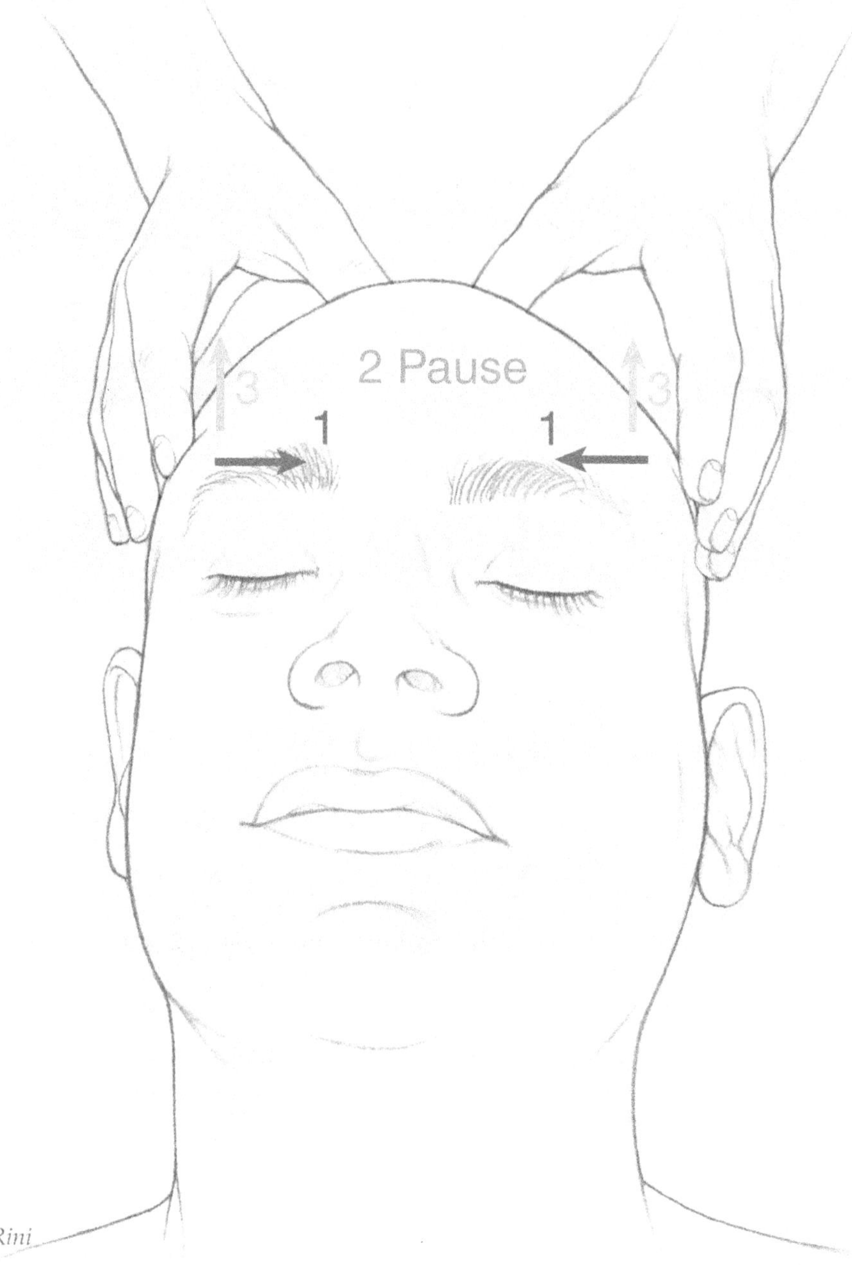

FIGURE 10-8 **Parietal release.** The hands are cradling the sides of the client's head with the thumbs resting on the sagittal suture. The direction of pressure has three steps. Step 1: Medial pressure. Step 2: Pause. Step 3: Pull superiorly (i.e., toward the head of the table) with 5 g or less pressure.

Recommendations for Optimal Use of the Craniosacral Approach

Asking the client to breathe or stretch during strategic pauses in CS massage helps create conscious awareness of changes that are occurring in the client's CT. It also helps to release some of the tension or pressure that can build up in response to such focused work. In addition, asking for feedback maintains interaction between therapist and client and can thereby increase the sense of safety and rapport. Asking for voluntary movement also facilitates the demonstration of self-help exercises that help maintain more lasting change.

If it seems as if the client is getting too spacey, too uncomfortable, or too involved in some emotional response to a CS touch, a good strategy is to bring her back to an

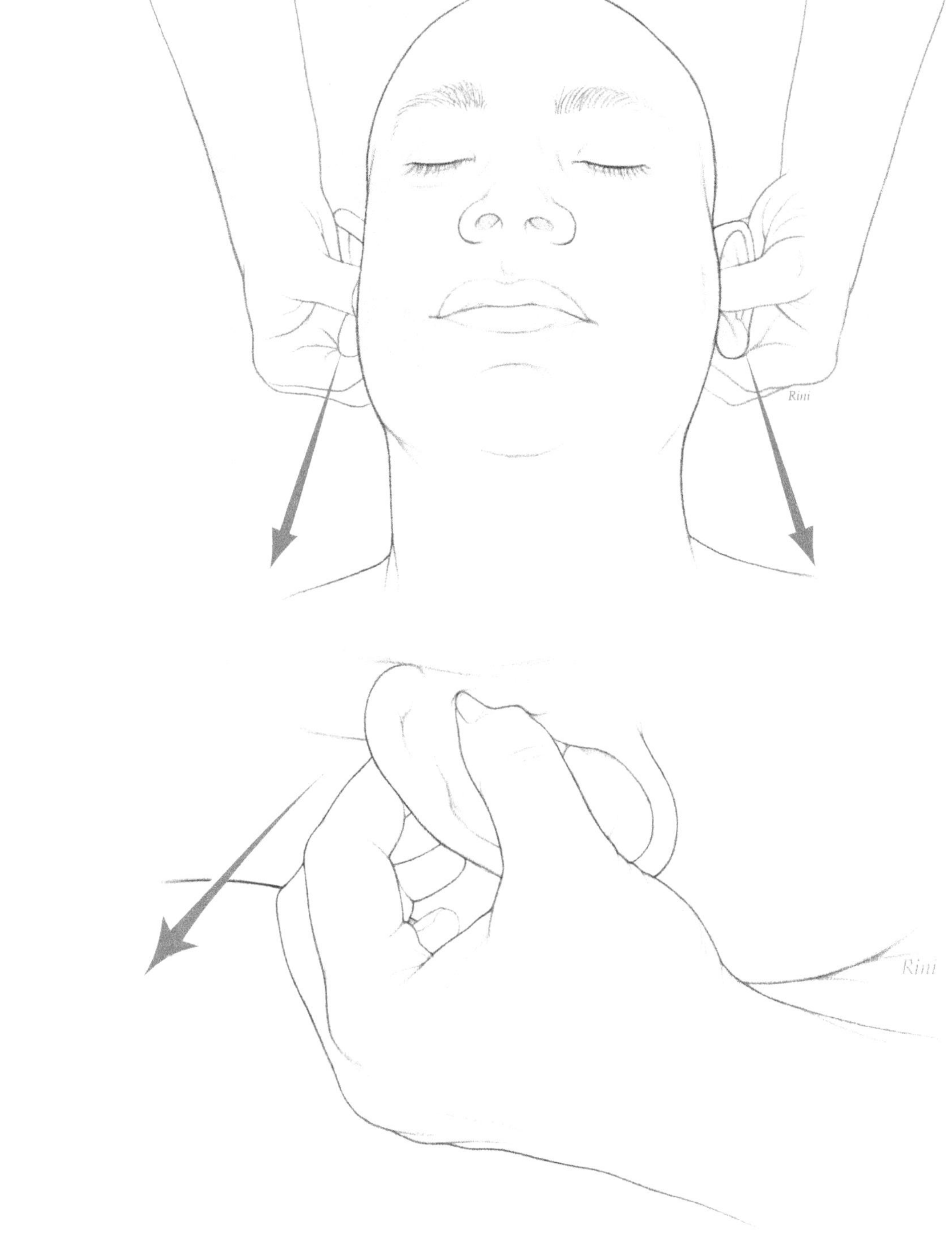

FIGURE 10-9 Temporal release. The thumb rests in the ear, making sure not to block off the canal. The index finger is behind the ear as close as possible to the bone. The direction of pressure is a diagonal pull toward the back of the client's shoulders. (**A**) Anterior view. (**B**) Lateral view.

awareness of her body. Some of the images that I use most in my practice are very simple suggestions. "Feel the table; feel the weight of your body on the table. Feel how your body is supported by the table." Suggestions such as these can help the client to focus on the comforting presence of her own weight. She can focus on her solidity and the support she can feel, as well as letting go enough to let her weight be supported by the table.

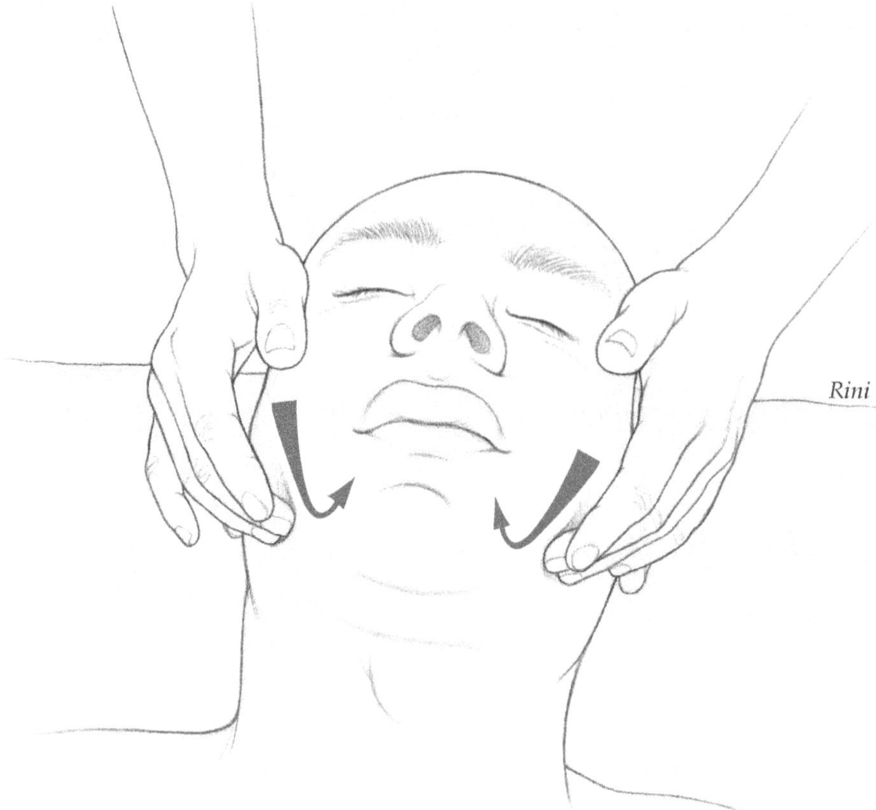

FIGURE 10-10 **Mandible release.** The fingers rest on the client's mental foramen, and the direction of pressure is inferior with a slight turn to the anterior to finish.

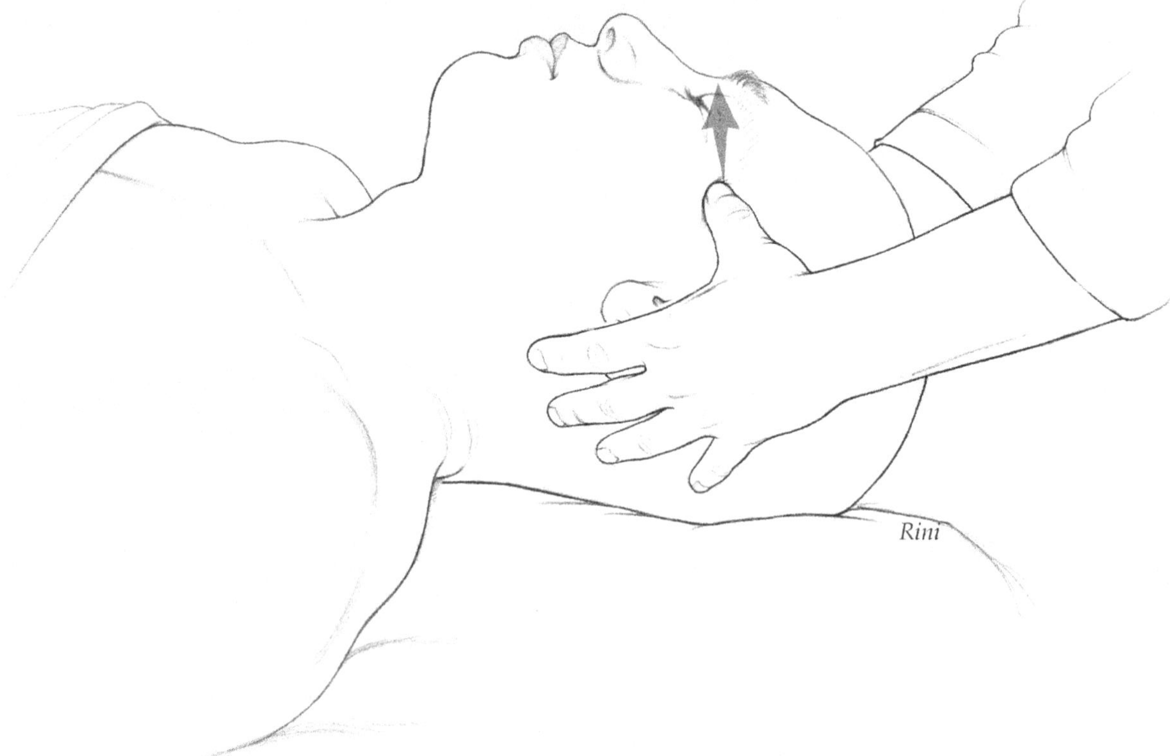

FIGURE 10-11 **Sphenoid release.** The thumbs rest on soft spots at the lateral corner of client's eyes, with the rest of fingers draping down toward the occiput. The direction of pressure is anterior.

TABLE 10-3 Craniosacral Techniques and the Intention that Guides Them

Technique	Description	Intention
Diaphragm and sacral releases	Find the bony landmarks and then ease off on pressure to 5 g or less. At this level, allow your hands to float in the direction of ease, the way the tissue wants to go.	Used to free up areas before "deeper" CS work; areas of focus can be sacral or pelvic, respiratory, thoracic, hyoid, and other diaphragms
Direction of energy	Send a message of healing intent. Draw on universal energy and sending "love" without a fixed agenda.	Can be used for any resistant or residual dysfunction, discomfort, or pain unless the client objects
Listening and following the CS rhythm or wave	Relax and open to experience the CSF wave; most easily felt on the cranium or sacrum.	Observing or normalizing the cerebrospinal rhythm; follows the Heisenberg principle that "observing will change the object that is observed"
Still point	Use 5 g of pressure as a barrier to quiet the CSF wave response and then let it reemerge; most easily induced on the cranium or sacrum.	Observing or normalizing the cerebrospinal rhythm; to encourage a more balanced or self-healing mode in the client
Sutural (cranial) releases	Find the bony landmarks and then ease off to 5 g or less of pressure. The vector of release is specific to the target suture.	Free up the zippers or sutural joints, so that the CSF can flow with less restriction

CS = craniosacral; CSF = cerebrospinal fluid.

The following recommendations for the use of cues can also help to optimize your CS work.

1. Stop every so often to let the client integrate changes that are happening.
2. Ask the client to feel how the releases affect a given area.
3. Ask the client to describe how an area feels after you have worked there. When the client has to put his sensations into words, it makes the sensations more real and memorable.
4. Use imagery to help the client visualize and reinforce sensations of release. The best images come from clients themselves. For instance, it would not be helpful to suggest the feeling of floating over a mountaintop if the client were afraid of heights.
5. When attempting to free up fascial or sutural restrictions or other restrictions preventing the free flow of CSR, focus on areas that move in a ratchety or discontinuous manner. Do not shy away from these areas; rather, select small movements that are easy for the body to make. Focus on finding the easy range so that the movements become more smooth and continuous.
6. Guide the client into breathing comfortably at his own pace. Guided easy breathing is particularly beneficial when addressing the fascia that surrounds muscles that move in inspiration or expiration (e.g., over the chest, neck, and upper and lower back).
7. Help the client comprehend the area you are working on. Show him a picture of the region from an anatomy chart or text. This engages conscious and voluntary aspects of healing into your session. He will better understand where you are working and actually see the unobstructed direction of the muscle fibers and fascia that lie in that area.

Craniosacral techniques can be directed to any region or segment of the body that requires attention. The key is to visualize how the physiological mechanisms of the CS system might affect the soft tissues that lie beneath your hands and to stimulate the fascia and CSF to trigger the body's own self-healing response.

Positioning, Draping, and Support

Craniosacral sessions are typically performed with the client fully clothed, so draping is not necessary for modesty. The CS client should be reminded to wear loose-fitting and comfortable clothes for the session. I prefer to cover the client with a top sheet and a blanket. This provides warmth, and the additional weight of the covers sends a signal of support and safety. If you are combining CS with other myofascial or Swedish approaches, it would be more convenient to have the client undress to her level of comfort; of course, a drape is then required.

When performing diaphragm releases (described in Chapter 8) over the pelvic and respiratory areas, keep the bottom hand underneath the bottom sheet and let the client know that you are doing this. For example, say "I am placing my hand underneath the bottom sheet under your sacrum."

When draping is called for, the sheet covers the body just as it does at the beginning and end of Swedish massage. No part of the body needs to be undraped for CS work. All hand holds can be performed over the top sheet and underneath the bottom sheet, when a bottom hand is required. Tell the client you are going to place your hand underneath the bottom sheet before doing so.

Use common sense. If holding the head to one side in the prone position makes your client uncomfortable, use a face rest. The entire 12-step protocol can also be performed in a supine position. After the first trimester, pregnant clients need to be placed on their sides. Other clients may prefer this position, too. Prop liberally if you use the side-lying position, as directed in Chapter 6.

Treatment Planning and Decision Making

When designing a session or series of CS sessions for a client, always begin with the needs of the client and a thorough history taking and intake procedure, as described in Chapters 5, 6, and 8.

Based on this information, identify a location of attention (e.g., spending most of the treatment session on the dural tube, lower fascial diaphragms, and sacrum to address a low back complaint), which is then modified as you work and feel how the tissues respond to the releases and direct you to new areas. If an area seems still and calm (but not stuck) at the outset, it is an indication that this region does not need additional work.

The CS approach is reputed to be an effective treatment for both recent and past injuries that have not healed correctly. Pain is a sign for caution. Although it is never appropriate to apply painful pressure, you can safely apply pain-free gentle pressure and movement (e.g., rocking) directly over an acute site. You can also move a painful area from a distant fulcrum (e.g., vibrating a painful back by means of rocking the belly), as long as it does not cause pain to the site.

Remember to attend to the whole body (in addition to targeted areas of focus). The CS approach requires curiosity and interest, and you may want to devote more time and attention to areas that initially seem blocked or stuck. Furthermore, it takes time to tap into dura or CSF or cranial or sacral bones and listen to where the movements stop or flow. You may wish to follow the sample protocol outlined below to stimulate healing in the client's whole body. Use the protocol as a jumping-off point to begin to listen to the cerebrospinal rhythm expressed by each individual. Feel free to emphasize different aspects of the protocol as you move your clients into greater stillness and self-healing with CS.

SAMPLE CRANIOSACRAL PROTOCOL: GENERAL SESSION

The protocol here includes various releases that can be used in CS work. It is important to remember that such charts can really only give a starting orientation for the application of the CS approach. Keeping your body relaxed as you work is the only way that you can effectively flow with and follow the rhythms of your client. Body awareness of your own discomfort will help you to modify your hand positions so that they are most effective. Keep your breath flowing, and when you become aware of tensions, let them go. If you cannot shift your body to be more relaxed, take a break from the position. Coach your client to do the same as you breathe deeply and shake off tensions. Then when you reconnect, you will be more fully present for your client and more available to identify the subtle shifts in the dura or CSF that can occur. Shifting out of an uncomfortable body position will help you to sense the very subtle shifts in the CSF or fascial motions. If your body is tense, you will be braced against the small movements and unable to register them. Moving with the flow of the CT allows you to listen to (and follow) the small movements of a client's body in the most effective way.

1. **Listening for cerebrospinal rhythm:** Can be performed anywhere on the body; however, most direct connections are at the cranium or sacrum. The purpose is to assess quality of movement, including symmetry, amplitude, strength, rate, imagery (e.g., colors or pictures), feelings, or sensations that emanate from the therapist, client, or both.
2. **Still point:** Used to bring the client to a state of "inner self." This state of quiet and inner peace is said to result in more balance and is said to be where self-healing can be activated.
3. **Sacral techniques—pelvic diaphragm, S1 to L5 (ligamentous), sacroiliac (SI) release (ligamentous):** Used to free restrictions in the sacrum.
4. **Fascial diaphragms—pelvic (same as pelvic diaphragm above), respiratory, thoracic inlet, hyoid, occipital base:** Used to free restrictions in the fascia.

5. **Dural tube release:** Used to free restrictions anywhere along the dura mater covering the spine and to synchronize the movements at the sacrum with the movements at the neck.
6. **Frontal release:** Frees the CT between the frontal bone and the parietal bones.
7. **Parietal release:** Frees the CT between the parietal bones and the temporal bones.
8. **Temporal release:** Further frees the CT between the temporal bones and the parietal bones.
9. **Sphenoid release:** Frees the CT between the sphenoid bone and the occiput.
10. **Mandibular release:** Frees up the CT at the jaw joint.
11. **Still point:** Brings the client back into a state of self-healing before closure.
12. **Closure:** Examples include simple holding of the head or feet; provides a sense of completion for the CS session.

SUMMARY

The CS approach has a distinct character that is especially useful for dealing with aches and pains that originate in the spine and head. CS practitioners meet resistance in the dura with a subtle touch and confidence in clients' abilities to heal themselves.

Important influences on the CS approach can be found in the work of osteopaths such as Still, Sutherland, Upledger, and Milne. Principles of osteopathy that inform CS massage include the concepts that the body is a whole, that structure and function are interrelated, and that the body is predisposed toward self-healing and self-organization. Sutherland applied the notion that structure and function are interrelated to the cranial sutures, which he believed existed to allow movement between the cranial bones and the free flow of CSF. Milne has carried on Sutherland's reverence for the spirit, heart, and art of CS bodywork, and Upledger has popularized the work and developed theories and descriptions about specific cranial and sacral movements.

Craniosacral manipulations include listening, inducing still points, direction of energy, sutural releases, and fascial releases such as the dural tube, sacral, and diaphragm releases.

Diaphragm releases and most sacral releases use gentle and slow pressure to access and follow a fluid CT movement into the direction of ease. This direction is palpable as the way the CT wants to move.

Keep your body attuned with your perception of the rhythm of the CSF when you listen to and follow or induce still points. Take time to pause and let the healing of the CSF rhythm sink into the client's consciousness. You need to incorporate breaks for the client's body to integrate the changes. Encourage breathing and questions. During pauses, cue the client to stretch and breathe to reinforce the conscious connection.

It is possible to release the spaces between the sutures. To perform these releases, rest your hand on the client's skull with 5 g or *less* pressure. If you do not understand how to free up a particular suture, do not attempt a release.

You can use all or part of the protocol mentioned in this chapter. Proceed through the protocol in the order provided, continuing as far down the list as you can in a 1-hour session. Even a full hour of listening to the cerebrospinal rhythm can be extremely satisfying and complete for the client if it is executed with attention, compassion, and care. Some non-CS massage therapists incorporate listening and still points at the beginning or end of a Swedish massage. Some therapists use CS techniques to identify areas to work with soft tissue manipulations or indirect or direct myofascial styles. You can customize your session as needed, in conjunction with other styles, for an eclectic massage.

Review Questions

1. Which of the following is *not* a principle of osteopathy as described by Still?
   a. The body is a whole.
   b. Function and form are interrelated.
   c. The body has a self-healing capacity.
   d. People need to be fixed.
2. Fluid is filtered out of the blood to become CSF in the __________ of the brain.
   a. arachnoid villi
   b. meninges
   c. dura mater
   d. choroid plexus
3. CSF is reabsorbed into the bloodstream in the __________ of the brain.
   a. arachnoid villi
   b. meninges
   c. dura mater
   d. choroid plexus
4. True or false: One phase of the CSR is extension or filling, which is characterized by the external rotation of the entire body and widening of the head.
5. True or false: The interval between the two phases described above is known as a still point. It can arise spontaneously or be induced by a CS therapist.

6. How much pressure do you use when executing the CS approach?

7. Name one place where the dura is attached to bone along the skull and spine.

8. Direction of __________ means taking the tissue in the direction that it wants to go.

9. The hand position for the __________ release is with your thumbs on the soft spots next to the lateral orbits of the eye and your little fingers reaching for the occiput.

10. Describe a characteristic of tissue release that you could feel (observe) to let you know that you have completed a cranial or diaphragm release.

REFERENCES

Avezaat CJ, van Eijndhoven JH. Clinical observations on the relationship between cerebrospinal fluid pulse pressure and intracranial pressure. Acta Neurochi (Wein) 1986;79:13–29.

Cardoso ER, Rowan JO, Galbraith S. Analysis of the cerebrospinal fluid pulse wave in intracranial pressure. J Neurosurg 1983;59:817–821.

Du Boulay G, O'Connel J, Currie J, et al. Further investigations on pulsatile movements in the cerebrospinal fluid pathways. Acta Radiol (Diagn) (Stockh) 1972;13:496–523.

Enzmann DR, Rubin JB, DeLaPaz R, Wright A. Cerebrospinal fluid pulsation: benefits and pitfalls in MR imaging. Radiology 1986;161:773–778.

Feinberg DA, Mark AS. Human brain motion and cerebrospinal fluid circulation demonstrated with MR velocity imaging. Radiology 1987; 163:793–799.

Frymann VM. A study of the rhythmic motions of the living cranium. J Am Osteopath Assoc 1971;70:928–945.

Green C, Martin CW, Bassett K, Kazanjian A. A systematic review and critical appraisal of the scientific evidence on Craniosacral Therapy. Joint Health Technology Assessment Series. Vancouver, British Columbia, Canada: British Columbia Office of Health Technology Assessment, 1999.

Greenman PE. Roentgen findings in the craniosacral mechanism. J Am Osteopath Assoc 1970;70:60–71.

Heifetz MD, Weiss M. Detection of skull expansion with increased intracranial pressure. J Neurosurg 1981;55:811–12.

Hubbard RP, Melvin JW, Barodawala IT. Flexure of cranial sutures. J Biomech 1971;4:491–96.

Kokich VG. Age changes in the human frontozygomatic suture from 20 to 95 years. Am J Orthod 1976;69:411–430.

Kostopoulos DC, Keramidas G. Changes in elongation of falx celebri during craniosacral therapy techniques applied on the skull of an embalmed cadaver. Cranio 1992;10:9–12.

Li J, He W, Yao J, Wen H. Possibility of observing the changes of cerebrospinal fluid pulse waves as a substitute for volume pressure test. Clin Med J (Engl) 1996;109:411–413.

Marzal JR. Craniosacral Therapy Level 1. San Francisco: Pacific Somatics Institute, 1993.

Milne H. The Heart of Listening. Vols. 1 and 2. Berkeley, CA: North Atlantic Books, 1995.

O'Connell JE. The vascular factor in intracranial pressure and the maintenance of the cerebrospinal fluid circulation. Brain 1943;66:204–28.

Pitlyk PJ, Piantanida TP, Ploeger DW. Noninvasive intracranial pressure monitoring. Neurosurgery 1985;17:581–584.

Sutherland A. With Thinking Fingers: The Story of William Garner Sutherland. Indianapolis, IN: The Cranial Academy, 1962.

Takizawa H, Sugiura K, Baba M, et al. Spectral analysis of cerebrospinal fluid pulse wave [English abstract]. No To Khinkwi 1983;35:1227.

Upledger JE, Vredevoogd JD. Craniosacral Therapy. Seattle, WA: Eastland Press, 1983.

Zablotny W, Czosnyka M, Walencik A. cerebrospinal fluid pulse pressure waveform analysis in hydrocephalic children. Childs Ner Syst 1995; 99:397–399.

SUGGESTED READING

Cohen D. An Introduction to Craniosacral Therapy—Anatomy, Function, and Treatment. Berkeley, CA: North Atlantic Books, 1995.

Part

IV

Integrating Myofascial Massage Into Practice

Chapter 11

Putting It All Together

OBJECTIVES

- Discuss integrating myofascial massage into bodywork practice.
- Identify psychological aspects of myofascial massage.
- Discuss empowering yourself and your clients.
- Explain how connective tissue and the client-therapist connection can be a source of healing and power.

CHAPTER OUTLINE

KEY TERMS

Inflammation: A programmed reaction of the body to tissue injury, in which blood and chemicals that increase fluid retention move to the injured tissues.
Acute: Stage of inflammation characterized by red, hot, swollen, and painful tissues.
Subacute: Stage of inflammation characterized by tissues that are "not so" red, hot, swollen, and painful.
Chronic: Stage of inflammation characterized by cold, white, or bluish-tinged tissues that are hard and generally not painful.
Mild, moderate, or severe: Stages of severity typically applied to an injury.

General rule of myofascial massage treatment: The milder or more chronic a condition, the more direct techniques are indicated, using more pressure or stretching against resistance. (Conversely, the more severe or more acute the condition, the more indirect and subtle techniques are indicated, as well as easy or passive exercise.)

Body armor: Hardening of soft tissues (i.e., muscles tensing and connective tissue becoming more dehydrated) to protect against physical or emotional pain.

Emotional release: Experience in which a client spontaneously expresses emotions during a massage.

Integration: Time (during a session or afterwards) when a client can absorb the effects of hands-on work and convert unconscious responses to conscious awareness.

Empowerment: Having a sense of control over your life and, more specifically, over your own healing process.

This chapter provides perspective on how to integrate the physical, psychological, conceptual, and spiritual lessons of Myofascial Massage. *In other words, this chapter will help you to synthesize all of the information you have learned about myofascial massage into a workable and inspiring massage practice that expresses you. It also provides suggestions for how to deepen your knowledge of myofascial massage.*

Frequently Asked Questions

After reading about the methods of myofascial massage introduced in this text, many students ask the following questions:

1. **How do you decide which approach would be best for a particular client?**

   See the section in this chapter called "Using Critical Thinking Skills During Assessment" to form a good working model of when to use what technique with a particular client.

2. **Some of the techniques in the neuromuscular approach "look" very similar to techniques in the direct connective tissue (CT) approach, and both can look similar to what are often termed "deep tissue" strokes. Are they all the same?**

   The three approaches are *not* the same. Although the application of strokes might look similar to an outside observer, all three approaches feel distinct for the therapist *and* the receiver of the massage. One of the main reasons for the different "feel" is the difference in intent. *Deep tissue massage* is a broadly used and ill-defined term that does not imply more than deep pressure into muscles. Neuromuscular therapists concentrate on the neuromuscular junction to reset muscle tone, as well as on the muscle itself. Direct CT therapists focus on the CT that surrounds specific muscles and the bodywide connections as felt in the pull (or movement) of the CT. Neuromuscular clients are likely to experience pressure that moves perpendicularly into the trigger points or large movements (stretching) against resistance as suggested by their therapist. Direct CT clients are likely to experience a shearing (diagonal) force as the therapist follows the line of the CT and their own micromovements pushing that force along.

3. **Can I mix approaches?**

   Mixing myofascial approaches with one another or with another type of massage is *not* recommended while you are still learning myofascial techniques. This is because it is so important to have a clear intent about what you are trying to accomplish with myofascial massage. (Paradoxically, although you want to hold a specific intent to help the client heal, holding an attachment to "fixing" the client, as discussed in Chapters 1 and 10, is counterproductive.)

   The four approaches have unique intents, and no myofascial intent is adequately described by muscle relaxation alone. Softening the CT between the sphenoid and occipital bones (craniosacral approach) is very different from stroking the hair (Swedish or relaxation massage), for example. When you do not maintain a clear intent, there is a tendency to get lost and just rub. This will probably feel good to the client, but it is not myofascial massage. Once you are proficient in the techniques and clear about what you want to focus on, it will become easier to switch from one approach to another as needed. Just be clear to keep an indirect CT intent (e.g., thinking about how the client's body and your own can move easier) when you jostle the leg, and a direct CT intent when following the client's tension line with direct pressure and coached micromovements.

4. **What if my client reacts emotionally to myofascial massage?**

   See the section in this chapter called "The Emotional Link: Psychological Considerations" and the subsection specifically devoted to understanding and knowing how to handle emotional release.

5. **Is it preferable to play music with myofascial massage?**
   Whether or not you play music depends on you and on your client's preferences. Some people prefer silence to better focus on their body rhythms (e.g., heartbeat, breathing, and cerebrospinal fluid [CSF] flow). Others think that music enhances the vibrational and pleasurable aspects of myofascial massage. It is good to offer clients some options and follow their preferences. Sometimes, even with input from the client, I have made the wrong choice (as indicated by a strong wince from the patient when the music begins), so I have had to make an adjustment during the course of a session. Changing the melody, volume, or rhythm can be seen as one more way of listening to and following the client's needs.
6. **Many workshops advertise "myofascial" as part of the title. How do I decide which workshops will best complement my personal myofascial style? In other words, how do I choose what to study and focus on in more depth?**
   See the section in this chapter called "What Do I Study Next?" If you merely learn "protocols and techniques" without developing critical thinking skills, you will not have the confidence to use your new "tools." To incorporate myofascial techniques effectively (and therefore to continue to use myofascial massage), it is important to develop the ability to determine which approach (or approaches) best meet your client's needs and how to implement them. It is also important to try out different approaches to see how they fit your individual practice style.

The Physical Link: Integrating Myofascial Massage Into Your Practice

To integrate myofascial massage into your current practice, you must develop critical thinking skills and a framework for deciding which myofascial approach may best suit your client's health condition, and know how to adapt your initial plan to best serve your client and yourself.

USING CRITICAL THINKING SKILLS DURING ASSESSMENT

This section outlines a critical thinking (decision-making) framework to help you decide which myofascial techniques to use in specific circumstances. Before creating a workable treatment plan, you must determine what conditions need to be addressed and accurately assess the extent of any damage (i.e., stage of inflammation and severity of injury). Only then can you choose myofascial approaches and techniques that suit your individual client.

An initial interview will help you decide on a treatment plan, and subsequent interviews will help you to evaluate the effectiveness of your treatment. During the initial interview, the client provides the following information:

1. **Chief complaint:** What is the primary reason the client is seeking massage? Most commonly, the chief complaint of clients who seek myofascial treatment is stress, pain, injury, or decreased range of motion (The Mainstreaming of Alternative Medicine, 2000).
2. **History:** When did the symptoms start? Was there an associated injury?
3. **Symptoms:** What makes the symptoms worse (e.g., certain positions or activities)? Does it get better after rest?
4. **Prior treatment:** Is there a diagnosis from a physician? What was the effect of treatment? Is the client taking medications?

After gathering this subjective information, you will objectively observe, palpate, and perform range of motion tests on the client. Only then are you prepared to characterize the stage and severity of the client's condition. Notice that you do not *diagnose* the condition, but merely characterize its stage and severity. Diagnosis is the actual naming of a disease or injury. In contrast, massage therapists make assessments of a condition based on signs and symptoms and then palpate the client's body to elicit confirming responses. If there is any doubt about suitability for treatment, the client should be referred to a primary care provider (e.g., physician or nurse practitioner) for a medical diagnosis.

Assessing the Stage of Inflammation

Inflammation is a programmed reaction of the body to tissue injury. Accurate assessment includes estimating the stage of inflammation (acute, subacute, or chronic) of any injury. The optimal myofascial approach differs for each stage of inflammation.

Redness, heat, swelling (edema), and pain are the hallmarks of acute inflammation. In the first 2 to 4 days after tissue is injured, blood flow and inflammatory chemicals that increase fluid retention increase in the injured region. This causes the area to become red, hot, and swollen. The injury itself or the pressure of the increased fluid in the region causes pain.

After the acute stage, blood flow to the injured area tends to decrease, and the injury can be categorized as subacute. The redness, heat, swelling, and pain also decrease, but pain occurs when the repairing tissue is overstretched.

Chronic inflamed tissue is colder, whiter, and harder to the touch than surrounding tissue. There is little pain unless palpation or stretch reinjures the tissue. Chronic conditions are found when an injury does not completely heal. The soft tissues are subject to reinjury (and resultant acute inflammation) or development of scar tissue.

Assessing the Severity of Injury

Another important part of accurate assessment is estimating the severity of the injury as either mild, moderate, or severe (sometimes called *marked*). With mild injuries, the tissue has suffered only a little damage. It heals quickly, with muscle tissue healing more quickly than ligaments or tendons, which are CT and thus have less of a blood supply. In moderate conditions, the tissue has suffered more damage and tends to heal more slowly than a mild injury. Severe (marked) injuries heal slowly and may require surgical repair.

APPLYING THE GENERAL RULE OF TREATMENT

The general rule of myofascial massage treatment is that milder, more chronic conditions indicate a need for more direct techniques with more pressure and stretch against resistance. Conversely, the more severe or more acute the condition, the more indirect, easy, and subtle techniques are indicated. Figure 11-1 provides a schematic representation of this general rule.

Important self-care options that enhance myofascial massage are the use of hot or cold water i.e., hydrotherapy), heat packs and pads, ice packs, rest, elevation, and prescribed at-home movements. When suggesting or using heat and cold, apply cold applications to reduce the temperature of acutely inflamed or severely damaged tissues and apply heat applications to increase the temperature and circulation in chronically inflamed or mildly damaged tissues. For subacute and moderate conditions, apply contrast applications (i.e., alternating heat and cold for a few minutes each, ending on the treatment that you want to emphasize).

When prescribing movements for the client to practice at home, suggest stretches against resistance (e.g., hatha yoga) for chronic (or mild) injuries and painless, nontaxing activity (e.g., enjoyable, gentle movements or swimming) for acute (or severe) injuries. Optimal self-care for subacute (or moderate) injuries lies between easy activity and resisted stretch, using pain avoidance as a guide. Figure 11-2 gives a visual guide to decision making about prescriptions for self-care.

In real life, clients often experience some overlap in an injury's stage of inflammation and level of severity. There are no absolute divisions between chronic, subacute, and

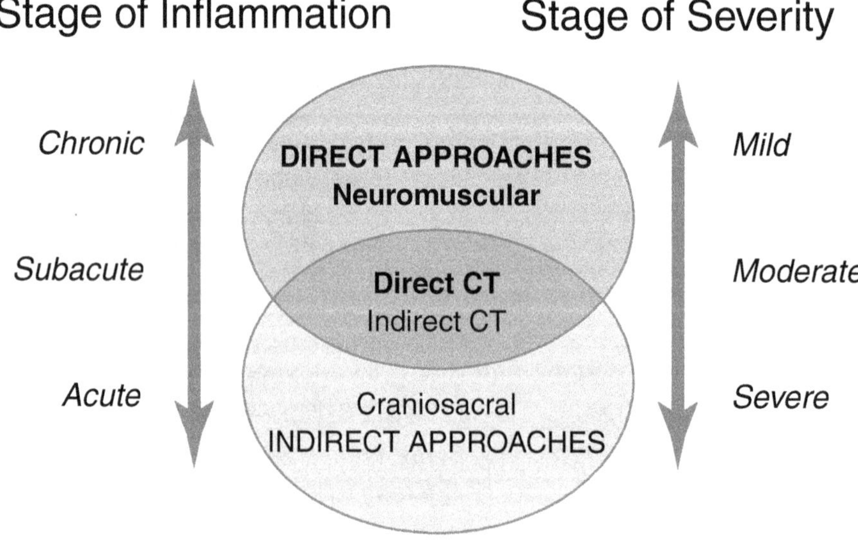

FIGURE 11-1 **Critical thinking schema for myofascial applications.** Note that suggested applications become progressively subtler as clients present with more acute (or severe) conditions.

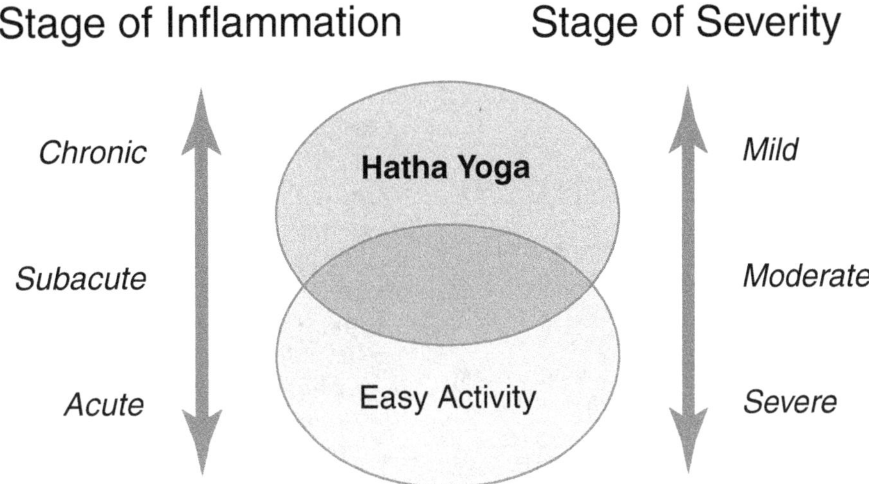

FIGURE 11-2 **Critical thinking schema for myofascial self-care.** Note that suggested self-care moves from resistive (hatha yoga) to following the direction of ease (easy activity) as clients present with more acute (or severe) conditions.

acute conditions, and you will often have to make a judgement call about whether to treat an individual client as if his soft tissues are acutely or subacutely inflamed. In ambiguous situations, *err on the side of conservative treatment.* Hence, if your client's low back feels a "little" hot, swollen, red, and painful and you do not know whether the condition is acute or subacute, assume it is an acute condition. That means you would avoid direct therapies (e.g., deep, direct pressure or resisted stretching) on the area that feels red, hot, swollen, or painful. On other areas that are not hot, swollen, red, or painful, direct therapies are *not* contraindicated and are, in fact, indicated.

Again, as always, *pain is a sign for caution.* If an application hurts the client, discontinue it and treat the injury more conservatively.

Decision making is also difficult when a client presents with a small band of hot and painful soft tissue within a larger cool and hardened but painless region. In this case, although direct CT or neuromuscular applications may be indicated for the larger area, direct therapies would be contraindicated for the smaller band within. Thus, you would be prudent to apply indirect or subtle techniques (indirect CT and craniosacral) as long as there is no resulting pain.

Similarly, you may notice that the damage in a targeted area may be considered mild, but within the mildly injured region, there is a small, severely damaged area. Again, in this situation, it is safe to use direct therapies (to the patient's tolerance) on the general area, but you should limit myofascial massage to indirect therapies on the severely damaged sector.

ADAPTING THE INITIAL TREATMENT PLAN

In some situations, you may have a "gut" sense that you should avoid direct methods, without knowing exactly why. Do not, however, ignore common-sense safety precautions to try out direct methods on severely damaged or acutely inflamed soft tissue. If a client requests that you avoid direct methods or any kind of work on a sensitive site, you must always respect that request. *Listen* to the voice of caution. Use common sense and, if in doubt, remember to *err on the side of conservative treatment.*

I choose my initial approach based on the intake interview, my "gut" sense, and any stated wishes of the client. This gives the client some control over the change that will occur. Some people want to feel the sense of strength and tension against resistance. Others crave a sense of ease. Still others prefer change to be almost imperceptible so that it seems more manageable. I finalize and sometimes totally revise my choice of approach and techniques after "listening and following" with hands-on palpation, which occurs in the course of the bodywork session. The client also helps to confirm whether the approach is relevant with body signals or verbal responses to queries.

WHAT DO I STUDY NEXT?

This text introduced you to four distinct myofascial massage approaches. Each approach attends to distinctly different sensory information and recommends distinctly unique ways of responding (i.e., techniques). Realizing this, the next step is to observe the experiential "flavor" as you work with each approach in practice and see what resonates. Determining what you want to specialize in or study more deeply requires reflecting on these experiences and asking the following kinds of questions:

- Do you like to find trigger points and release them? (*neuromuscular approach*)
- Do you like the feeling of falling toward the fascial line of resistance and matching resistance with pressure, while simultaneously coaching your patient into precise micromovements? (*direct CT approach*)
- Do you like to keep your own body moving in easy rhythmic patterns? (*indirect CT approach*)
- Do you prefer to follow very small, subtle, precise, but almost nonperceptible movements of the CSF? (*craniosacral approach*)

It can be difficult to decipher what advanced myofascial workshops really offer. Much of the confusion results from the imprecise language that various workshops use for approaches, styles, and techniques. Hopefully, this text has provided more precise language to describe myofascial methods, approaches, and techniques, so that you can feel more prepared to evaluate and categorize the brand names. For example, now you know that some myofascial styles with different names may be essentially the same (e.g., Rolfing and structural integration). You also know that the same technique may be addressed by different names in different workshops (e.g., skin rolling is a type of pétrissage).

The Emotional Link: Psychological Considerations

We are psychological creatures, as well as physical ones, from the day we are born until the day we die. In addition to releasing physical tensions, myofascial massage can be a tool to release unhealthy emotional patterns. Although psychological issues were mentioned in Chapters 5, 6, 8, and 10, as they related to various myofascial approaches, it is useful to discuss in more detail psychological considerations that are likely to arise in myofascial massage.

Myofascial massage, like any bodywork, can alter a person's emotional responses by disrupting patterns of muscular tension intended to inhibit emotions (Greene and Goodrich-Dunn, 2004). Insofar as myofascial massage specifically targets the myofascia, which comprises the armor of an emotional coping defense, myofascial therapists must be especially prepared for psychological sequelae. The *psychological rule of myofascial massage* is to be prepared for clients to have an emotional response without an agenda that emotional responses are necessary or even desirable in therapeutic treatment.

STRESS REDUCTION AND TENSION RELIEF

One of the most profound and broad-based mechanisms of any massage is the relaxation response. Muscle tension is the premier symptom of the stress response, and massage therapy is the best technique to diminish it (Seaward, 1994). Releasing tension through massage often brings relief, a feeling of well-being, and a heightened sense of somatic awareness.

A complicating factor of healthy stress reduction is that muscle tension can also be used to protect against pain. In massage jargon, protective tension is referred to as body armor. The purpose of the armor is to defend against threatening sensations or feelings. Thus, release of protective tension without adequate warning (generally meaning applying myofascial techniques too quickly or with too much force) can actually create distress (emotional, physical, or both).

The protective role of muscle tension is behind this book's continuing emphasis on searching for protective tension in tissues and using that level of tension as a guide. It is important to touch the edge of protective tension without crashing through. Protective tension is felt as resistance to pressure or as a barrier to movement. Using tension to guide direct therapies (neuromuscular and direct CT) means meeting and matching resistance without pushing through it. Using tension to guide indirect therapies (indirect CT and craniosacral) means providing an impetus for movement, letting the client's body move as far as it comfortably can, and following as the body returns in the direction of ease.

EMOTIONAL RELEASE

Emotional release is a phenomenon in which a client, during a therapeutic massage, begins to spontaneously express emotions. Emotional release can manifest as laughter, tears, tremors, or whole-body contractions; however, signs can also be barely detectable, manifesting only as a shift in breathing or a change in color (Greene and Goodrich-Dunn, 2004). Any time a pattern of tension is shifted, there is a potential for emotional release. Because myofascial massage is so effective in shifting unwanted patterns, the potential for emotional release is strong.

Signs of emotional release include:

- Laughing
- Crying
- Talking a lot
- Twitches or quick movements
- A motion that moves through the whole body like a wave
- Goosebumps
- Shivering
- Report of warmth
- Headaches
- Nausea
- Wincing, grimacing, shrugging, or other gestures and facial expressions (adapted from Greene and Goodrich-Dunn, 2004)

I have found that unpleasant emotional reactions are more likely to occur when physical tension is released abruptly or unexpectedly. To minimize the unexpected, it is imperative to read client signals (e.g., twitches, sighs, and grimaces) and maintain open communications at all times. Receivers of myofascial massage cannot be allowed to "zone out" as in Swedish massage. Explain to new clients the benefits of providing feedback. Most myofascial clients quickly become motivated to execute micromovements, breathe as directed, respond to specific queries, and even initiate requests when therapists relate that these responses will help them feel better faster. If your client remains noncommunicative, you must revert back to other forms of massage. Note, however, that specific queries are *not* persistent open-ended questions that keep asking the same thing. For example, when the therapist finishes massaging a region, it not as helpful to ask the open-ended questions, "Do you feel alright? Do you feel alright now?" as opposed to a more specific query such as, "Does this leg feel complete?"

Integration

As soon as the myofascial therapist perceives that a therapeutic change is taking place (either through tissue softening or some other clue as discussed in the paragraph above), it is important to allow time for the client to integrate the change. For the therapist, **integration** is a time for slowing down or backing off from a pressure or even taking hands off the body, while coaching the client to breathe easily or stretch in a way that feels good.

Because Swedish massage students are usually directed *never* to break physical contact during a session, the concept of taking your hands off for a therapeutic response may seem foreign. In myofascial work, pausing so that the client can breathe or move into the change actually promotes real contact between the client and therapist. Integration allows time for the patient to absorb the effects of hands-on work and shift her body awareness accordingly. Therapists can coach the client to breathe to take in the new way of being or to move in a way that makes the shift feel right and complete. At the same time, therapists can stretch out their own kinks or breathe fully to be more fully present when their hands next meet the client's myofascia.

Guidelines for Responding to Emotional Release

There is a huge difference between an emotional release that arises spontaneously and the deliberate stimulation of release by the therapist. Setting an expectation that emotional release is necessary or desirable leads to "fixing" instead of *listening* to clients.

Although myofascial therapists should never enter into a session with the mindset that a certain client needs an emotional release, they should be prepared to help clients cope with the process if it occurs. Guidelines to help therapists prepare for this eventuality follow:

1. **When a client displays emotional behaviors such as laughing, crying, or excessive talking, truthfully examine your own reactions as the situation is unfolding.**
   In other words, look inside silently to "seek your own truth" (e.g., "How do I feel about this?"). If you find that you are fearful, angry, or otherwise not present in the moment and you cannot trust that these feelings will resolve, you are no longer serving as support for the client experiencing the emotional release. If this is the case, do not get angry with yourself; instead, recognize your feelings and calmly but confidently guide the session to an end. Some safe ways to guide clients back to physical awareness include asking them to focus on:
   - The *breath*
   - The *weight of the body* and the feeling of that weight being supported on the table
   - Some other comforting *aspect of physicality*, such as air brushing over the closed eyelids or the sound of the music in the background
2. **Explore your own feelings about emotional release.**
   Before letting a situation catch you by surprise in the middle of a session, do some homework to prepare for the eventuality of emotional release. Greene and Goodrich-Dunn (2004) suggest examining your responses to questions such as:
   - What kinds of emotions do I feel *comfortable* with?
   - What kinds of emotions cause me to feel *uncomfortable* or threatened?
   - What level of *intensity* of emotional expression can I tolerate?
   - What *beliefs* do I have about emotions and emotional release?

3. **Avoid judging the client.**

   Because emotional displays are not usually under conscious control (Greene and Goodrich-Dunn, 2004), it is important to avoid judging the client. Judgement can cause the client to tighten his tissues and block his breathing in an effort to stop the process that is evoking your negative reaction. According to Greene and Goodrich-Dunn (2004), judgement can also reinforce a client's defensive patterns and stimulate anxiety, fear, shame, humiliation, guilt, dissociation, anger, despair, emotional paralysis, depression, confusion, or feelings of rejection.

4. **Observe and avoid judging yourself.**

   When a client reacts in an unexpected way, you must evaluate the situation and see whether it feels safe to continue or not. If you do not feel comfortable or safe in seeing if you can ride it out, it is best to guide the bodywork session to an end as just suggested. Your client will not benefit from your feelings of guilt or shame that you did not "stick it out." If you do decide to continue with the session, your confident manner will convey that emotional release is a normal occurrence and you are not overwhelmed, frightened, or repelled. This provides a sense of safety that "contains" the process so that emotional release does not feel abnormal, uncontrollable, or endless.

5. **Maintain your scope of practice.**

   It is imperative to avoid psychotherapeutic intervention in the context of myofascial massage. The scope of practice for a bodyworker does not include psychotherapy. (Note: If you are a licensed mental health professional, your scope of practice may well include psychotherapy. Even then, my personal recommendation is to separate your services as a myofascial therapist from your work as a psychotherapist. Keeping the practices separate ensures that clients know what to expect when they contract for services and provides a more defined therapeutic experience.) Specifically, avoiding psychotherapeutic intervention means refraining from giving advice, offering solutions, making interpretations, asking psychological questions, or probing into a client's personal life.

6. **Promote "grounding" in the physical world.**

   Emotional reactions can disorganize and disrupt a person's ability to function in the physical world. Strategies for bringing clients back into physical reality ("grounding") focus on the *here and now.* For example, you might suggest that the client tell you the approximate time of day. Or you might ask the client to describe concrete details about the surroundings, such as the color of the walls or small objects in the room.

   At the end of the session, look at the client's eyes to ascertain if she is focusing and not staring off into space. Some clients need help getting off the table. Verbal suggestions (e.g., "Turn to the side and then let your legs slide off the table as you sit up") or touch (e.g., offer an arm for the client to pull herself up or put a supportive hand on her back as she moves to sit up) are a good way to provide support. After the client is standing, suggest that she feel her feet contacting the floor. When the client seems stable in the standing position, you might also ask her to walk around the room. Offer a drink of water. Physical activities such as walking or eating help ground the client. Suggestions to experience breathing can be helpful at any time (e.g., "Feel the breath as it flows in and out of your nostrils" or "Focus on the movement of your chest as it rises and falls with each breath").

7. **Put a sense of completion on the emotional release.**

   The way that you say goodbye and end the session is important. Clients may need to return to work or to fulfill a social obligation (although neither is particularly recommended after an intense emotional experience!). When emotional release occurs toward the end of a session, facilitate a good transition by noting the time verbally (e.g., "We are nearing the end of our time together") and helping the client "wind down" the release before the allotted time runs out. Being "thrown out" too quickly into the world after an emotional experience can be scary and disorienting. An uncompleted emotional experience may leave your client so unfocused that it would be dangerous for her to drive home.

   If there is time and the client has had an emotional release, she may want to talk a little about the experience. If there is not enough time right then (or if the client is not inclined to talk), provide an open invitation to talk about what might have felt uncomfortable and what felt beneficial about the experience and set aside some time at future sessions to do so.

REFERRALS

Myofascial massage therapists should be able to make appropriate referrals when psychological issues arise that are outside their scope of practice. Therapists may want to make a referral during the initial interview if they determine that the prospective client might be better served by a mental health professional. Also, issues may arise in the course of a session that require the attention of a mental health professional. To be prepared for these situations, myofascial therapists need to have a referral listing on hand.

A good directory includes one or more of the following healthcare professionals: physicians, psychiatrists, psychologists, clinical social workers, psychotherapists, and licensed personal counselors. In addition, it may be useful to refer to specialists who work with abuse, addiction, chronic pain and illness, death and dying, or other specific issues. It may also be helpful to refer clients to support groups, such as Alcoholics or Narcotics Anonymous, shelters, or hospice. Building a strong referral base takes time and persistence. Although you may not have a personal connection with all of the contacts, making phone calls and attending promotional programs provide ways to get to know more about the professionals or organizations you wish to recommend. Even if you rarely call upon the network that you have developed, referrals can provide an invaluable resource for you and your client.

The Spiritual Link: Empowerment

Empowerment means having a sense of control over your life and, more specifically, over your own healing process. In other words, empowerment means being in touch with your own "power." I believe that it is important to promote empowerment in clients because it brings them into contact with their body's inner wisdom. It is my experience that seasoned myofascial clients do seem to be "in touch" with their bodies more than clients who seek other styles of bodywork. Empowerment is also important for massage therapists so that we can perform our bodywork services confidently and well, free from the unreasonable burden of having to "fix" our clients or ourselves.

STRATEGIES FOR EMPOWERING YOUR CLIENTS

Two therapist behaviors that empower myofascial clients are specific, informed touch and communication that reinforces success.

Specific, Informed Touch

Skilled myofascial touch spotlights the exact areas where tensions (or ease) reside. Precise kinesthetic information stimulates healing and optimizes tissue functioning. Specific touch is informed by attention to the anatomy and physiology of the living myofascial unit and palpation that involves listening to and feeling what is really there.

In basic massage programs, students learn to apply strokes to muscles. In contrast, every stroke in myofascial massage takes the interrelated structure and function of muscles, fascia, and nerves into account. Following myofascial movements and pulls relies on knowing the tissue structure (i.e., anatomy) that lies underneath your hands. Palpation and pressure also depend on knowledge of how tissues function normally and under stress (i.e., physiology).

By listening to and following the feel of the fascia, a myofascial therapist's sensitive hands can pinpoint the level, depth, and degree of movement that is most beneficial for a specific client. What exactly the therapist "listens to" depends on the myofascial approach chosen. With the craniosacral approach, the focus is on the dural tube and the flow of CSF within. In the neuromuscular approach, the therapist "listens to" muscles and their reactions to neural input. In the direct CT approach, the therapist listens to fascial resistance, and in the indirect CT approach, the therapist focuses on fascial ease of movement.

Communication That Reinforces Success

Myofascial bodywork also involves precise communication about how to create movement in areas that seem stuck and how to create ease where it is constricted. Clear communication about successful movements and breathing contributes tangibly to tension release. Guided visualizations that include concepts such as "letting go" and feeling "support" also reinforce the client's work to become healthy and strong.

In the direct CT approach, effective communications skills are essential to promote a client's success. While outlining the edge of "stuck" fascia, the therapist verbally coaches the client in micromovements that help the fascia move. During pauses, the therapist prompts bigger movements and breaths to help the client mimic the hands-on work that immediately preceded the pause. Effective stretches and breathing on the exhale can be further reinforced with hatha yoga assignments to practice at home, as discussed in Chapter 7.

In the indirect CT approach, therapists apply jostling to match the client's body rhythm—this communicates without words what easy, free movement feels like. Ease is also reinforced with strategically timed questions that prod a client to experience her body moving freely. At-home suggestions to follow through with exercise that brings a sense of ease further reinforce the experience.

EMPOWERING YOURSELF

Incorporating myofascial ideas and techniques into practice can also prove empowering for the massage practitioner. In fact, you may already be noticing benefits as you work. Personally, practicing myofascial massage has lead me to a greater sense of connection among body parts and between body and soul, increased body awareness and improved body mechanics, refined communication skills, a better awareness of and sensitivity to movement, and a heightened desire to accept myself and grow. These benefits are discussed in Chapter 1.

One Therapist's Experience: The Experience of Listening and Following

Many times in my myofascial classes, I have related the following story to illustrate the importance of listening to and following your client and yourself. This strange event really happened in a massage session, and I love to tell about the experience because it so clearly demonstrates the value of listening to your client's body wisdom when you are stumped about what to do.

"In the middle of her first massage session with me, J declared without warning, 'Bring me a spoon.' I was confused, to say the least, and to tell the truth, confounded by her statement. This was by far the most unusual request I had ever heard during a massage session, and it certainly caught me off guard. 'Bring me a spoon.' What a strange request! To comply would require me to take my hands off my client and actually leave her in the room alone to go get the spoon. I inquired of J, 'Do you want me to stop the massage?' and 'What do you want the spoon for?' and she replied in a more animated, and perhaps slightly agitated voice, 'No, get me a spoon, I need something to put my energy in.' Well, this didn't really make sense to me on a conscious level, but I kept my composure and asked myself a few silent questions. 'Do I feel safe? Is it okay to continue the session? Can she be left in the room by herself? Is this person crazy?' My inner answers were a clear 'yes' to the first three questions and a distinct 'no' to the last. So, I decided to go ahead and get that spoon, even if it made no sense in the context of my therapeutic treatment plan. Knowing full well that I was going against standard massage practice to break contact with the client and certainly to leave the treatment room, I told J that I was going to get the spoon now, and asked whether she needed anything else. 'Good,' J said, '. . . and make sure the spoon is not an especially good one.' So I went into the other room and found a spoon, not a really good one, and brought it back to J. And she took that spoon and proceeded to wind the handle around and around itself three times (Figure 11-3). Then J asked me to continue the massage, which I did. When the massage session was over, J was calm and relaxed as she explained again that a lot of energy 'came out' during the first massage and she just needed some object into which she could channel that excess. She had never experienced this kind of need for a spoon before, but she knew exactly what she needed this time.

J came back for several more massages, and nothing dramatic happened in any one of them. She always seemed pleased with her progress in the sessions. I still marvel that J was strong enough to bend that spoon handle into a tightly wound coil, and I keep the spoon to this day as a reminder to listen to and follow the wisdom of my clients. I also use it as a reminder to avoid judging my client and myself and to remember to truthfully examine my own reactions as the situation is unfolding. I'm very happy that I had the presence of mind to check in with myself to find out if it felt okay in my gut to continue the massage and to make sure that the environment still felt safe.

A lot of people ask me if J bent the spoon with some kind of psychic power, and the answer is no—she used sheer physical force to curl it around itself. I can attest that I surely don't have the strength to coil a spoon handle—I had to try it for myself."

The Big Picture: Speculations

Reflection on empowerment leads me to speculate on sources of "power" in myofascial massage. What makes myofascial work so compelling?

CONNECTIVE TISSUE AS A SOURCE OF POWER

My personal practice of myofascial massage has led me to the kinesthetic sense that one source of power lies in the physical matter of CT itself. For example, the CT can feel as

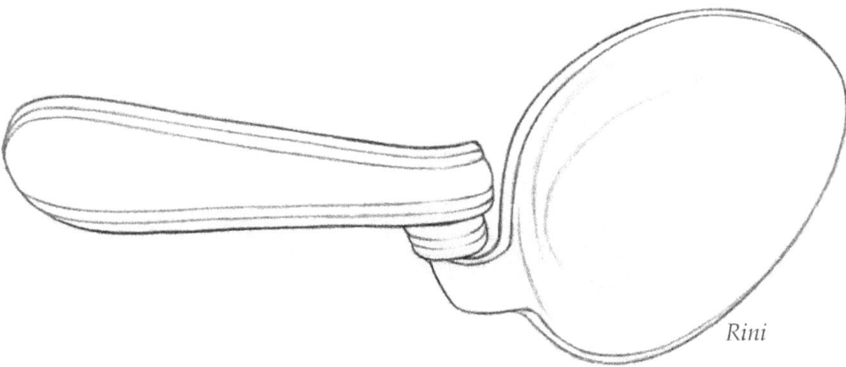

FIGURE 11-3 Bending the spoon.

if it is tangibly pulling the direct CT practitioner into the line of fascial movement. As another example, the CS therapist can often detect a palpable cranial pressure, as if he were pulling strings inside the client's head. I envision each individual's CT as having a nonphysical extension that goes past the physical body like some sort of energy field and that individual CT force fields interact with other CT force fields to create a therapeutic effect. Figure 11-4 illustrates this model.

This model helps explain why intent is so powerful in myofascial massage. My therapeutic intents manifest as a direction in the flow of my energy field, so for maximum therapeutic benefit, my thoughts must be "in line" with my physical line of force as I interact with the client's myofascia. I must clearly know what I am doing and why, or I will diffuse the power of my physical manipulations.

My theory may be simply an extension of Oschmann's (2000) "living matrix" schema. Oschmann describes the fascia as part of a living matrix, which extends out as CT to the farthest reaches of the body and into the cytoskeleton and DNA of every living cell. His salient points are:

1. All organ systems of the body (e.g., circulatory, nervous, and musculoskeletal systems and the digestive tract) are defined with a covering of CT.
2. CT extends throughout the human body and into the innermost part of each cell.
3. CT determines the overall shape of an individual organism (as well as the detailed architecture of its parts.)
4. All movement is created by tensions carried through the CT fabric. Chronic static tensions in the CT fabric may limit movement.
5. Each tension causes the crystalline structure of CT to generate electronic signals (i.e., piezoelectricity).
6. Piezoelectric signals make up an information system that travels through CT and can signal from any part of the body to any other part. (This signaling system is separate from and independent of the nervous system.)

Oschmann (2000, after Froelich, 1988) postulates that piezoelectric signals radiate through the living matrix and are radiated into the environment. He describes the signals as laser-like and able to integrate complex metabolic processes such as growth, injury repair, and defense. Each cell, tissue, organ, and individual coordinates its activities by vibrational frequencies. By manipulating vibrational signals through pressure and movement upon the CT, myofascial therapists can influence the self-organizing and self-healing capacity of an individual down to the level of every living cell.

The piezoelectric field can be described as concentric rings of vibrations moving out from the body. Imagine the circular wave pattern formed on the surface of a lake when a stone is thrown into the water. Every event produces a new set of vibrations, so that when a myofascial therapist contacts fascia, the energy ripples as if another stone were thrown into the lake. Therapeutic intent creates its own ripple in the flow of the energy field, and maintaining clarity about what you are doing and why keeps that ripple in synchrony with the waves of your physical manipulations.

Furthermore, piezoelectric fields attract water to the specific area of fascia being contacted, and water is an excellent conductor of electricity. (Do you remember your mother's caution to get out of the river during an electrical storm? This is because she did not want you to get shocked in the water.) This water-attractive quality of piezoelectric fields is important because areas that have been traumatized, diseased, or under continued stress become dehydrated. Interstitial fluids and ground substance tend to flow away from these regions (Reddy et al, 1979), resulting in "biologically older" CT. In contrast, water molecules are attracted to a myofascially induced piezoelectric signal, and CT becomes rehydrated, softened, more pliable, and "biologically younger."

Other myofascial mechanisms of action include mechanical stretching of the fascia itself and resetting nerve receptors that regulate muscle tension. In Young's (1957) model of CT, environmental stresses such as trauma or chronic postures reorient the direction of collagen fibers in the fascial web. For example, in response to chronic structural or emotional tensions, CT fibers "bunch up" at the ends where tendons and ligaments attach to bones. This

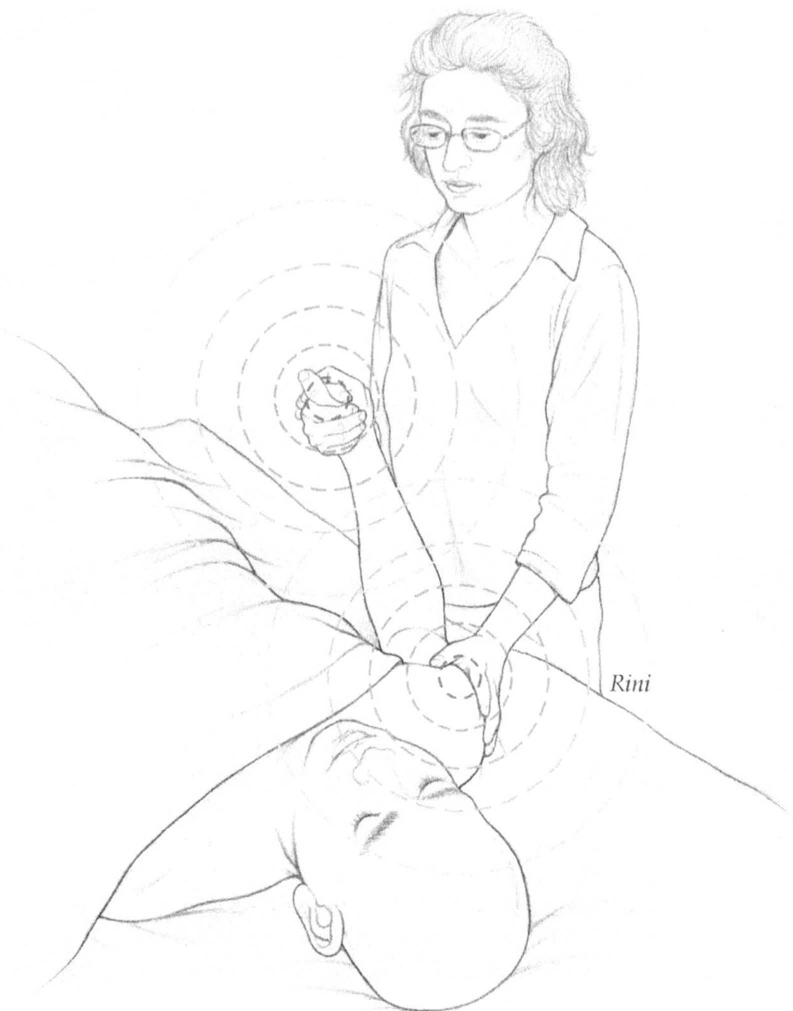

FIGURE 11-4 **Energetic model of connective tissue (CT).** This model shows CT extending past the physical body like an energy field and the interaction between two individual CT force fields.

shortens the tendon or ligament, tightens the affected muscles, and strains the joints. Myofascial massage manually softens these "bunched up" regions, enabling chronically tightened muscles to relax. In addition, myofascial massage alters the input to sensory receptors that register touch, pressure, or stretch. Guided breathing, imagery, active movements, and direct questions that require a verbal response further alter the sensory input and help override habitual neural responses, with a resultant change in muscle tone.

THE THERAPIST–CLIENT CONNECTION AS A SOURCE OF HEALING

Thus, the power of myofascial massage lies not in any special technique or approach per se but in using myofascial skills to *listen to and follow* the tissues. All of the approaches to myofascial massage presented in this text foster the ability and motivation to palpate in this open, curious, and nonjudgmental way. When a protective tension is met and purposefully followed (direct methods) or when a natural rhythm of ease is elevated to importance (indirect methods), the client's body can learn to let go. Myofascial approaches also foster patience, precision, and clarity about what you are doing with the soft tissues and why.

A good myofascial therapist paces communication with touch so that the client can match verbal information with a "felt sensation." This coupling of skillful talk with focused touch (rather than any elaborate technique, style, or approach) leads to deeper client awareness and drives therapeutic change (Seem, 2004). Thus, the accomplished myofascial therapist is also a skilled health educator who facilitates healing with knowledge. This is in contrast to the not-so-skilled therapist, who may give what appears to be a correct treatment but undermines its effectiveness with insensitive comments. (Berating the client for not being able to "relax" is my favorite example of this.)

In myofascial massage, the connection between client and therapist is a primary source of healing. The practitioner works to listen and observe and be present in ways uncommon to everyday living, and the myofascial client works actively to be more integrated and whole. From the moment the client enters the room and all throughout the myofascial session, the focus is on partnership and respect rather than on matching the client to some preconceived clinical condition.

When a therapist *listens* and *follows,* information about the movement or lack of movement in the fascia is revealed. By carefully and mindfully tracing and prodding the fascial pathways, myofascial massage brings a person into deep contact with the protective nature of his CT. In this way, the massage becomes more than a series of relaxation techniques or treatments; instead, it stimulates the client's body to remember how to restore appropriate functioning. Like other bodywork, myofascial massage leads to an alleviation of symptoms, but it is also an iterative process in which the client learns to regain and manage his health.

Treating muscles as disconnected entities divides a person. This perspective tries to "fix" people as if they are broken toys; it dissects clients into symptoms and divorces people from their own bodies. In contrast, listening to and following the "living matrix" taps into the protective and healing capacity of CT. Working from the myofascial perspective leads to respect for the body as a source of all the information necessary to make ourselves "whole."

SUMMARY

Myofascial massage is really about listening to and following the information that is embedded in a client's myofascial tissues. Four different approaches to myofascial "listening" have been described in this text, with enough detail so that any and all of the approaches can be practiced with confidence. Although all myofascial approaches are based on listening, the techniques that make up the various approaches look very different to outside observers. Pressure, movement, and intent vary depending on the approach. Choosing the optimal myofascial approach for a specific client depends on any injuries the client has and the stage of inflammation and severity of the condition. Choosing a path of subsequent study depends on the student's personal experiences with using each approach.

As myofascial massage releases protective tensions in the soft tissues, it engages the client's normal stress relief response and occasionally engages an accompanying emotional release. Stopping, slowing down, and waiting for the client to integrate therapeutic change allows protective responses to shift gradually while the client's CT learns to protect in more adaptive ways.

Myofascial bodywork entails a faith borne out of experience that bodies really do carry their own wisdom about how to heal. This experiential understanding is empowering for the client and therapist alike.

The power of myofascial work stems partially from working directly with the CT, which extends outward to the farthest boundaries of the body and inward to a person's very core. Another source of the power lies in the therapist–client connection that this kind of bodywork induces. The connection can be tangibly felt by experienced practitioners as a pull toward the client and a sense of greater relaxation within the therapist's own body, a sort of "settling in" to what is right. I speculate that this is caused by an electromagnetic force field created by the CT itself.

Analyzing the living matrix into mechanical parts isolates the activities of muscles, fascia, and nerves. It is hoped that the study and practice of myofascial massage will heal this split and increase the comprehension of connection within the human body and between bodies in the physical world.

Review Questions

1. The soft tissues are hot, red, swollen, and painful in the __________ stage of inflammation.
   a. acute
   b. subacute
   c. chronic
   d. last

2. The protective tensions that the body holds onto is/are called __________.
   a. the myofascial trigger point
   b. the body armor
   c. shearing
   d. spasms

3. __________ is a phenomenon in which a client, during a therapeutic massage, begins to spontaneously express emotions.
   a. Crying
   b. Asking to stop the session
   c. Emotional release
   d. Transference

4. Because emotional displays are not usually under conscious control, it is important to avoid __________ the client. This can cause the client to tighten his tissues and block breathing in an effort to stop the process.

a. touching
b. hugging
c. judging
d. observing

5. True or false: Always stick to myofascial indirect therapies when your client has a chronic and mild condition.
6. True or false: Two therapist behaviors that empower myofascial clients are specific, informed touch and communication that reinforce success.
7. Name two ways that myofascial techniques can be empowering for clients.
8. Name one way that myofascial techniques can be empowering for practitioners.
9. After finding the general area through knowledge of the fascial anatomy and physiology, ________ to and ________ the CT feel for more specific and accurate palpation.

REFERENCES

Froelich H. (ed.). Biological Coherence and Response to External Stimuli. Berlin: Springer Verlag, 1988.

Greene E, Goodrich-Dunn B. The Psychology of the Body. Baltimore: Lippincott Williams & Wilkins, 2004.

Oschmann JL. Energy Medicine: The Scientific Basis. Edinburgh, UK: Churchill Livingstone, 2000.

Reddy NP, Cochran G, Van B. Phenomenological theory underlying pressure-time relationship in decubitus ulcer formation [abstract no. 4885]. Federation Proceedings 1979;38:1153.

Seaward BL. Managing Stress. Boston: Jones and Bartlett Publishers, 1994.

Seem MD. Acupuncture Imaging. Rochester, VE: Healing Arts Press, 2004.

The mainstreaming of alternative medicine. Consumer Reports 2000; May:17–25.

Young JZ. The Life of Mammals. New York: Oxford University Press, 1957.

SUGGESTED READINGS

Benjamin BE, Sohnen-Moe C. The Ethics of Touch. Tucson, AZ: Sohnen-Moe Associates, 2003.

Cousins N. Anatomy of an Illness. New York: W. W. Norton, 1979.

Gerber R. Vibrational Medicine. Santa Fe, NM: Bear and Company, 1988.

Oschmann JL. Energy Medicine: The Scientific Basis. Edinburgh, UK: Churchill Livingstone, 2000.

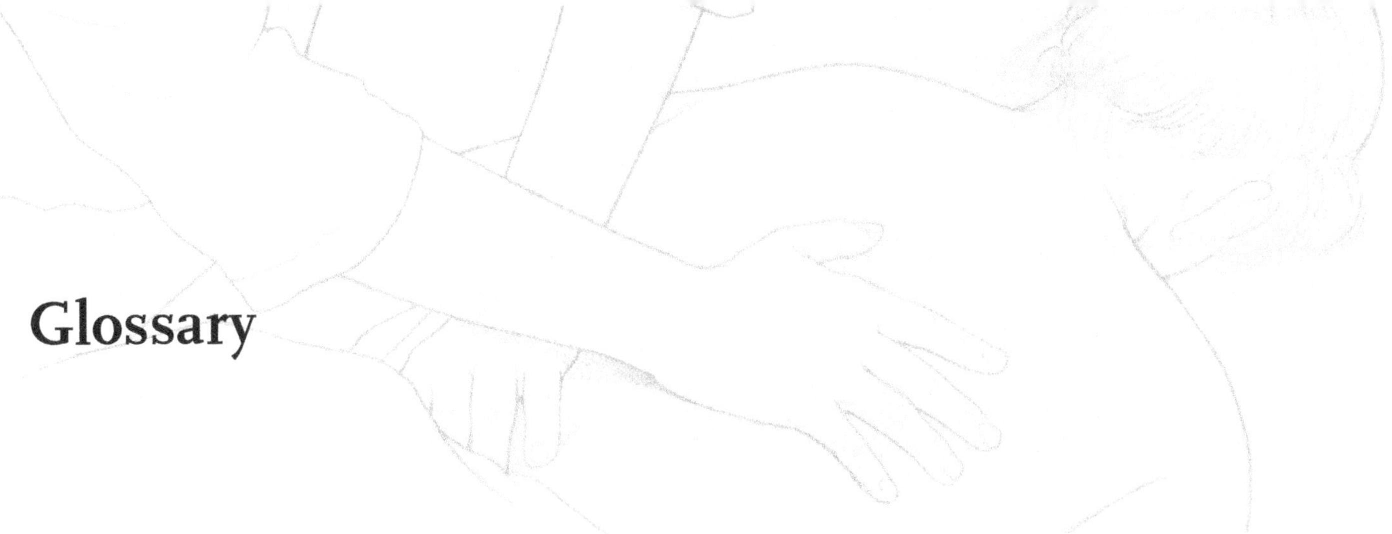

Glossary

Actin: Primary protein component of thin myofilaments.

Active trigger points: Hypersensitive areas that are painful without stimulation. Active trigger points are very tender and produce referred pain upon palpation.

Acupuncture points: Precise points (tsubos) along meridians as specified by traditional Chinese medicine.

Acute: Stage of inflammation characterized by red, hot, swollen, and painful tissues.

Aponeuroses: Flattened sheaths of connective tissue that connect muscle to flat bones.

Arachnoid villi: Outpouchings located throughout the cerebral cortex where cerebrospinal fluid is reabsorbed back into the bloodstream.

Asanas (asans): Physical postures used in hatha yoga; can include standing poses; forward, backward, and lateral bends; spinal twists; and seated, reclining, and inverted poses.

Autonomic nervous system (ANS): Functional division of the nervous system through which automatic motor responses are sent primarily to organs via their smooth muscles and glands; these responses may be either sympathetic (fight or flight) or parasympathetic (rest and repose).

Axon: Long extension of the neuron that carries information away from the cell body to another neuron, a muscle, or a gland.

Ayurveda: Sanskrit term meaning knowledge of the way to live or knowledge of longevity. A comprehensive system of health care that emphasizes the interrelatedness of body, mind, and spirit and seeks to restore an individual's innate harmony. Therapies include foods, herbs, and lifestyle changes, as well as asanas (postures), pranayama (breathing practices), and mantras (sacred sounds) specific to a patient's unique constitution.

Body armor: Hardening of soft tissues (i.e., muscles tensing and connective tissue becoming more dehydrated) to protect against physical or emotional pain.

Brain: Largest and most complex organ of the nervous system. It is made up of approximately 100 billion neurons and neuroglia that together interpret, regulate, and coordinate information.

Cell body: Part of the neuron that contains the nucleus and the organelles needed to sustain cell metabolism.

Central nervous system (CNS): The brain and spinal cord.

Cerebrospinal fluid (CSF): An extract from the blood that circulates around, cushions, and provides nutrients for the brain and spinal column.

Choroid plexi: Braids of capillaries located in spaces (ventricles) within the brain where blood is filtered and refined into cerebrospinal fluid.

Chronic: Stage of inflammation characterized by cold, white, or bluish-tinged tissues that are hard and generally not painful.

Compression: Technique applied to superficial fascia; pumping the muscle (and surrounding fascial layer) against the bone.

Connective tissue (CT): Tissue that provides structure and holds the body together. CT is composed of a small number of cells embedded in a matrix (mother substance) of fibers and a solid, semisolid, or liquid ground substance. The five types of CT are loose CT, dense CT, cartilage, bone, and blood.

Contractility: Shortening of muscle tissue in response to stimulation by an electrical charge.

Contraction: Period during which the thick (myosin) and thin (actin) myofilaments slide past each other.

Contract relax (CR): Muscle energy technique identical to post-isometric relaxation, except that the muscle is *not* taken into greater lengthening after the first resistance barrier.

Contract relax antagonist contract (CRAC): Muscle energy technique in which the therapist alternates performing post-isometric relaxation and then reciprocal inhibition.

Cool down: A session of light to moderate tapering-off activity after more vigorous exercise, often consisting of the same exercises used in the warm-up.

Craniosacral approach: An orientation to myofascial massage in which the therapist applies very light pressure at the cranium, sacrum, and spine to free restrictions in the dura mater and balance the flow of cerebrospinal fluid. Used to relieve pain in the head, spine, and pelvis and release trauma throughout the body. Also called craniosacral technique, Craniosacral Therapy, sacrocranial work, CS, and CST.

Craniosacral rhythm (CSR): One complete cycle of flexion and extension.

Cross-fiber friction (transverse friction, Cyriax friction): Soft tissue mobilization technique used to prevent or soften adhesions in the contractile tissue between the ligaments and the underlying bone and to smooth roughened surfaces between tendons and their sheaths. To apply, move the client's skin over the underlying tissue in a direction perpendicular to the muscle fibers.

Deep direct connective tissue massage: The direct connective tissue approach applied to deep fascia (dense or collagenous connective tissue surrounding muscles, tendons, or ligaments).

Deep fascia (dense connective tissue): Fascia that surrounds individual muscle fibers, fiber bundles, and whole muscles, as well as tendons attaching muscles to bones and ligaments joining together bones.

Deep pressure (ischemic compression): Sustained pressure on a trigger point (8 to 10 sec up to 1 min).

Dendrites: Neuron projections that receive signals from the outside environment, inside the body, or from another neuron.

Direct CT approach: An orientation to myofascial massage in which the therapist releases muscle tissue by using sustained pressure with coached micromovements on the connective tissue (or fascia).

Direction of ease: Moving in the direction that the body wants to move or moves most easily, or moving back from a point of restriction.

Direct method: A myofascial massage approach or technique that focuses on meeting resistance in the tissues with an equal and opposite force.

Dura mater: The outermost band of the three-layered connective tissue sac (meninges) that surrounds the brain and spinal cord. Sometimes refers to the entire sac. Also known as the dura.

Dural tube (dura): The outer layer of connective tissue that surrounds the brain, spinal cord, and cerebrospinal fluid; sometimes (incorrectly) used synonymously with meninges.

Elasticity: Ability of a muscle to return to its normal resting length after being stretched.

Emotional release: Experience in which a client spontaneously expresses emotions during a massage.

Empowerment: Having a sense of control over your life and, more specifically, over your own healing process.

Endomysium: Thin connective tissue sheath that wraps each muscle fiber.

Endoneurium: Thin connective tissue sheath that wraps each individual axon or dendrite.

Epimysium: Connective tissue sheath that wraps an entire muscle.

Epineurium: Connective tissue sheath that wraps the entire nerve.

Excitability: Reactive quality of all muscle tissue in response to an electrical or chemical stimulus.

Exercise: Purposeful movement or physical activity, including formal activities such as team sports, dance, and games, and less formal activities, such as walking, jogging, and swimming. Can refer to large muscle activities or nontaxing, specific small muscle movements.

Extensibility: Stretchability beyond a muscle's normal, resting length.

Extension: Emptying, contraction, narrowing, or inward rotation of the body corresponding with the decreased amount of cerebrospinal fluid filtering into the system.

Fascia: Two specific types of connective tissue: loose connective tissue (superficial fascia) and dense connective tissue (deep fascia).

Fascial release: Indirect connective tissue technique that takes areas of horizontal stress on the superficial fascia into a direction of ease (the way it wants to move).

Fascicles: Bundles of muscle fibers.

Flexion: Filling, widening, expansion, or outward rotation of the body corresponding with an increased amount of cerebrospinal fluid filtering into the system.

Flopping: Indirect CT technique; a type of shaking by which a limb is bounced in a controlled way onto the massage table.

General rule of myofascial massage treatment: The milder or more chronic a condition, the more direct techniques are indicated, using more pressure or stretching against resistance. (Conversely, the more severe or more acute the condition, the more indirect and subtle techniques are indicated, as well as easy or passive exercise.)

Hanna Somatics Education (HSE): Indirect connective tissue style; hands-on method for teaching voluntary, conscious control of the neuromuscular system to clients suffering from involuntary, maladaptive reflex disorders.

Hatha yoga: Branch of yoga that emphasizes the practice of physical postures called asanas (asans) and breathing exercises called pranayama.

Ice friction (intermittent cold): Slow application of ice over soft tissue with unidirectional parallel strokes.

Indirect CT approach: An orientation to myofascial massage in which the therapist releases muscle tissue with movement in the form of jostling, compression, or traction applied to the connective tissue (or fascia). Indirect techniques move up to a restricted point (but not beyond) and then move back from that boundary.

Indirect method: A myofascial massage approach or technique that focuses on meeting a resistance by softening into a sense of ease.

Inflammation: A programmed reaction of the body to tissue injury, in which blood and chemicals that increase fluid retention move to the injured tissues.

Integration: Time (during a session or afterwards) when a client can absorb the effects of hands-on work and convert unconscious responses to conscious awareness.

Jostling: Indirect connective tissue technique; a rhythmic type of vibration applied with the whole body that moves the client's body or body part as far as it can easily go, then allows it to return.

J stroke: A more forceful soft tissue mobilization technique performed to release skin restrictions or adhesions that do not respond to skin rolling. This stroke is used in localized areas only.

Latent: Short period of time that elapses after the initial nerve impulse and before the muscle begins to shorten.

Latent trigger points: Hypersensitive areas that are not ordinarily painful but upon palpation are tender and may produce referred pain.

Matrix: Noncellular part of connective tissue containing fibers and a solid, semisolid, or liquid ground substance.

Meninges: Three connective tissue layers that together form a sac that surrounds and protects the brain and spinal cord.

Micromovements: Very small regular movements made by the client, usually in response to coaching by the massage therapist. Used to enhance lengthening and release of the client's soft tissue.

Mild, moderate, or severe: Stages of severity typically applied to an injury.

Motor end plate: Location on the sarcolemma where the somatic motor neurons meet the muscle.

Motor fibers: Nerves that transmit information from the brain or spinal cord to effect responses in muscles, glands, or other nerves.

Motor unit: A somatic motor neuron and all of the muscle fibers to which it connects.

Movement reeducation: Any style of bodywork or active exercise that is used to reeducate the client's body to optimize functionality, increase range of motion, and make unconscious movement conscious. Some popular movement reeducation styles include Hanna Somatics Education, Trager, Feldenkrais method, Alexander technique, Rubenfeld Synergy, and Aston Patterning.

Muscle energy techniques (METs): Set of procedures requiring client to voluntarily contract a specific muscle in a specific direction against (or with) a specific force applied by the therapist.

Muscle fibers: Individual muscle cells.

Muscle sculpting (longitudinal friction, deep effleurage): Technique that uses deep effleurage or longitudinal friction to lengthen the myofascial in the direction parallel to muscle fibers and/or the epimysium surrounding the whole muscle.

Muscle spindle: Spindle-shaped proprioceptor within skeletal muscles that monitors the muscles' degree of stretch.

Myelin: Lipid-insulating coat of neuroglia that surrounds some axons.

Myofascia: A type of deep fascia that is bound to muscle tissue. The term is sometimes used to specify only the fascia that is bound to the muscles and is sometimes used to refer to the entire unit of muscle and fascia.

Myofascial (MF) massage: A type of bodywork that focuses on the myofascial unit, including muscle, connective tissue, and the neuromuscular junction.

Myofascial Release: Trademarked style of manual therapy that includes indirect connective tissue, direct connective tissue, and soft tissue mobilization techniques.

Myofilaments: Microscopic threads that make up the myofibrils of muscle fibers. There are two types, thick and thin.

Myosin: Primary protein component of thick myofilaments.

Nerve impulse (action potential): Electrical message transmitted by nerves.

Neuroglia (glia): Cells in the nervous system with a connective function; they insulate, bind, support, and protect the neurons and help the neurons transmit their messages more efficiently.

Neuromuscular approach: An orientation to myofascial massage in which the therapist focuses on local muscular or neural dysfunctions, including trigger points, ischemia, inflammation, hypertonia, and neural impingement. The thumb or finger glides or drags to detect taut bands or muscular nodules and ischemic compression to treat trigger points. Also called neuromuscular therapy (NMT) or neuromuscular techniques.

Neuromuscular junction: Region at which an electrical impulse is transferred into a muscle.

Neuromuscular Therapy (neuromuscular techniques; NMT): Trademarked style that focuses on local dysfunctions, including trigger points, ischemia, inflammation, muscle hypertonia, and nerve impingement.

Neurons: Nerve cells that send and receive electrical impulses.

Perineurium: Connective tissue sheath that wraps groups of axons or dendrites.

Peripheral nervous system (PNS): The cranial and spinal nerves.

Perimysium: Connective tissue sheath that wraps groups of muscle fibers (fascicles).

Piezoelectricity: A property of connective tissue whereby it conducts electricity when compressed.

Post-isometric relaxation (PIR): Principle in MET by which the therapist lengthens the target muscle up to a point of mild resistance. Holding that position, the therapist coaches the client to voluntarily resist for 8 to 10 seconds. As the client relaxes, the therapist takes the muscle into a greater stretch and repeats the process two more times, ending on a stretch/relax.

Prana: Life energy that travels freely throughout the body.

Pranayama: Breathing exercises that enhance the flow, effectiveness, and balance of asanas. Sometimes considered a meditation practice.

Pressurestat theory: Upledger's explanation of how movement of the cranial bones is necessary to accommodate the cerebrospinal fluid pulsations as the fluid is filtered into the system and then is reabsorbed.

Proprioception: Information about the position of muscles, tendons, and ligaments in space. Relayed by nerve receptors in the muscles, joints, and fascial sheaths.

Ratchet model: Model attributing to myosin a swiveling head that acts like a ratchet to pull the sarcomere together and cause muscles to contract.

Reciprocal inhibition (RI; antagonist contract): Principle in MET by which the therapist inhibits the reciprocal (or antagonist) muscle to the one he or she want to target.

Refractory: Period when a new nerve impulse cannot cause the muscle to contract again.

Relaxation: Period during which the myofilaments return to their separated state.

Rocking: Indirect connective tissue technique; can involve up and down, side to side, or circular motions.

Rolfing: Bodywork style that aims to realign the structural components of the body for enhanced function. Usually requires 10 or more sessions to realign the whole body.

Sarcomere: Functional (contracting) units of a muscle fiber.

Scraping: Technique applied to superficial fascia; involves scraping bony or ligamentous areas with your thumb, knuckles, or fingers and imagining that you are smoothing the surface, as if you were shaving off ice.

Sensory fibers: Nerves that transmit information from the external or internal environment to the brain or spinal cord.

Shaking: Indirect connective tissue technique; a type of vibration, beginning with lifting and pulling and followed with a downward or sideways motion that warms joints and prepares muscle groups, joints, or limbs for more focused bodywork.

Skeletal muscle tissue: Muscle that is attached to the skeleton through the connective tissue. It moves bones and stabilizes the body.

Skin rolling: Technique applied to superficial fascia. A type of pétrissage in which the tissue just beneath the skin is grasped between thumb and forefingers and held until a movement of fascia (release) is felt by the therapist.

Sliding-filament theory: Description of skeletal muscle contraction as a chain of physical and chemical reactions ending in actin and myosin myofilaments sliding toward each another.

Soft tissue mobilization: More aggressive direct CT approach techniques; includes cross-fiber friction and the J stroke.

Somatic motor neurons: Nerve cells that carry impulses related to muscle movement or glandular secretion.

Spinal cord: The part of the central nervous system that extends from the base of the occiput to the low back.

Spinal cord reflexes: Automatic reactions to a stimulus that involve at least three neurons: a sensory neuron, an interneuron, and a motor neuron.

Still point: When the cranial wave stops; still points can occur spontaneously without intervention or can be induced in response to specific craniosacral techniques.

Stimulus period: The core of the exercise workout or period of most intense activity.

Stretching: Technique applied to superficial fascia; involves mechanically lengthening the muscle and fascia in a line between your hands.

Stripping: Neuromuscular technique that is a type of deep effleurage that travels down the length of the muscle fiber while maintaining depth.

Structural integration (postural integration): Bodywork style that is similar to Rolfing, but instructors are not certified by the Rolf Institute.

Style: A bodywork modality that is trademarked or so popular in massage culture as to be designated by a unique brand name (e.g., Myofascial Release, Trager, or Swedish massage).

Subacute: Stage of inflammation characterized by tissues that are "not so" red, hot, swollen, and painful.

Superficial direct CT massage: The direct CT approach applied to superficial fascia (i.e., loose connective tissue underneath the skin).

Superficial fascia (loose connective tissue): Fascia that lies just beneath the surface of the skin.

Synaptic cleft (synapse): The extracellular space between two neurons or between a neuron and the muscle fiber or gland it affects.

Technique: Massage stroke or manipulation. A mechanical description of what is actually being performed on the client's body.

Tender points: Hypersensitive areas that do not cause increased tightness or radiating pain in surrounding areas. Release of a tender point does not cause a release in other areas.

Thixotropy: A property of connective tissue whereby it can sometimes change form from thick and hard to more pliable and soft.

Traction: Indirect connective tissue technique; longitudinal stretching that pulls connective tissue in the direction of the muscle fiber and follows tiny movements to achieve a release.

Trager Approach: Trademarked indirect connective tissue style that aims to release psychophysiological areas of holding or guarding.

Trigger point (trigger zone, trigger spot, trigger area, TrP): Hyperirritable area that is locally tender and may refer pain, tenderness, other autonomic phenomena or proprioceptive changes when pressed. Trigger points produce weakness and prevent complete lengthening in the muscle and may elicit a local twitch response upon compression.

Vibration: Neuromuscular technique in which the therapist presses into the trigger point and then adds an up-and-down trembling motion.

Warm-up: A session of light to moderate activity, including stretching, done before serious exercise or, in some cases, as a stand-alone exercise period.

Yoga: Sanskrit word from the root *yug* (to join, yoke, or concentrate together). A method or discipline that seeks to join the body, mind, and self (soul) or the union between the individual self and the transcendental self.

APPENDIX A

Intake Form/Massage History Questionnaire

Please complete this brief questionnaire so that I may better understand your history regarding massage. This will enable our work together to be more effective. ***All information is kept in strict confidence.***

Name ______________________________ Date ____________ Date of Birth ____________ Phone ____________

Address ______________________________ City ____________________ State ________ Zip ________

Referred by (if applicable) ____

Y N Have you had a professional massage before?

Y N Are you taking any drugs or medications? If yes, explain here: ______________________________

Y N Are you currently under the care of a health care practitioner? If yes, note name below and briefly describe nature of care.

Health Care Practitioner's Name ______________________________ Phone ____________

Reason for Care ____

Y N Do you have a particular part of the body which needs special attention? if yes, where?

____

Y N Do you have part(s) of your body where you wish to avoid massage? if yes, where?

____

Please mark X if you have experienced any of the following, and mark C if the condition is current:

______ circulation problems
______ heart disease
______ high (or low) blood pressure
______ varicose veins
______ contagious disease
______ joint swelling or inflammation
______ open cuts/sores
______ chemotherapy
______ diabetes
______ other

______ broken bones (recent?)
______ osteoporosis
______ skin allergies or skin conditions
______ recent illness or injury
______ lack of feeling in parts of your body
______ migraines
______ headaches
______ lymph node removal
______ arthritis

______ pregnancy
______ anxiety
______ history of abuse
______ depression
______ mental or emotional diagnosis
______ trouble sleeping
______ cancer
______ radiation
______ seizures

The purpose of massage is to maintain good health and physical condition. I understand that licensed massage therapists (LMTs) may not diagnose or treat patients and that massage does not take the place of a doctor's care. Either the LMT or the client may terminate the session if either experiences discomfort during the massage. Discomfort may include (but is not limited to) physical pain, sexually suggestive behavior, or personal remarks or requests. Payment is due at the time of the appointment, and 24 hours' notice is requested to avoid payment for a missed session. My initials signify that I understand and agree to these policies. __________ Initial here

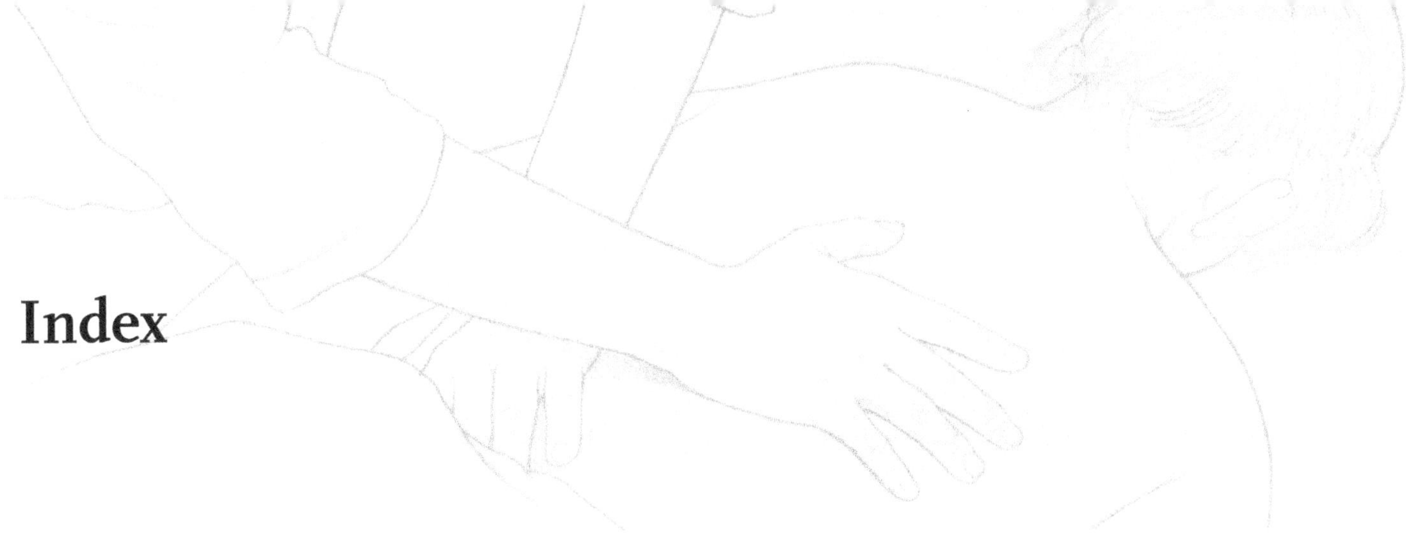

Index

Page numbers in *italics* denote figures; those followed by a t denote tables.

D

E

J

K

L

M

CPSIA information can be obtained
at www.ICGtesting.com
Printed in the USA
BVHW060257210721
612085BV00006B/147